BLOOD IS LIFE

A History of Hematology

Jan Jansen, MD, PhD

ISBN: 978-163848053-2

Copyright: © 2022 by Jan Jansen

Cover Images

Membrane fluorescence *hairy cell*
Sickle cells *bone-marrow harvest*
Van Leeuwenhoek *Blundell's paper*

LIST OF CHAPTERS

	page
Foreword	1
INTRODUCTION	3
BONE MARROW AND STEM CELLS	7
TECHNOLOGY	23
RED BLOOD CELLS	53
Hereditary anemias	57
Thalassemia	57
Sickle cell anemia	65
Hereditary spherocytosis	73
G6PD deficiency	78
Acquired anemias	87
Iron-deficiency anemia	87
Pernicious anemia	91
Acquired hemolytic anemia	100
Aplastic anemia	106
WHITE BLOOD CELLS	127
Leukemia	137
Acute Lymphoblastic Leukemia	141
Acute Myelogenous Leukemia	147
Chronic Myelocytic Leukemia	153
Chronic Lymphocytic Leukemias	156
Myelodysplastic syndromes	174
Myeloproliferative disorders	180
Primary myelofibrosis	182
Polycythemia vera	184
Essential thrombocythemia	186
Other MYPROS	187
Lymphoma	191

Paraproteinemias	212
STEM CELL TRANSPLANTATION	223
PLATELETS	245
Hereditary platelet disorders	249
Glanzmann's disease	249
Von Willebrand's disease	251
Giant platelets disorder	253
Acquired platelet disorders	254
Idiopathic thrombocytopenic purpura	254
Thrombotic thrombocytopenic purpura	257
COAGULATION	261
Bleeding disorders	274
Diffuse Intravascular Coagulation (DIC)	278
Thrombosis	279
TRANSFUSION	285
Blood groups	296
Blood products	302
Red cells	302
Platelets	303
Granulocytes	306
Infectious complications	308
Non-infectious complications	316
Hemolytic transfusion reactions	317
Febrile transfusion reactions	318
Graft-versus-host disease	320
Transfusion-related acute lung injury	321
CONCLUSIONS	324
BIBLIOGRAPHY	329
INDEX	332

Biographical sketches

	page
Ernst Neumann	20
Georges Hayem	48
Paul Ehrlich	49
Jon van Rood	51
Maxwell Wintrobe	83
Ernest Beutler	85
John Dacie	120
Georges Mathé	123
William Crosby	124
Ilya Mechnikov	135
Rudolf Virchow	168
Jean Bernard	169
Eugene Cronkite	172
William Dameshek	188
Henry Kaplan	210
Don Thomas	243
Kenneth Brinkhous	283
Karl Landsteiner	321
Patrick Mollison	323

ACKNOWLEDGEMENTS

The comments and criticisms of my colleagues Luke Akard (Indianapolis, IN), Eva Bromfield-Jansen (Amstelveen NL), Erik de Jong (Amsterdam, NL), Leo McCarthy (Indianapolis, IN), Koen van Besien (New York) and Ferry Zwaan (Goedereede, NL) are gratefully acknowledged. They helped me focus, and tried to prevent errors in content and use of language. All remaining errors are mine alone.

The members of the nursing and laboratory staff with whom I had the privilege collaborating, both in the Netherlands and the USA, enabled us to practice our medical profession with expertise and empathy. Their contributions cannot be over-emphasized.

My family endured my many absences during nights and weekends. They were always understanding and supportive. Retirement has solved the absence problem. I am grateful for their support.

The author also acknowledges the workers in the field of hematology for their longevity. Out of the 199 persons, who were born after 1900 and whose biographical data were mentioned in this book, at least 52 (26%) lived for ≥90 years. Hematology must indeed be a healthy profession!

"Those who cannot remember the past, are condemned to repeat it."
  Jorge (George) Santayana (1863-1952)

or

"History is something that never happened, written by a man who wasn't there"
  Rámon Gómez de la Serna (1888-1963)

Your choice!

Introduction

FOREWORD

This history tries to follow the various developments in hematology. It is not a scientific study, and does not choose who was right or who was wrong. The historical trends will likely show whose contributions have mattered most. Certain important developments (*e.g.*, monophyletic versus dualistic theories about stem cells; immunological typing of lymphocyte populations; reticulo-endothelial system) are mentioned more than once, to fit into the appropriate chapters.

The chapters were chosen to follow the hematology training and clinical practices of continental Europe. Thus, coagulation and blood transfusion are considered parts of hematology. In England and North America these disciplines are part of clinical pathology.

Even though an attempt has been made to describe all fields of hematology, the personal preference of the author has led to certain fields (malignancies, anemias, stem-cell transplantation) to receive more attention than some other fields (*e.g.*, coagulation, transfusion). Hematology has too many subspecialties nowadays for a single author to equally review all fields. Developments after the year 2010 will be mentioned only infrequently.

Short biographical sketches have been added of giants in the history of hematology. These are printed in *cursive*.

Unlike my earlier historical studies, a reference will not be added for each fact or statement; that would have created too many pages of references (80[+]?). Instead of individual references, a bibliography has been added that lists books and articles that have been most helpful for this historical study. Wikipedia was extremely helpful for biographical data (*e.g.,* date of birth and death, *etc.*).Maxwell Wintrobe's *Blood Pure and Eloquent* from 1980 gave a great overview of the history of many disciplines within hematology. Each chapter also gave a list of original references. I used this out-of-print book extensively for my historical review.

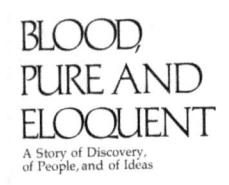

Gerrit A. Lindeboom (1905-1986), my first teacher in Internal Medicine, stressed the importance of the history of the profession we were embarking upon. He was an expert on Herman Boerhaave (1668-1738), whom Albrecht von Haller (1708-1777) called *Communis Europae preceptor (*teacher of all Europe). Via his pupil Alexander Monro (1697-1767), Boerhaave influenced the founding of the Edinburgh Medical School. This school, in turn, influenced American medicine via Benjamin Rush (1746-1813), who studied in Edinburgh UK and later published medical education books from Philadelphia PA. Six degrees of separation?

Names of cities lesser known than Paris, Berlin, London, or New York, will be followed by two letters that indicate either the country or, in case of the USA, the State. This list is the first page of the index (*p.333*).

INTRODUCTION

Hematology is the science that studies blood, blood-forming tissues and blood diseases. Blood and hematological tissues include red blood cells, hemoglobin, blood proteins, bone marrow, white blood cells, platelets, blood vessels, spleen, lymph nodes, and the mechanism of coagulation.

The famous German poet/author Johan Wolfgang von Goethe (1749-1832) wrote the popular line "Blut ist ein ganz besondrer Saft" (Blood is a special juice) in 1808. He could not have been more correct.

Most religions forbid the consumption of blood. Judaism states "the life of the flesh is in the blood" (*Leviticus 17:11*) and man "shall not eat flesh with its life, that is its blood" (*Genesis 9:4*). Islam considers the consumption of blood to be "haram" (forbidden). Buddhism recommends a vegetarian diet and rejects the consumption of meat and blood. Hinduism in its Vedic books prohibits the eating of whole blood.

On the other hand, Judaism, Islam and Hinduism all support the slaughter of animals as sacrifice to God, with the dashing of blood against the altar as a sanctification ritual (*Exodus 24:6-8*). Christianity worships the execution of Jesus as a cleanser of sins (*1 John 1:7-9*). In the secular world, the Egyptians advocated blood baths for rejuvenation. Gladiators in Rome would drink the blood of slain adversaries to acquire their strength. Even spectators were known to participate.

Blood is Life

Despite the various religious instructions, blood is treated as a delectable food product in many countries/cultures: *blood sausage* and *black pudding* in Great Britain, *boudin noir* in France, *morcilla* in Spain, *Blutwurst* in Germany, *kaszanka* in Poland, *sundae* in Korea, *blood tofu* in China, *gyurma* in Tibet, and in North America and South America blood products for consumption are named depending on which European culture has been dominant.

In ancient history, blood diseases were not known. Obviously, when (too) much of the blood was lost in warfare, the soldier died, but why was unknown. Blood diseases were not really known because blood could not be studied.

The Jewish faith prescribes circumcision (*Brit Milah*) for all male babies of 8 days of age (*Genesis 17:10-13*). The Babylonian Talmud, however, teaches that if a woman had 2 or 3 sons who had died from circumcision, subsequent boys should not be circumcised. When the woman had 3 sisters who also lost sons to circumcision, her son should not be circumcised. It clearly indicated the presence of a bleeding disorder that affects boys, but is caused by a problem in the mother, not the father. The great Jewish philosopher and physician Moses ben Maimon (Maimonides; 1135-1204) in Cordoba SP, instructed that in these cases circumcision should be postponed, to see whether the boy would be healthy and not suffer from bleeding episodes. The Talmud and Maimonides preceded

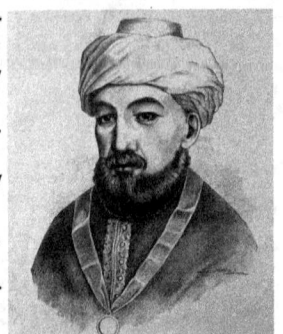

Maimonides

Introduction

the description of hemophilia by many centuries. The first modern description of this bleeding condition, only called *hemophilia* after 1828, was made in 1803 by John Conrad Otto, a physician in Philadelphia PA. He traced it back to a woman who settled near Plymouth NH in 1720.

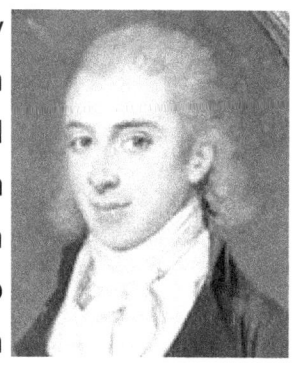

John Otto

The three Synoptic Gospels report on a woman who had already been bleeding for 12 years (*e.g., Mark 5:25-34*), despite attempts by many doctors to heal her. Depending on the translation, it was an "issue of blood" (King James version), a "flux of blood" (Wycliffe version), or "hemorrhages" (NRSV). We do not know whether it was a gynecological (metrorrhagia?) or a hematological disorder.

Since Galen (130-200 CE) and perhaps already since Hippocrates (c.460-c.370 BCE), the doctrine of the four humors: blood, phlegm, black bile, and yellow bile, dominated medical thinking until at least the 17th century. Even now some of the terms survive: sanguine, phlegmatic, melancholic, and bilious! Undoubtedly, people who were malnourished were judged as "pale", but the underlying anemia was not recognized. Bloodletting (Phlebotomy) as therapy was already practiced in the days of Hippocrates. The practice continued into the 19th century. It probably contributed to the immediate cause of death of America's first President: "being bled to death".

Blood is Life

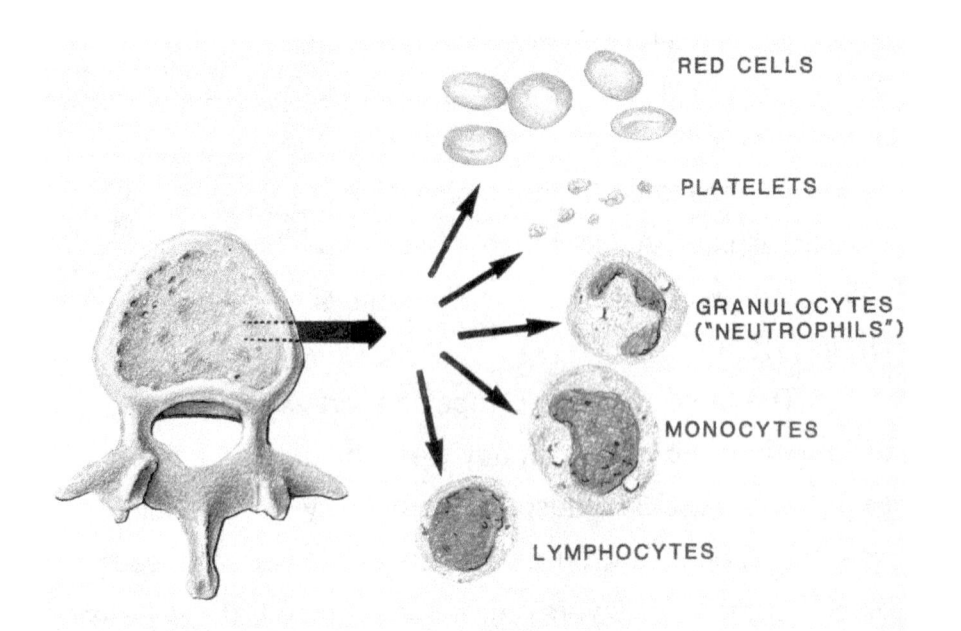

BONE MARROW

PERIPHERAL BLOOD COMPONENTS
(greatly enlarged)

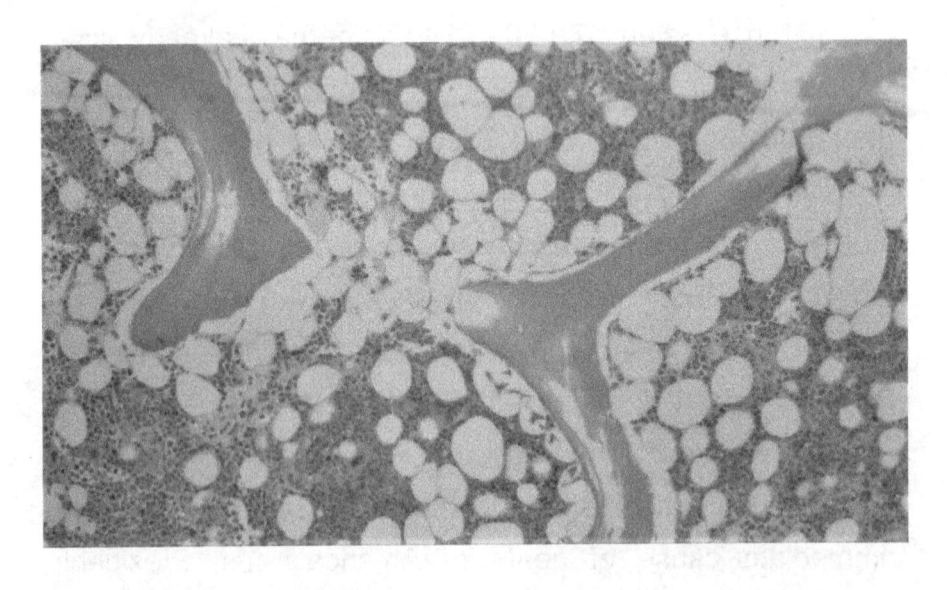

- RED CELLS
- PLATELETS
- GRANULOCYTES ("NEUTROPHILS")
- MONOCYTES
- LYMPHOCYTES

Normal Bone-Marrow Histology

BONE MARROW & STEM CELLS

Both Hippocrates (ca.460– ca.370BCE) and Galen (129-ca.200) believed that the function of bone marrow was to nourish the bone. In the Middle Ages, bone marrow was primarily known as a delectable food product or as a source of warmth and energy. Shakespeare stated that "Love melts the marrow". In 1868, Ernst Neumann in Königsberg, East Prussia (now Kaliningrad RU) postulated, on the basis of microscopy, that the bone marrow was important for the production of red blood cells. Neumann (*p.20*) did post-graduate studies in Prague, and in Berlin with Rudolf Virchow (*p.168*). He also postulated a common stem cell for all hematopoietic cells, and that the production of red cells was continuous. He concluded that at birth all bone marrow is red (producing blood cells), but with age the blood-producing marrow contracts toward the center of the body, leaving the more peripheral parts with yellow fatty marrow. Around the same time, the recent medical graduate Giulio Bizzozero (1846-1901) in Pavia IT postulated that the bone marrow was not only responsible for production of red cells, but also of leukocytes. In 1870, Neumann reported that acute myelogenous leukemia started in the bone marrow, not in the spleen as suggested by others. In his "monophyletic concept" of a single

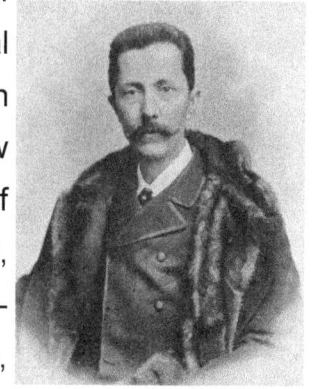

Giulio Bizzozero

stem cell for all hematopoiesis he was supported by Claude Bernard in France, by Bizzozero in Italy, and by Alexander Maximow and Artur Pappenheim in Germany; the latter believed that his *lymphoidozyt* was so primitive that it could be the ancestor of all blood cells. This monophyletic origin was actively opposed by Rudolf Virchow, Paul Ehrlich, and Georges Hayem, who all wanted to maintain the "dualistic concept" (splenic vs lymphatic). One of the most verbal dualists was the authoritarian Otto Naegeli in Switzerland, who described the myeloblast in 1900, and remained convinced that he, and perhaps only he, could differentiate morphologically between myeloblast and lymphoblast. Even in 1931, he still wrote that he had substantiated Ehrlich's dualism. It took until the 1940's for Neuman's concept to be fully accepted.

Competing theories of the origin of red cells suggested disintegration of white cells, production by platelets, release from scavenger cells, or production by fat globules in the liver! It was difficult for many scientists to give up on their pet theories, and to accept that red cells originated from nucleated cells in the bone marrow.

The lack of good blood and bone-marrow staining techniques obviously made the study of hematopoiesis far more difficult. Furthermore, it was unclear how the red cells would lose their nucleus: disintegration or extrusion? Artur Pappenheim (1870-1916) in Berlin tried in 1896 to bring both options together: degeneration, fragmentation and then extrusion. It did not become completely clear until the 1950's, when Bessis' group in Paris documented expulsion, which probably occurred at the marrow-blood barrier.

The function of the red blood cells was also unclear. Otto Funke, who studied in Leipzig and Heidelberg GE, discovered hemoglobin by crystallizing it in 1851, and he called it "Blutfarbstoff". Felix Hoppe-Seyler (1825-1895), considered by many to be the father of biochemistry, described the optical absorption spectrum of hemoglobin and its two distinctive absorption bands in 1858. He recognized the binding of oxygen to hemoglobin to form oxyhemoglobin and confirmed the difference in color of arterial and venous blood.

Between 1913 and 1923, Ludwig Aschoff (1866-1942) at the University of Freiburg GE, developed the concept of the "Reticulo-Endothelial System" (RES) as a system of specialized cells that clear colloidal vital stains. He, and Schilling-Torgau, who described the first case of monocytic leukemia, believed that these leukemic cells derived from the RES. In 1923, Otto Ewald in Heidelberg GE described a case of leukemia that he called "leukemic reticuloendotheliosis". We now assume that his was probably also a case of monocytic leukemia. Ewald thought these cells were "reticulum cells", the ancestors of lymphoblasts, histiocytes, and myeloblasts. In 1914, Ernst Neumann drew a picture of the "great lymphocyte stem cell", which he believed to be the stem cell for the post-embryonic and embryonic development of erythropoiesis and leukopoiesis; it was already responsible for the blood formation

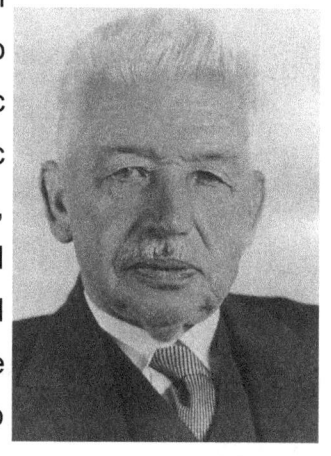

Ludwig Aschoff

in the fetal liver, as suggested in 1846 by Ernst H Weber (1795-1878) in Leipzig GE. Alexander Maximow (1874-1928) claimed, in 1909, that in the peripheral blood "gemeinsame Stamzellen" (common stem cells) were present among the lymphocytes that had, or could regain, pluripotency.

Surprisingly, little was done in this field for almost 50 years. More attention was paid to study the bone-marrow morphology by postmortem aspiration or biopsy. After some unsuccessful attempts, Laird Morris of San Francisco CA introduced a drill to perform biopsies from tibial marrow in patients in 1922. The same year, Seyfarth in Germany developed a puncture needle for open biopsy of the sternum. Arinkin in Leningrad RU performed the first sternal aspiration in 1927. Some investigators recommended needles with a guard (*e.g.*, Klima and Rosegger in 1935), but Grunke still recommended a short lumbar needle with the help of a wooden mallet on the sternum

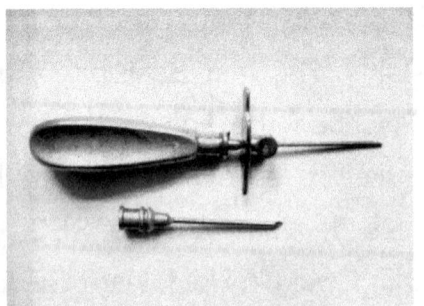

Klima sternal needle

in 1938! Until 1940, many aspirations from the sternum were done without local anesthesia. Even in the mid 1980's, I have seen older hematology colleagues do a sternal tap, in a very slick way, without local anesthesia, claiming that the local anesthesia was equally painful; I never had the courage to try this myself. Sometimes the sternum was punctured completely, and even some deaths from puncturing the heart were reported. Especially in myeloma and/or osteoporosis, the risk of puncture of the sternum was considerable. I remember being taught first to rub over the sternum: if it was very tender, a different site for the aspiration should be sought. The Westerman-Jensen needle, reported in 1964, was a modified Vim-Silverman liver-biopsy needle with finger grips and an obturator. The biopsy was performed using a small incision of the skin. Occasionally, a wooden mallet was used to move the needle through the cortex. This biopsy needle often led to crushing of the specimen.

A major improvement was the Jamshidi needle of 1971. Khosrow Jamshidi, an Iranian hematologist, designed

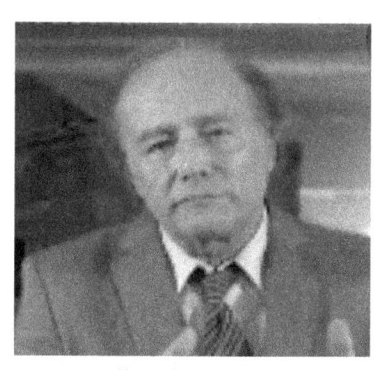

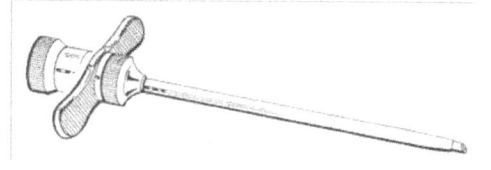

Jamshidi needle

Khosrow Jamshidi

a needle that was tapered radially towards the cutting tip, allowing the biopsy sample to freely enter the lumen without crushing the tissue. These biopsies were typically taken from the posterior iliac spine and did not require a skin incision. A completely different approach was the electric drill introduced by Rolf Burkhardt (1920-2018) in 1966 in Munich GE. An incision was made over the anterior iliac crest, and the local periosteum was numbed and cleared of fat and muscle. Then a funnel was held by an assistant. The operator used an electric "core" drill to obtain a biopsy of 1.8 cm length and 4mm diameter. The specimen was taken out with a fetcher.

The large specimen gave superior morphology, especially after methyl-methacrylate embedding. However superior the morphology may have been, the several days' turn-around time (up to one week) was a negative for clinical care. Decalcification of bone-marrow biopsy specimens did not give equally beautiful morphology, but took considerably less time to get answers.

The issue of stem-cell research did not truly come up until after World War II. The experience with mustard gas in World War I had shown that it could cause, in addition to chemical blisters, severe leukopenia with marked decrease in the production of myeloid cells in the bone marrow. This was confirmed in World War II, even though mustard gas had been banned by the Geneva Protocol in 1925. For example, in 1943 German bombers attacked allied shipping in Bari, Italy, releasing mustard gas from bombs in the wrecked John Henry cargo ship. Many military and civilian victims died, from chemical blisters or from bone-marrow damage. The secret reports of the disaster were only declassified in 1959! During the war, physician Louis Goodman (1906-2000) and pharmacologist Alfred Gilman (1908-1984) studied the effects of mustard gas and its less toxic derivative mustine (nitrogen mustard), after assignment to this task by the military. Their nitrogen mustard became the start of cancer chemotherapy.

Radiation had also been shown to damage bone marrow production. In 1922, Danish radiologist Jan Fabricius Møller observed that the bleeding tendency of guinea pigs exposed to total-body irradiation, did not occur when the limbs were shielded with lead. In that setting, the platelet count did not decrease dramatically. Marie Sklodowska Curie (1867-1934), a Polish investigator mainly working in Paris, discovered the elements Radium and Polonium, and introduced the term "radioactivity". She died from bone marrow failure, possibly caused by her careless handling of radioactive products. After World War II, with its conclusion by nuclear bombs on Hiroshima and Nagasaki, the interest in the effects of radiation on bone-marrow function markedly increased. In 1949, Leon Jacobson (1911-1992), who had participated in the Manhattan Project at the University of Chicago and later became the Chairman of Medicine there, rediscovered the effect of shielding part of the body during total-body irradiation (TBI). His group shielded the spleen of mice before otherwise lethal TBI. They documented that in mice the spleen is a hematopoietic organ. They confirmed this by injecting spleen cells after lethal TBI. Egon Lorenz and Delta Uphoff at the National Cancer Institute (Bethesda MD), were capable of rescuing mice after TBI by injecting bone-marrow cells from mice of the same strain in 1952.

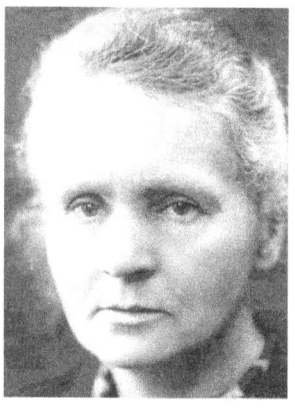

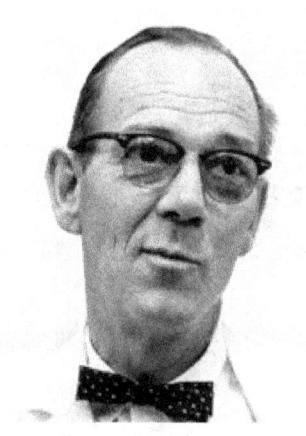

Marie Curie

Leon Jacobson

Interestingly, both the Chicago and NCI groups believed that the salutary effect of spleen or bone-marrow injection was humoral rather than cellular! The next couple of years saw a vivid discussion about the nature of the rescue. Ultimately in 1956, Charles Ford (1912-1999) of the Harwell group in England, showed that the repopulation event was cellular: they found chromosome translocations from the donor spleen cells after injection into irradiated CBA mice. They introduced the term "radiation chimaera" for an animal carrying a foreign hematopoietic system. The mouse experiments opened the way for human bone-marrow transplantation (*p.223*). Edwin Osgood (1899-1969) in Portland OR, developed the theoretical basis of stem-cell proliferation with asymmetric division: providing a new stem cell and a maturing cell.

A major development in the study of stem cells came from Toronto CN. Ernest McCulloch (1926-2011) graduated from medical school at the University of Toronto, and then continued his education at the Lister Institute in London. He joined the Ontario Cancer Institute at Princess Margaret

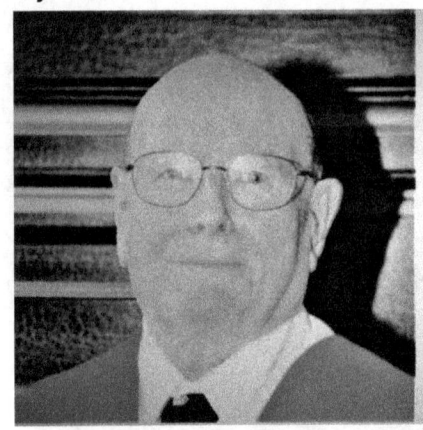

Ernest McCulloch   *James Till*

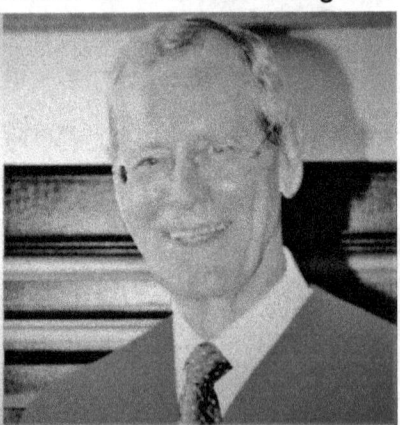

Bone Marrow and Stem Cells

Hospital in 1957. His major interests were normal hematopoiesis and leukemia. He started to collaborate with James Till (b.1931), a biophysicist who had his PhD from Yale University. In 1960, when they studied bone-marrow transplantation in mice after TBI, they observed visible nodules in the spleens of the mice. They speculated that each nodule arose from a single marrow cell, perhaps a stem cell.

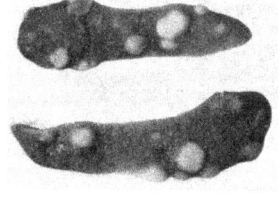

CFU-s

They showed that indeed each nodule arose from a single cell, which they called CFU-s (*colony-forming unit, spleen*). They also showed that these cells were capable of self-renewal, which was important for the functional definition of stem cell. Dirk ("Dick") van Bekkum (1925-2015) in Rijswijk NL enriched the cells that form CFU-s from mouse bone marrow in 1971, and called these cells

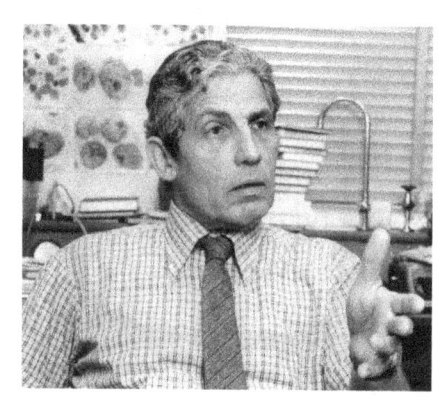

Dick van Bekkum 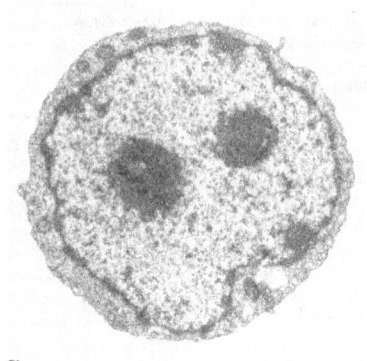   *CMOMC*

"CMOMC" (*Cells Meeting Our Morphological Criteria*). He also believed these cells to be stem cells.

Blood is Life

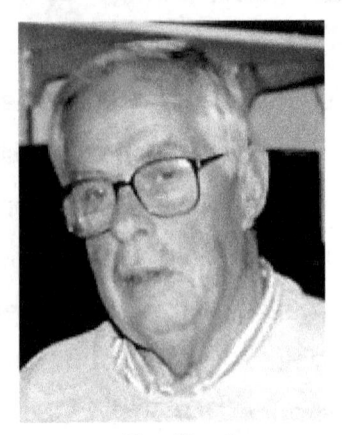

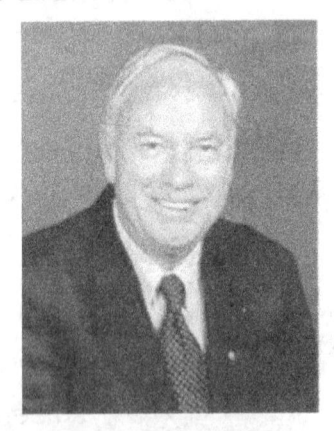

Ray Bradley   *Donald Metcalf*

In 1966 in Melbourne AU, Ray Bradley (1923-2013), a physiologist who had studied cell cloning as a visiting scientist at NIH (Bethesda, MD), and Donald Metcalf (1929-2014), a physician who studied blood formation and leukemia, developed an *in-vitro* technique to grow mouse bone-marrow cells in semi-solid agar. The growth required a colony-stimulating factor (CSF). The growing cell was named "*Colony-forming unit, culture*" (CFU-c). In the same year, Dov Pluznik and Leo Sachs at the Weizmann Institute in Rehobot IS were able to grow clones of normal mouse mast cells using a CSF.

    Then in 1970, Beverley Pike and William Robinson in Denver CO, who had learned bone-marrow cultures in Melbourne, were able to grow human bone marrow in agar, using a feeder layer of peripheral-blood leukocytes. These colonies were almost exclusively granulocytic. The cells giving rise to CFU-c (or CFU-GM) in humans, proved quite similar to the CMOMC in mice. At the Ontario Cancer Institute, Norman Iscove used methylcellulose instead

BFU-E   CFU-E

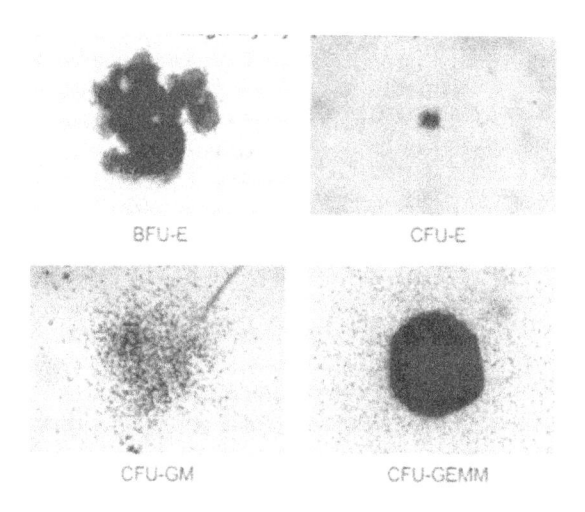

CFU-GM   CFU-GEMM

of agar, and he used a conditioned medium obtained from human leukocytes. While at the Basel Institute of Immunology in 1976, he also was able to grow erythroid early (*BFU-e*) and later (*CFU-e*) colonies by adding erythropoietin to the cultures. When PHA-stimulated leukocyte-conditioned medium was also added, colonies consisting of granulocytes, erythrocytes, macrophages and megakaryocytes (*CFU GEMM*) could be distinguished after 3 weeks.

In 1977, Michael Dexter (b.1945), who had been a visiting fellow with Malcolm Moore at Sloan-Kettering Cancer Center in New York, and who was now part of Laszlo Lajtha's (1920-1995) group at the Paterson Institute for Cancer Research in Manchester UK, showed that bone-marrow cells could proliferate in long-term cultures for many weeks: *Dexter cultures*. Lajtha had graduated from medical school in Budapest HU and came to England in 1947, first to Oxford and later to Manchester. Malcolm Moore (b.1944) had gone in the opposite direction. He obtained his PhD from Oxford University in 1967, and then went to work with Donald Metcalf in Melbourne. He worked primarily on colony stimulating factors there. This resulted later in his work with granulocyte colony-stimulating factor (*G-CSF*), marketed as filgrastim. In 1974, he joined Sloan Kettering Cancer Center in New York as Head of the James Ewing Laboratory of Developmental Hematopoiesis

It had become evident, through all these international collaborations, that bone marrow contained stem cells that were responsible for continuous blood-cell production, just as had been claimed by Ernst Neumann around 1870.

But where do these hematopoietic stem cells come from? In the earliest embryogenesis, the inner cell mass has embryonic stem cells (*ESC*) that can differentiate into any embryonic cell type. These pluripotent stem cells will ultimately differentiate into ectoderm, endoderm, and mesoderm. ESC were for the first time obtained from a mouse embryo by Martin Evans (b.1941) and Matthew Kaufman of Cambridge University UK, and by Gail Martin (b.1944) of San Francisco CA in 1981. Eight years later, the Cambridge group was able to modify ESC, leading to the first "knockout mice". In 1989, the group of James Thomson (b.1958) in Madison WI derived ESC lines from human blastocysts. They recognized their pluripotency and capacity of self renewal.

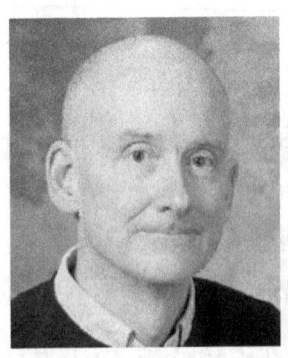

James Thomson

Bone Marrow and Stem Cells

The use of human blastocysts created the anticipated ethical problems. The George W. Bush administration allowed funding to support research with only the by then known approximately 60 ESC lines. Several of these cell lines "petered out" over the years. The Obama administration removed the restrictions in 2009. Around the same time, the FDA gave approval for the first phase-I trial of ESC for spinal-cord injuries.

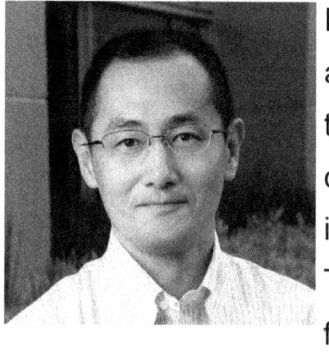

By 2006, Shinya Yamanaka (b.1962) and colleagues in Kyoto JA were able to induce pluripotent stem cells from cultures of adult mouse fibroblasts: induced pluripotent stem cells (*IPSC*). This was done by the introduction of four specific genes, including *Myc*.

Shinya Yamanaka

The next year, both Yamanaka and Thomson did this also with human fibroblasts, introducing the four pivotal genes with either a retroviral or a lentiviral vector. In 2008, IPSCs were also derived from keratinocytes and in 2010 from peripheral blood cells. Catharine Verfaillie (b.1957) of Louvain BE, while working in Minneapolis MN, claimed in 2002 that her adult derived stem cells were multipotent (*MAPC*). For opponents of abortion this was obviously a God send. Unfortunately, her results could not always be repeated by other groups, and questions arose about her scientific methods. For tissue repair, such MAPC would obviously be attractive, but much still needs to be learned about them.

Franz Ernst Christian Neumann *was born in 1834 in Kônigsberg, East Prussia (now Kaliningrad RU). He was the son of the physicist Franz Ernst Neumann (1798-1895). He received his medical degree in Kônigsberg in 1855, and continued his studies in Prague CZ and in Berlin under Rudolf Virchow. Then he returned to Kônigsberg to become Head of the Pathological Institute. His main interests were in hematology, and in 1868 he documented that erythropoiesis originates in the bone marrow. Neumann also postulated a common stem cell for all hematopoietic cells. The next year he described the "lymphoid marrow cell" as the source of erythropoiesis, but also as a cell capable of self regeneration. In additional studies, he identified the bone marrow as the source of AML and of pernicious anemia. In 1882, he recognized that at birth all bone marrow is red, but that with advancing age the blood producing contracts toward the center of the body, leaving the more peripheral bones with only yellow (fatty) marrow: "Neumann's law". In his conclusions, he was supported by Giulio Bizzozero in Italy, Claude Bernard in France, and Alexander Maximov and Artur Pappenheim in Germany, but he was opposed by Georges Hayem in France, and Rudolf Virchow and Paul Ehrlich in Germany. The latter all believed in the dualistic origin of*

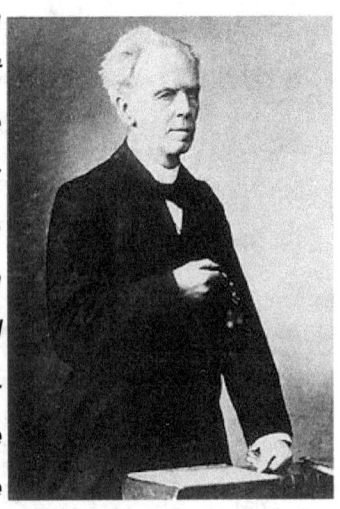

splenic and lymphatic blood cells. In 1912, Neumann further developed his stem-cell theory, claiming the "great-lymphocyte-stem-cell" (probably similar with the lymphoid hemoblast of Pappenheim), as the stem cell for post embryonic and embryonic development of red-cell and white cell production. It took about 50 years before Neumann was shown to have been completely correct. Just like Immanuel Kant, Ernst Neumann spent his entire career in Königsberg. He died there in 1918. In 1995, the International Society of Experimental Hematology introduced the Ernst Neumann award and Donald Metcalf, another stem cell giant, became its first recipient, more than 80 years after the monophyletic concept had been suggested by Neumann.

Neumann's 1868 paper

Blood is Life

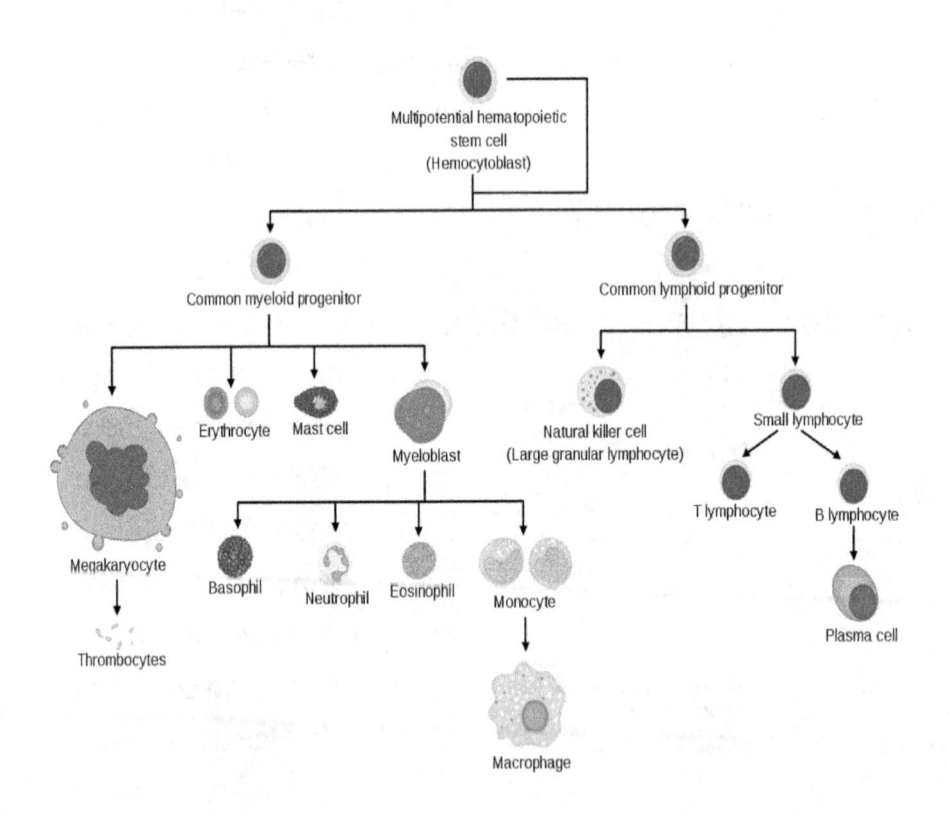

Normal Human Hematopoiesis (current understanding)

22

TECHNOLOGY

To understand blood and its diseases, technology to study blood specimens is required. The first instrument to study blood was the microscope.

Magnifying glasses, derived from eyeglasses, were introduced in the 13th century. Zacharias Janssen (1585-ca.1632), perhaps together with his neighbor Hans Lippershey in Middelburg (province of Zeeland NL), was the first to make a compound microscope: he combined lenses between 1590 and 1618 to make the first telescope/microscope. Many different opinions still exist as to who actually built the first microscope. Other important persons in the early development of microscopes were Cornelis Drebbel (1573-1633), a Dutch expatriate and inventor of the submarine, and Robert Hooke (1635-1703), both in England, and Galileo Galilei (1564-1642) and Marcello Malpighi (1628-1694), a physician and biologist in Bologna, both in Italy.

Jan Swammerdam (1637-1680) was probably the first to see and document red blood cells. He helped his apothecary father in Amsterdam with his curiosity collection, and studied Medicine at the Leiden University NL and then in Paris. He focused his microscopic studies mainly on insects.

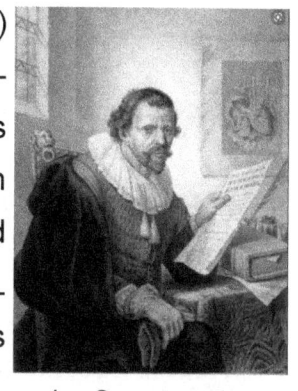

Jan Swammerdam

Blood is Life

He saw red blood cells in 1658 and described them in his notebooks; these were published many years later. The first published report about red blood cells came from Antonie van Leeuwenhoek (1632-1723) in 1674 in a letter to Christiaan Huygens (1629-1695). Van Leeuwenhoek was a lay person and linen-drapery shopkeeper in Delft NL.

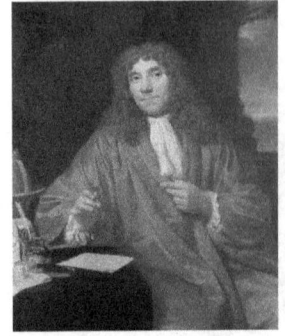

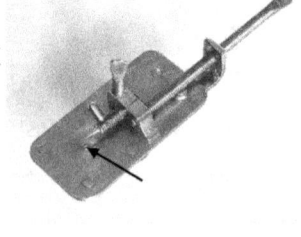

Facsimile of Van Leeuwenhoek's microscope. Arrow indicates the lens (Boerhaave Museum, Leiden)

Antonie van Leeuwenhoek

He was also an amateur scientist and excelled in lens making. The best of his microscopes, with only a single minute biconvex lens, had a magnification power of 275x, or even 500x? He mainly studied microbes ("animalcules" = tiny animals), as reported in many letters to the Royal Society in London. He also reported on red blood cells and estimated their size ("diameter of <1% of a grain of sand") in 1675. Marcello Malpighi (1628-1694) in Italy had seen red cells already in 1661, as documented in a letter that was not published until 1687. During the next 2 centuries, little progress was made, since focusing light on the specimen was difficult. When electric lamps became available for illumination, August Köhler (1866-1948) in Jena GE, working for Carl Zeiss AG, optimized microscopic resolution by evenly illuminating the field of view (*Köhler illumination*). In the early 19th

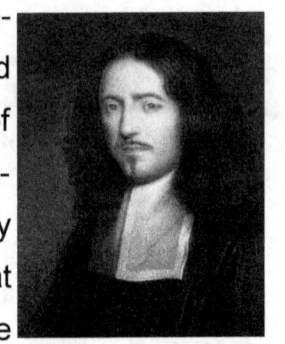

Marcello Malpighi

century, achromatic lenses became available to limit the effect of chromatic and spherical aberration. Yet, it remained difficult to get beyond 1,500x magnification.

To image unstained transparent samples, Frits Zernicke (1888-1966) of Amsterdam NL developed phase contrast microscopy in 1933, and Georges Nomarski (1919-1997) of Warsaw PO introduced differential interference contrast illumination around 1955.

For the study of blood cells, staining techniques were of the utmost importance. Unstained blood smears showed red blood cells and some transparent cells. Joseph Lieutaud (1703-1780) reported these "globuli albicantes" for the first time, but William Hewson (1739-1774), of northern England, studied their nuclei (which he called "central particles") and the lymphatic tissues, better. He published his findings around 1770-1773. He also determined that red blood cells were not globular, as reported by Van Leeuwenhoek, but discoid. He mistook the central part of the red cell for its nucleus. He suggested that all blood cells came from the lymphoid organs. Many Anglophones (and especially William Dameshek; *p.188*) consider him to be the father of hematology.

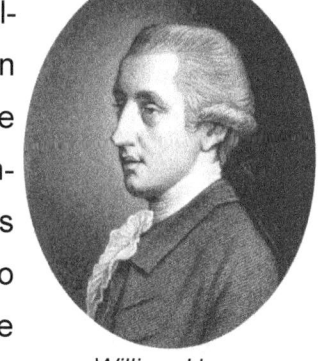

William Hewson

More information about white blood cells became available, when in the mid-19th century cases of leukemia were reported with large numbers of white cells in the blood stream. In 1845, cases were reported almost simultaneously from Scotland and from Germany. John Hughes Bennett (1812-1875) in Edinburgh reported on a 28-year-old man with splenomegaly and many white cells in the blood stream. He made drawings of the peripheral blood smear (*p.138*) and proposed the name "*leucocythaemia*". In the same year, Rudolf Virchow (*p.168*) in Berlin reported on a woman with a 4-year history of poor health and with abdominal swelling. She died 4 months later and was found to have large numbers of white cells ("pus cells") everywhere in the body. For the disease of his 50-year-old patient, he introduced the name "*leukemia*". Virchow also saw that not all white blood cells looked the same. Many were granular and had irregular nuclear shapes. Others were agranular and had mostly rounded nuclei. When the new disease leukemia became accepted, he proposed to subdivide the disease into two types: "splenic" leukemia, and "lymphatic" leukemia.

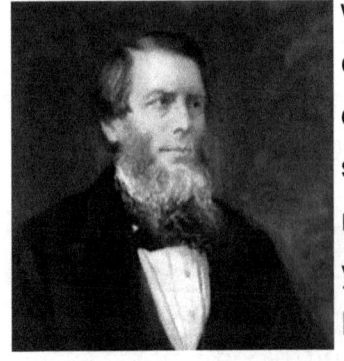

John Hughes Bennett

Further distinction between the various white blood cells (leukocytes) became only possible, when Paul Ehrlich (*p.49*) introduced staining of thin air-dried blood smears with aniline dyes in 1877. These dyes had just been discovered in the rapidly developing German chemical industry. His triacid stain changed blood morphology and hematology dramatically. Ehrlich also reported the myelocyte as an early form of the granulocyte. He did not pay any attention to lymphocytes, since they did not have stainable features.

In 1891, Dimitri Romanovsky (1861-1921) in St. Petersburg RU improved on the triacid stain of Ehrlich by using a combination of eosin Y and "aged" (demethylated) methylene blue, creating a distinctive shade of purple, the *metachromatic* or *Romanovsky effect*. Two variants became popular in 1902: May-Grünwald-Giemsa stain and Wright's stain. The latter is primarily used in North America, the former in the rest of the world. This difference was caused by the fact that aniline dyes from Germany could not easily be obtained in the New World during World War I. For the most recent 100[+] years, staining techniques of blood and bone marrow smears have remained basically unchanged.

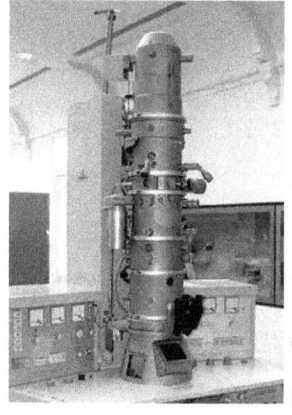

The electron microscope was introduced in the early 1930's by the Siemens company in Germany to allow magnifications of >1,000-1,500x (resolution of about 0.2 micrometers, determined by the wave length of the light source). The far smaller wave length of the electron beam allowed resolutions up to 0.05 nanometers (magnification up to 10,000,000x). In the 1950's, the group of Marcel Bessis (1917-1994) in Paris was important for hematological studies with electron microscopy, using ultrathin tissue sections. He described the ultrastructure of the various

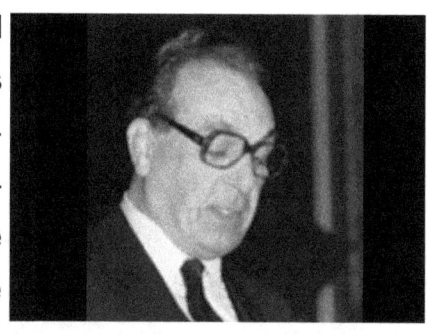

Electron Micoscope

Marcel Bessis

blood cells in his 1957 booklet *Microscopie de phase et microscopie électronique des cellules du sang.*

The fluorescence microscope was developed in 1911, simultaneously by Heinrich Lehmann in Jena GE and Carl Reichert in Vienna AT, to study the properties of organic substances. A specimen is illuminated with light of a specific wavelength, which is absorbed by the fluorophore/chromophore, causing it to emit light of a longer wavelength. A filter separates the illuminating and emitted lights. Common fluorophores in hematology initially were fluorescein isothiocyanate (FITC; green) and rhodamine isothiocyanate (TRITC; red); many additional fluorophores were added later. Fluorescence microscopy in hematology was used primarily to study antigens on or in blood cells. Antibodies (polyclonal or monoclonal) were conjugated to a fluorophore to detect the proteins on the surface of the cell, or inside the cell.

All the techniques discussed so far, were used to study individual blood cells. Additional important information can be obtained by determining the concentration of cells or proteins in the blood stream.

An important measurement is the hemoglobin (Hgb) level, used to diagnose anemia. Even though experienced clinicians can reasonably well estimate the degree of anemia from inspection of the hand palms (of non-construction workers!), or even better the conjunctivae, a laboratory test was still worthwhile. The simplest test was to absorb a drop of blood into a linen cloth, and compare the color with that of a healthy person. Wilhelm Türk (1871-1916; Vienna AT) claimed to be less than 5% off with this method in 1904. Theodor Tallquist (1871-1927; Porvoo Fl) absorbed a drop of blood into filter paper and compared it to colored paper in 1903. This method is still in use, particularly for prenatal care in Third-World countries. This WHO hemoglobin color scale (HCS) has an acceptable level of precision. A far more recent, and far more expensive, variant of the Tallquist method is the hemoglobin test strip (*e.g.*, Aimstrip®).

In 1879, the English neurologist William Gowers (1845-1915) had compared diluted blood with a solution of picrocarmine in glycerin, as suggested by Rajewski in 1874. Two comparison tubes were available, one for day light and the other one for artificial light. Hermann Sahli (1858-1933) was a Swiss internist, who trained at the University of Bern but continued his education in Leipzig GE. He worked there for a period under Karl Weigert, the cousin and inspirator of Paul Ehrlich. After return to Bern, he became Professor of Medicine. In 1902, he developed the hemoglobinometer. A sample of blood was treated with hydrochloric acid, and the developing brown color of hematin hydrochloride was compared to the color of standards. The test tube is diluted with distilled water until the color matches the standard as closely as possible. The box he developed contained a hemoglobin pipette (0.02ml capacity), the graduated hemoglobin tube, and the comparator box with the brown glass standard. The Sahli hemoglobinometer can still

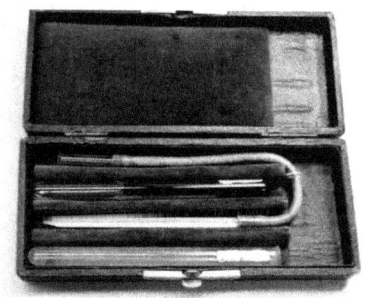

Sahli Hemoglobinometer

be used in places where more automated machines are not available. It is not clear whether it is any better than the simpler Tallquist method.

An alternative method to diagnose anemia (or polycythemia) is the hematocrit. The word hematocrit comes from Greek and means "to separate blood" (αίμα = blood; κριτης = judge). It represents the volume percentage of red blood cells, normally 41-50% for men and 36-44% for women. The simplest test is to let anticoagulated blood settle, but that may take quite a while. Charles Thackrah (1795-1833) in Leeds UK had calculated in 1819, that clotted blood could express about 40% of serum by weight. In 1929, Maxwell Wintrobe (*p.83*) developed a simpler technique by spinning anticoagulated blood in capillary tubes in a centrifuge (*microhematocrit*). Especially surgeons used to prefer the hematocrit (Ht) over the hemoglobin (Hgb); I never quite understood why. Modern automated analyzers do not measure the actual hematocrit anymore, but calculate it from the number of red blood cells and their mean cell volume (MCV). Automated analyzers provide Hgb, MCV and number of red cells, from which the other red cell parameters can be calculated: Ht (MCV x number of red cells), MCH = mean cell hemoglobin (Hgb/number of red cells), and MCHC = mean cell hemoglobin concentration (Hgb/Ht).

The size of blood cells can be easily measured with a micrometer in an eyepiece of the microscope. The introduction of achromatic lenses after 1830 had markedly improved microscopy.

Technology

The first attempts to enumerate red cells and white blood cells were very laborious: the method of Karl Vierordt in 1852 took more than 3 hours! Alfred Donné (1801-1878) in Paris taught clinical microscopy classes, to counter-act the many clinicians who did not understand the importance of this instrument. Slowly the opinion about studying the components of blood started to change.

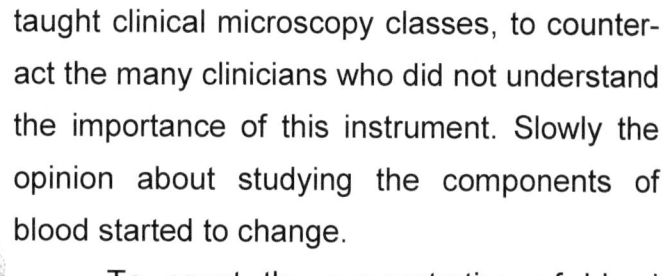

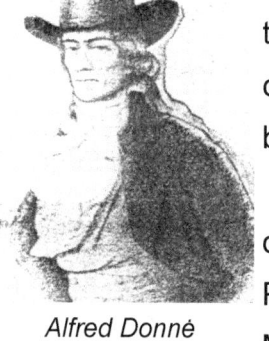

To count the concentration of blood cells, Louis-Charles Malassez (1842-1909) in Paris developed the hemocytometer. Dr. Malassez, born in the Départment Nièvre, studied Medicine in Paris and worked later with Claude Bernard. He was mainly an anatomist and histologist. In 1874, he described a chamber to count red blood cells. The chamber consisted of a thick glass microscopic slide with a rectangular indentation to create a precision-volume chamber. Georges Hayem (p.48) produced his own hemocytometer and dilution fluid, consisting of an isotonic solution of sodium chloride, sodium sulfate, mercuric chloride and distilled water. Many modifications of the chamber were made for different applications. William Gowers in London developed his hemocytometer that did not require calibration of the microscope with ocular rulings in 1877. The improved Neubauer hemocytometer of 1922 consisted of nine 1x1mm squares, each of 0.1mm

Alfred Donné

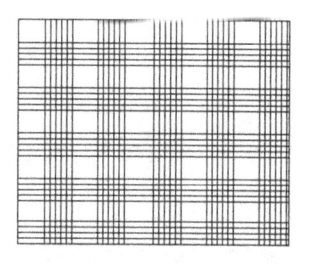

Malassez Hemocytometer

Neubauer Hemocytometer

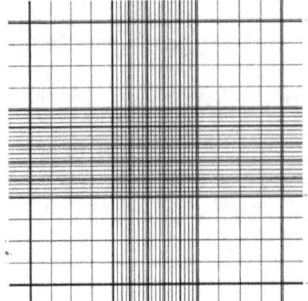

depth. The corner squares, mostly used for counting white blood cells, were subdivided into 4 squares of 0.25x0.25mm each (volume 0,00625mm^3). The central square, used for red blood cell counting, was subdivided into 25 squares of 0.2x0.2mm each (volume 0.004mm^3). The special coverslip is positioned on the surface of the counting chamber, in such a way that Newton's rings indicate proper contact. The blood sample is diluted appropriately and applied to the edge of the coverslip; the sample is sucked into the void by capillary action. Then a microscope is used to count the necessary squares. Trypan blue can be added to the sample, if the viability of the white blood cells needs to be determined.

In 1934, Andrew Moldavan in Montreal CN designed a photoelectric apparatus to count individual cells flowing through a capillary tube that was mounted on a microscope stage. Wallace Coulter (1913-1998) was an electrical engineer from Little Rock AR, who, together with his brother Joseph, patented the Coulter principle in 1953. Particles pulled through an orifice, concurrent with an electrical current, produce a change in impedance that is proportional to the volume of the particle. Coulter had already discovered this principle in the 1940's; it

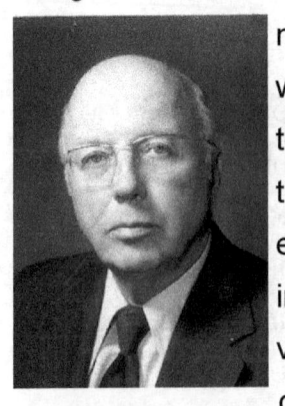

Wallace Coulter

was partly based on Moldavan's studies. Coulter developed the technology, spurred by the nuclear bombs released upon Japan, to produce equipment that could measure blood values rapidly and on a large scale. His first commercial Coulter counter for hematology purposes (model A) came out in 1954, and had a production of 300 instruments. This model A was designed not for red blood-cell counts, but for white blood-cell counts. Once the value of the instrument had been established, subsequent editions had more capabilities and fewer problems (*e.g.*, model FN from 1968). These counters are now necessary tools in hematology, and provide a complete blood count (red cells with their parameters, white cells with their differential, and platelets with size distribution).

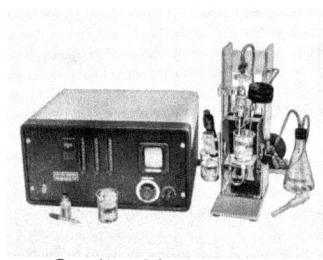

Coulter Model A

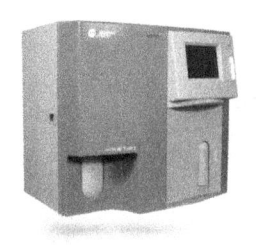

Coulter model FN

In 1968, Wolfgang Göhde (b.1940) and Wolfgang Dittrich of the University of Münster GE developed the first fluorescence-based flow-cytometry device, which was commercialized as the ICP11 by Phywe AG in Göttingen GE. This technique was called "*Impulszytophotometrie*", and the device was soon followed by similar devices from Bio/Physics Systems (later Ortho Diagnostics) and Becton Dickinson

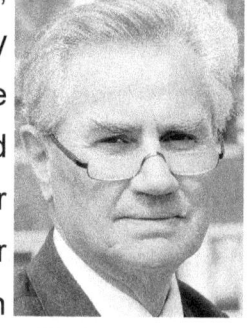

Wolfgang Göhde

(BD). The immunologist/geneticist Leonard Herzenberg (1931-2013) at Stanford University, in collaboration with his wife Leonore ("Len and Lee"), developed the fluorescence-activated cell sorter (FACS) that combined flow cytometry with cell sorting in 1969. He teamed up with Becton Dickinson and the name FACS became a registered trademark. The cell-sorting technology had been developed by Mack Fulwyler (1936-2001) of Los Alamos National Laboratories, NM. He combined the Coulter Counter with the ink-jet oscillograph, invented by Dick Sweet in 1965. The basis of flow cytometry and cell sorting is that cells suspended within a high velocity fluid stream, pass through a laser beam in a single file. When labeled with fluorescent markers the light from the laser is absorbed and then emitted in a band of wavelengths. Detectors and analog-to digital conversion convert analog measurements of forward scattered light and side-scattered light as well as dye-specific fluorescence signals into digital signals. The computer can express them either in linear or logarithmic amplification.

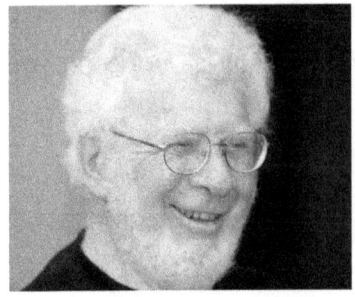

Len Herzenberg

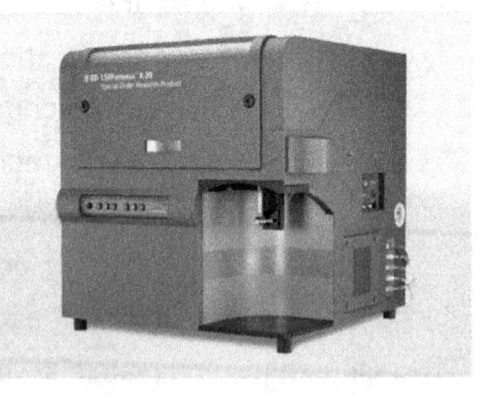

*BD LSRFortessa X-20
4 lasers– 18 signals*

Technology

Walther Flemming (1843-1905), a physician biologist in Kiel GE, was the first to see animal chromosomes, using the newly introduced aniline dyes in 1882. Chromosomes received their name from Wilhelm von Waldeyer-Hartz (1841-1923) in Berlin (1908). Forty years earlier, Karl von Nägeli (1817-1891) in Zürich SU likely had already seen them in plants. Although Gregor Mendel (1822-1884), the priest biologist in Brno CZ, had studied genetics in pea plants by 1866, his work was only rediscovered in 1900, by several investigators *(e.g.,* botanist Hugo de Vries (1848-1935) of Leiden University). De Vries introduced the term *pangenes*, later shortened to *genes* by Wilhelm Johannsen (1857-1927) in Copenhagen DE. Johannsen also coined the names *genotype* and *phenotype*. Walter Sutton (1877-1916) in New York, and Theodor Boveri (1862-1915) in Würzburg GE, both developed the "chromosome theory of inheritance", now called the *Boveri-Sutton chromosome theory* and introduced *cytogenetics* in 1903. Developments were not fast. Hans de Winiwarter (1875-1949), a gynecologist in Liège BE, reported in 1912 that men had 47 chromosomes and women 48. In 1923, Theophilus Painter (1889-1969), a zoologist in Austin TX, studied the testicles of men in an insane asylum who had been castrated, or even executed by hanging (!). He reported 48 chromosomes even though, two years earlier, he had reported 46. He also introduced the X and Y chromosomes. The next year, Grigoriii Levitsky (1878-1942) in Kiev RU formulated the term *karyotype*. In 1946, Albert Fisher of the Jackson Labs in Maine, showed that cells could be grown in tissue culture. T.C Hsu (1917-2003) in Austin TX reported in 1952, that cultured cells were better suited for studying chromosomes. He produced metaphase drawings of all 48(!) human chromosomes. A laboratory error resulted in the swelling of the chromosomes in hypotonic saline, called the *"hypotonic shock"*. By 1955, Charles Ford and John Hamerton in Harwell UK pretreated cultured cells with colchicine, to destroy the mitotic spindle apparatus and accumulate dividing cells in metaphase. Then finally in 1955, Joe Hin Tjio (1919-2001), an Indonesian cytogeneticist working in Lund SW with Albert Levan(1905-1998), proved that humans have 46, not 48, chromosomes. Thus, one paper overturned a dogma of 30 years! In 1959, Jérôme Lejeune (1926-1994), working in Paris with Raymond Turpin (1895-1988), documented that children with Down's syndrome had an extra 21st chromosome. Studies documenting 45XO in Turner syndrome and 47XXY in Klinefelter syndrome followed. Chromosome studies in malignancy started in 1960, when Peter Nowell and David Hungerford found the Philadelphia (Ph') chromosome in Chronic Myelogenous Leukemia (CML; *p.155*).

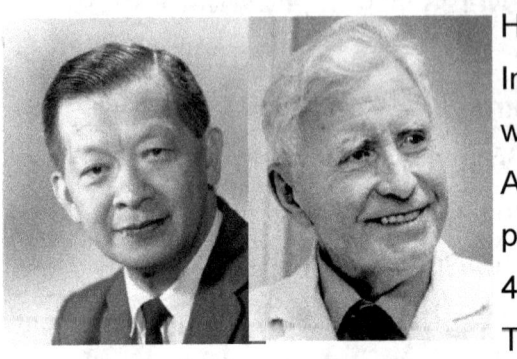

Joe Hin Tjio   *Albert Levan*

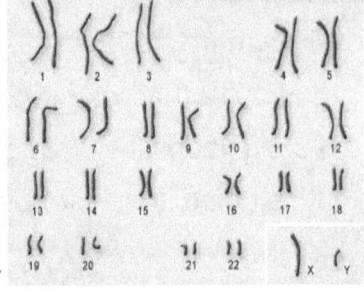

Normal human chromosomes

Technology

In the same year, Peter Nowell also demonstrated that the kidney-bean extract phytohemagglutinin (PHA), used to separate red and white blood cells, stimulated lymphocytes to divide. This *mitogen* permitted peripheral blood cells to be studied, often eliminating the need for bone-marrow aspiration to obtain dividing cells. Torbjörn Caspersson (1910-1997) in Stockholm SW introduced fluorescent quinacrine banding in 1968, allowing each chromosome to be identified. The fluorescence would "quench" rapidly. This was resolved three years later, when Máximo Drets and Margery Shaw in Ann Arbor MI introduced Giemsa-banding.

In 1969, Mary Lou Pardue and Joseph Gall of Yale University introduced a method for detecting specific DNA fractions. Their technique involved the hybridization of a radioactive test DNA in solution to the stationary DNA of a cytologic preparation, followed by autoradiography. This was an *in-situ* application of the Southern blot. Edwin Southern (b.1938), a molecular biologist at Oxford University UK, published a method to detect specific DNA sequences in 1975. He combined the transfer of electrophoresis-separated DNA fragments to a filter membrane, and subsequent fragment detection by hybridization with radioactive probes. The disadvantage of the radioactive *in-situ* hybridization was the long exposure period needed for autoradiography. Then in the mid 1980's, biotin labeled DNA probes were put into practice; these could be labeled with different fluorochromes, leading to the **F**luorescent **I**n **S**itu **H**ybridization (FISH) technique. The signal intensity of fluorescence was greater than with immunochemical stains such as horseradish peroxidase.

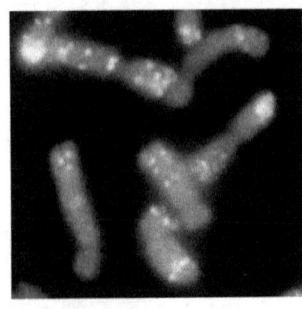

Repetitive sequences in FISH

The next types of blot all referenced to Edwin Southern and were called northern blot, western blot, *etc*. The northern blot was introduced to quantify RNA In 1977. Again, the autoradiography was time consuming; furthermore, a large quantity of RNA was necessary for detection. Then in 1983, Kary Mullis (1944-2019) of Cetus Corporation in Emeryville CA developed the polymerase chain reaction (PCR). He received part of the Nobel Prize in Chemistry for this invention in 1993. The PCR rapidly replaced the northern blot as the method of choice for RNA detection and quantification (reverse transcriptase PCR; RT-PCR). In this procedure, the RNA template is first converted into a complementary DNA (cDNA) using reverse transcriptase. The cDNA is then used as a template for exponential amplification. In combination with fluorescent DNA-labeling techniques, it is now the standard as real time PCR.

Leonard Landois (1837-1902) in Greifswald GE documented blood incompatibility between species in 1873. Jules Bordet (1870-1961), the Belgian immunologist who was working at the Pasteur Institute in Paris, showed that hemolysins were produced after heterologous (now called xenogeneic) transfusion in 1895. Paul Ehrlich reported 5 years later that part of these hemolysins were already existing before the heterologous transfusion . That same year, Karl Landsteiner (*p.321*) in Vienna AT showed that incompatibility also existed between the red cells and serum of healthy, non-transfused, humans. His ABO system was the start of *immunogenetics*, the study of genetically determined polymorphisms with immunological techniques. Peter Gorer (1907-1961) in London studied a tumor system in mice, and he introduced tissue and transplantation antigens in 1937. His studies mostly used red cells for the serological tests. These transplantation antigens in mice were called the H antigens by George Snell (1903-1996), who worked at the Jackson Laboratories in Bar Harbor ME. The serological tests with red-cell agglutination were cumbersome. Peter Medawar (1915-1987) in London, by many considered the "father of transplantation" for his studies of acquired immunological tolerance, had already shown in the 1940's, that leukocytes also carry transplantation antigens. Bernard Amos (1923-2003), who would later go to Duke University NC, had, while still in London in 1953, shown that the H antigen system could also be found on leukocytes

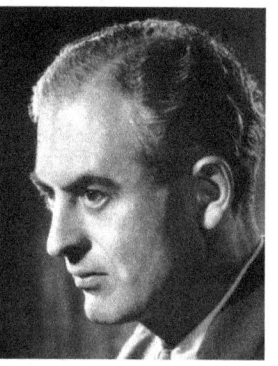

Peter Medawar

(leukocyte agglutination). In the same year, Jean Dausset (1916-2009) in Paris found agglutination of donor leukocytes by the serum of a multi-transfused patient. This allo-antibody reacted with only a fraction of donors. In 1958, he reported that leuko-agglutinins appeared in the blood of a patient who had received multiple small transfusions from the same donor; he called the antigen MAC (later HLA-A2). That same year, Jon van Rood (*p.51*) at Leiden University and Rose

Payne (1909-1999) at Stanford University, both detected leuko-agglutinins in the sera of women after pregnancy. These pregnancy-induced leuko-agglutinins proved to be more persistent than the transfusion-induced agglutinins. The leuko-agglutinin technique proved not always reproducible, and a major improvement occurred when Paul Terasaki (1929-2006) in Los Angeles CA, introduced the microcytotoxicity technique in 1964. The transplantation antigen system, located on chromosome 6, and called the Human Leukocyte Antigen (HLA) system in 1967, proved extremely complex. The antigens were divided into class I molecules (A, B, C) that were detected with antisera, and class II antigens (D) that were identified by the mixed-lymphocyte culture (MLC), introduced by Fritz Bach (1934-2011) in New York in 1964. These class II antigens could also be identified with serology after 1977. With newer immunological and genetic testing, an increasing number of alleles were reported. Many of these alleles were unique. The HLA-genotype of each human consists of two haplotypes, one inherited from the mother and the other from the father. For transplantation purposes, the chance that a full sibling is

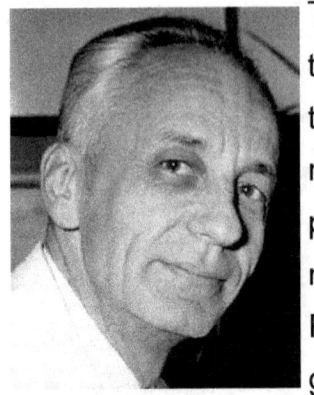

Jean Dausset

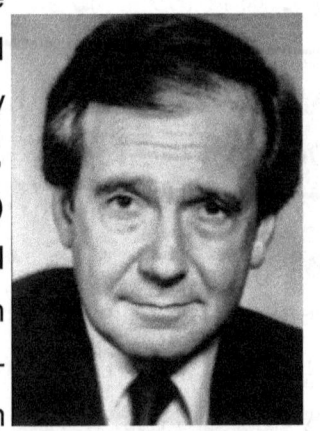

Fritz Bach

Technology

HLA identical is $1-3/4^x$ (x=number of full siblings) x100, meaning that with 1 sibling the chance is 25%, and with 8 siblings 90%.

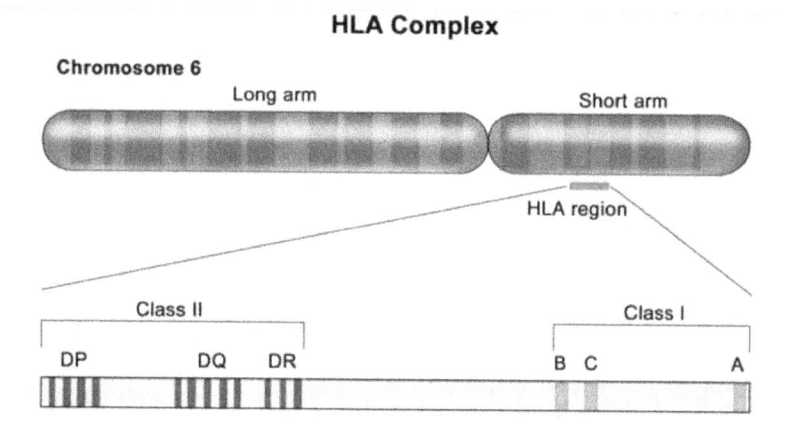

HLA Complex

Chromosome 6

To study the fate of red blood cells in the circulation, Winifred Ashby (1879-1975), born in England but working in Rochester MN, studied blood-group-O red cells transfused into blood group-A recipients. She made suspensions of post-transfusion blood in anti-A serum in 1917-1921. The unagglutinated blood-group-O cells survived for 100 days in a healthy man, but much shorter in a patient with cancer. Several other groups confirmed her findings in the 1930's. In 1950, Seymour Gray (1911-?) and Kenneth Sterling (1920-1995) at Harvard were able to label autologous red-blood cells with ^{51}Cr, a harmless label that emits gamma rays. Not only did it allow the determination of survival of red cells, but also their place of destruction. This

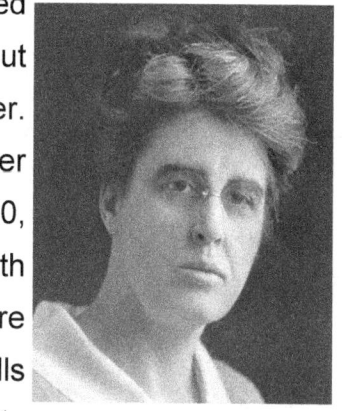

Winifred Ashby

technology was also used to measure total RBC volume. The disadvantage of ^{51}Cr was that it slowly eluted from the red cells (about 1% per day). An alternative was ^{32}P used to label diisofluorophosphanate (DFP), introduced by Jacob Cohen (1915-1969) in Rijswijk NL in 1954. My first appointment after training was in the J A Cohen Institute for Radiopathology and Radiation Protection in Leiden, named after this untimely deceased radiobiologist. The DF^{32}P bound irreversibly to red cells, with no elution. Both labeling techniques confirmed a red-cell survival time of about 120 days. In hemolytic anemia, the red-cell survival was obviously much shorter. Other radioactive isotopes used were ^{59}Fe, ^{14}C glycine, and ^{99}Tc. More recent analyses can also use flow cytometry (1988). A blood specimen is labeled with NHS-biotin, injected and the labeled red cells stained with fluorochrome conjugated (strept)avidin.

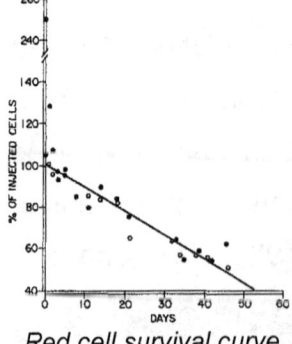

Red cell survival curve (60% survive 40 days)

Similar techniques could also be used for the study of platelet survival. ^{51}Cr and DF^{32}P were useful, but ^{111}In was thought to be superior: shorter half-life, higher photon yield and greater affinity for platelets. In addition, ^{111}In can be used at lower platelet levels than ^{51}Cr (1988). With all techniques, the lifespan of platelets in a healthy individual was only 7-10 days.

To study bleeding tendency, the bleeding time was introduced in 1910 by William Duke (1883-1945) of Johns Hopkins. He showed that the interval between the start of bleeding after a small incision in an earlobe and the cessation of bleeding was relatively constant. When fewer circulating platelets were present, the bleeding time increased proportional to the decrease in platelets. Jacques Roskam (1890-1977) in Liège BE questioned the reliability of this test in 1921: the effect of platelets on the bleeding time was influenced by the age of the blood, the surrounding plasma, and any associated diseases. In young healthy individuals the earlobe bleeding time should be between 2 and 5 minutes. Andrew Ivy (1893-1978) and colleagues in Chicago IL punctured the ventral side of the forearm after a blood-pressure cuff was inflated to 40 mm Hg in 1941. Ivy was an interesting physiologist. He served as a medical expert at the 1947 Nuremberg trials. He claimed to have written the Nuremberg Code on Human Experimentation almost single-handedly! Then in 1951, he stunned the medical world by proclaiming a cancer cure named Krebiozen, that turned out to be a hoax.

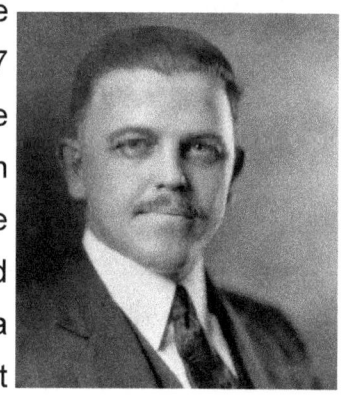

Andrew Ivy

Harold Mielke and colleagues in Los Angeles CA improved the Ivy bleeding time in 1969, by using a template that standardized the puncture/cut. Normal values are between 2 and 8 minutes. The bleeding time was mostly abandoned after the appearance of HIV. In addition, it did not have any predictive value for surgical bleeding (1991), and it had rather limited reproducibility.

Blood is Life

To test the entire coagulation system, Hellmut Hartert (1919-2003) in Heidelberg GE introduced *Thromboelastography* (TEG) in 1948. This technique, used mainly in surgery and anesthesiology, simultaneously tests coagulation, platelet function and fibrinolysis. TEG determines the speed and strength of clot formation, which depends on the activity of the various parts of the coagulation system. The device also measures clot lysis.

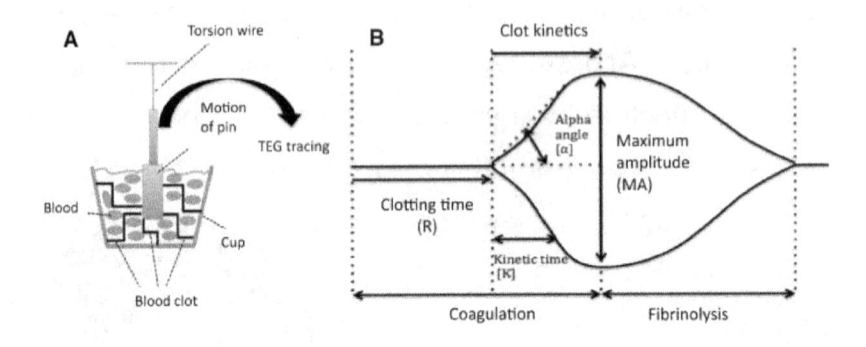

Thromboelastography, showing the different phases of coagulation

Platelet aggregation studies were introduced shortly after the first description of platelets by microscopy in the 1870-1880's. In 1872, the German-Swiss pathologist Friedrich Zahn (1845-1904) found thrombi of alternating brighter layers of platelets mixed with fibrin, and darker layers of red cells, called the "*lines of Zahn*", in places where rapid blood flow was present before death. Giulio Bizzozero in Italy saw that platelets ("*Blutplättchen*") clump together at sites of vessel damage in 1881. He described the changes that platelets undergo after exposure to foreign surfaces, forming "white thrombi". The technique to measure platelet aggregation did not become available until 1962, when both Gustav Born (1921-2018) in London and John O'Brien (1914-2002) in Portsmouth UK, developed platelet aggregometers. This

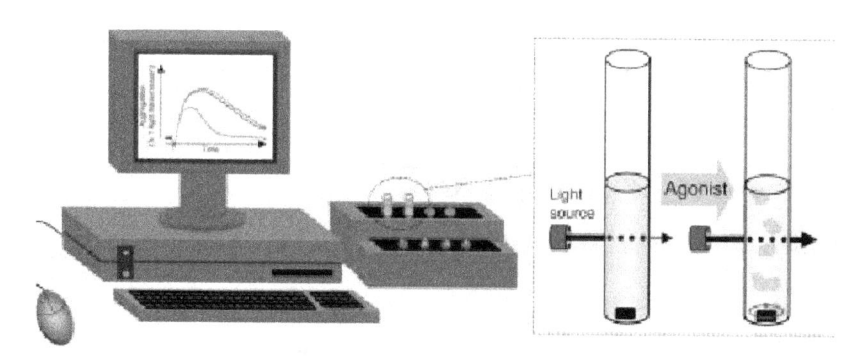

Platelet aggregometer

simple technique involved stirring a suspension of platelets in the presence of a platelet activating factor, and measuring the clumping of platelets by monitoring the changes in light transmission. Adenosine diphosphate (ADP), thrombin, and later also ristocetin (1977), were used as platelet activating factors.

To study the extrinsic pathway of coagulation, organic chemist/physician Armand Quick (1894-1978), in 1932 still in New York before his move to Milwaukee WI, developed the test named after him. This one-stage test measured the clotting time of decalcified plasma after the addition of thromboplastin and calcium: the *prothrombin time* (PT).

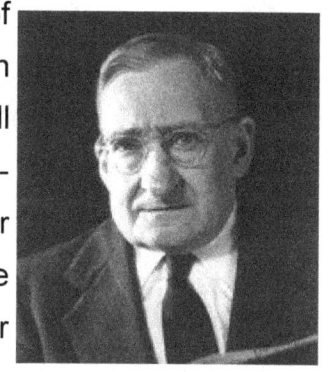

Armand Quick

Blood is Life

This test became of extreme importance for the treatment of patients with oral anticoagulant therapy and for monitoring liver failure. It was simplified by using a metal hook to detect the first clot. More automated techniques were developed: the simple fibrometer or far more sophisticated devices. A problem was standardizing the thromboplastin that used to be made from cadaver brains. Less responsive commercial thromboplastins led to larger doses of anticoagulants, with an increased risk of bleeding. Standardization began with the Manchester Reagent in England in 1962, followed by the British Comparative Thromboplastin (BCT) in 1970. Then in 1983, Tom Kirkwood (b.1951) in Manchester UK reported on the WHO International Normalized Ratio (*INR*) for calibrating thromboplastins. The standard was the average of the PT of 20 healthy individuals.

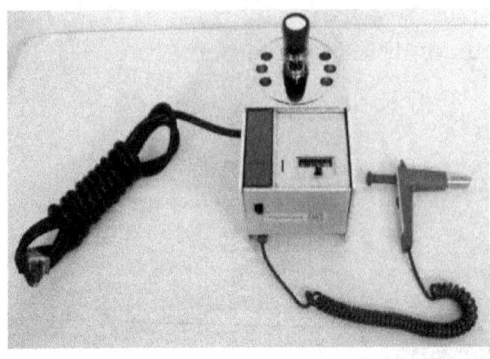

BBL 60415 Fibrometer

Emil 'Fredi' Loeliger (1924-2017)'s group in Leiden NL, and several other groups, confirmed the results. The INR became rapidly accepted as the standard. The goal is to achieve an INR of 2.0-3.0 for oral anticoagulation. Recently, point-of-service devices that use test strips have been introduced, (*e.g.*, Coaguchek XS by Roche; 2009).

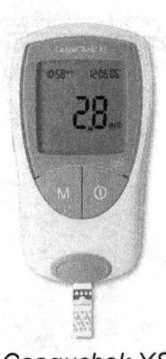

Coaguchek XS

Technology

To study the intrinsic and common pathways, the *Partial Thromboplastin Time* (PTT) was introduced. The group of Kenneth Brinkhous (1908-2000; *p.283*) in Chapel Hill NC reported it as the kaolin-cephalin clotting time (KCCT), since kaolin and cephalin were historically used in the test. Blood was drawn into a blue vacutainer tube (blue color for his University of North Carolina!) that contains citrate. The plasma at 37°C is mixed with excess calcium and an activator (kaolin, silica, celite, or ellagic acid) is added. The normal values vary between 30 and about 50 seconds. Because an activator is used, PTT is also called aPTT (*activated partial thromboplastin time*).

D-dimer is a useful recent test to study fibrin degradation. Plasmin degrades the cross-linked fibrin and exposes the D-dimer antigen. The name derives from the two D fragments of the fibrin protein joined by a crosslink (late 1970's). In the late 1980's, a latex-bead test for the terminal plasmin digestion product fragment, D-dimer-fragment-E complex, was developed. Automated special analyzers record the rate at which antibody-coated particles aggregate in response to D-dimer antigen. Next an ELISA test was introduced (2002). Even a whole blood agglutination test, not requiring sophisticated instrumentation, was marketed in 1990. The various tests are used in the diagnosis of deep venous thrombosis (DVT), pulmonary embolism (PE), diffuse intravascular coagulation (DIC), and many other diseases (*e.g.*, sickle-cell anemia, cytokine-release syndrome *etc.*).

Georges Hayem was born in Paris in 1841. He studied Medicine there, with a special interest in Internal Medicine and Hematology. He became a Professor of "Therapy and Materia Medica". He was associated with Hôpital St. Antoine and held the chair of Clinical Medicine for 18 years. His interests in hematology concerned the origin of leukocytes and erythrocytes. He adhered to Paul Ehrlich's dualistic theory (splenic versus lymphatic), in opposition to Neumann's monophyletic theory of a single hematopoietic stem cell.

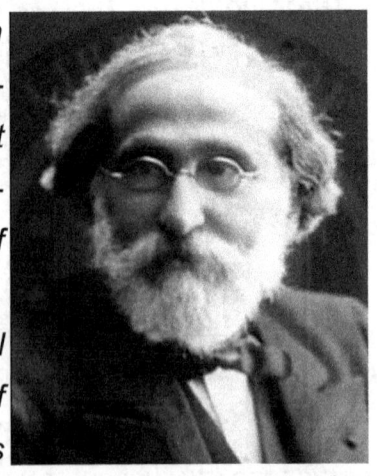

Hayem was the first to make accurate blood counts of platelets, and he developed the mercury chloride, sodium chloride and sodium sulfate solution used for dilution of blood prior to counting red cells in a hemocytometer. He described cases of acquired chronic jaundice in 1898. When Georges Fernand Widal (1862-1929) in Paris described similar cases ten years later, the disease became known as the Hayem

Hayem's Hematology text book (1878)

Widal syndrome: acquired hemolytic anemia. In other fields of internal medicine, he described cases of chronic interstitial hepatitis in 1874, and he introduced an intravenous saline solution for the treatment of Asiatic cholera. He died in 1933. In France, he is considered the father of hematology, just like William Hewson is in some Anglophone countries

.

Paul Ehrlich was born in 1854 in Strehlen, a small town in upper Silesia, Prussia (now Strzelin PO). He went to the Gymnasium in Breslau, and subsequently studied Medicine in Breslau, Strasbourg, Freiburg and Leipzig. During his medical studies, he already developed the triacid stain that revolutionized the study of peripheral blood and bone-marrow smears (p.25). He was influenced for this work by his cousin Karl Weigert, who owned one of the first microtomes. After graduation he joined the Charité Hospital in Berlin in 1882, focusing on histology, hematology, and staining techniques. In 1886, he completed his habilitation, comparable to a PhD, in Medicine. He reported the first case of acquired aplastic anemia in 1888, the same year he had to recover from tuberculosis in Egypt. Upon his return, he joined Robert Koch (1843-1910) at the Berlin Institute of Infectious Diseases; he worked on tuberculin as a testing agent and started the

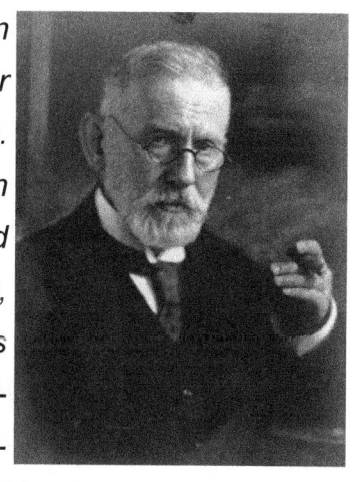

*Division of Serum Research and Testing (*Institut für Serumforschung und Serumprüfung*) in 1896. Here, he did his first experiments on immunization (creating ricin-proof mice), and he postulated that "inherited immunity" was conveyed by antibodies from mother to baby. He also studied autoimmunity, calling it "horror autotoxicus". He collaborated with Emil A Behring (1854-1917) on the diphtheria antitoxin, which earned Behring his Nobel prize in 1901, but Ehrlich was left out. Behring also was honored with Prussian nobility, becoming Von Behring. The Institute for Serum Research and Testing moved in 1899 to Frankfurt am Main and was renamed the Royal Prussian Institute for Experimental Therapy. He postulated that cell protoplasm contains special structures with chemical side chains to which the toxin binds. If the cell produces a surplus of side chains, they may be released into the blood as antibodies. For his work on humoral immunology he was awarded the Nobel Prize in 1908 together with Ilya Mechnikov (p.133), who worked on cellular immunology. In 1909, Ehrlich and Sahachiro Hata (1873-1938) discovered the first drug targeted against a specific pathogen,* Treponema Pallidum, *as therapy for syphilis (Arsphenamine). The drug was marketed as Salvarsan in 1910 by Hoechst AG, and became soon the most widely prescribed drug in the world. Ehrlich also postulated that a toxin for a disease-causing organism could be delivered coupled to a selective agent: the magic bullet ("Zauberkugel"). Paul Ehrlich died in 1915. His stellar reputation suffered before and during the 1930's, because of raging* *antisemitism, but the* Frankfort *Institute for Experimental Therapy, of which he was the first director, was named after him in 1947.*

Johannes Josephus ("Jon") van Rood *was born in 1926 in The Hague NL. After World War II, he studied Medicine at the Leiden University. During his Internal Medicine residency, his turn came to medically supervise the Blood Bank, where Aad van Leeuwen was one of the technologists. Aad became an important contributor to his HLA work. Van Rood's interests in blood banking continued, and he started studying non-hemolytic transfusion reactions. His group was able to prevent these reactions by removing the leukocytes from the transfusion products. In 1958, a multiparous woman, who had never been transfused before, developed a non-hemolytic transfusion reaction after a single red cell transfusion. This led the group to conclude that the pregnancy had induced leukocyte allo-antibodies. Those antibodies reacted with the white cells of her husband and some of her children. Studies of families and the use of the first computer in the Netherlands, allowed the distinction of various clusters. This all contributed to the new area of Human Leukocyte Antigen (HLA) typing. Van Rood also studied HLA's influence on the outcome of renal transplantation. Survivors and their organ donors showed an*

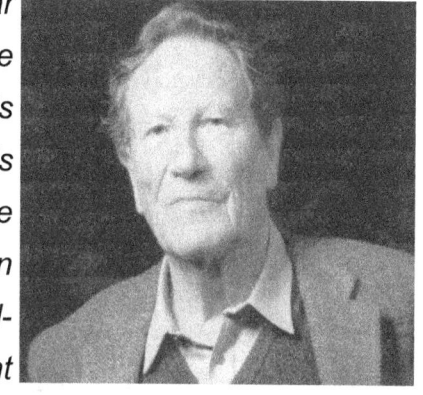

unusual leukocyte-antigen compatibility. In 1967, he founded Eurotransplant *which helped the exchange of donor kidneys based on histocompatibility between 75 collaborating centers in 6 European countries. This Registry was expanded to also find platelet donors and unrelated bone-marrow donors (*Europdonor*). Actually, the Van Rood group claimed to have saved the first patient in the world through HLA typing. A patient with severe aplastic anemia was bleeding in 1964, and had extensive leukocyte antibodies. They HLA-typed the extended family and were able to identify suitable donors; the patient survived. Van Rood's group also introduced the use of leukocyte depletion of transfusion products, to avoid allo-immunization (1975). In 1973, Van Rood and Bruno Speck were the instigators of the* European Bone Marrow Transplant Group (EBMT), *which rapidly was joined by centers from all over Europe. He was also one of the founders of the* World Marrow Donor Association *in 1994; the WMDA's headquarters is still in Leiden. Van Rood retired in 1991, but remained active. He contributed to the field of the influence of allogeneic cells on the T- and B-cell repertoire, and its possible effect on the outcome of transplantation. This led to the concept of NIMA (non-inherited maternal antigens) and its effect on GvHD after haploidentical sibling donor allografts or cord-blood transplants. Van Rood died in 2017, at age 91.*

RED BLOOD CELLS

The overwhelming majority of cells in the peripheral blood are red cells (*erythrocytes*). Because of their color and abundance, they were recognized first when blood could be studied with the earliest microscopes in the second half of the 17th century. Several investigators documented them, but Antonie van Leeuwenhoek first reported them (*p.24*). He believed that they were globular and had the size of "less than 1% of a grain of sand". William Hewson (*p.25*) discovered that the red cells were discoid, but he considered their center to be the nucleus. Hewson believed that all blood cells, including the red cells, originated in the lymphatic system. Not everybody believed in the existence of red cells. The French physiologist Francois Magendie (1783-1855) used regular water to dilute blood in 1817. He then claimed that the red blood cells seen by others were in fact air bubbles! This was not the only time he was wrong. He also was an avid practitioner of vivisection. His experiments in Paris led to the "Cruel Treatment of Cattle Act 1822" in England.

Rudolf Virchow (*p.168*) held the dualistic view of blood cell production (splenic versus lymphatic), but in 1868 Ernst Neumann (*p.20*) in East Prussia and Giulio Bizzozero in Italy demonstrated that in the adult organism the bone marrow is the main site of all blood production. The fight between the monophyletic and dualist concepts continued for decades and was rather fierce. Georges Hayem (*p.48*) accused

Ernst Neumann of "encumbering science" by ill-founded statements. Similar harsh views were uttered later by Otto Naegeli in Zürich SU.

Around the end of the 19th century, it was generally accepted that red cells were produced by the bone marrow. The early stages of erythropoiesis in the bone marrow involved cells that had a nucleus (erythroblasts), whereas the circulating red cells did not have a nucleus. In 1958, Marcel Bessis in Paris elucidated this change. He showed the existence of erythroblastic islands in the bone marrow. These islands, positioned around a macrophage, produce maturing erythroid cells. Upon leaving the islands, the erythroblasts are enucleated (into the macrophage) and become reticulocytes. The process from committed stem cell to circulating red cell takes about 7 days. The mature red cells of healthy individuals circulate about 100-120 days as demonstrated with survival studies (*p.42*). Every second, the bone marrow produces about 2.4 million new red cells (2.1 x 10^{11} per day). The aging red cells undergo changes in their plasma membrane, and become susceptible to phagocytosis by spleen and liver macrophages (*eryptosis*).

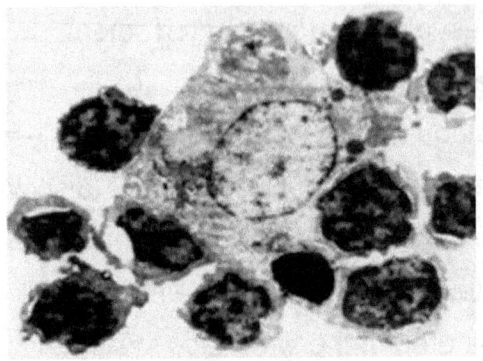

Erythroblastic island

The function of red cells remained a mystery until almost the late 19th century. In 1820, a medical dictionary still opined that red cells had nothing of importance.

Red Blood Cells

Sven G Hedin (1859-1933) in Lund SW demonstrated that the red-cell membrane was semi-permeable in 1897. The next step was to document that red cells had extensive metabolic activity, in particular glucose consumption and utilization. The biochemist Otto H Warburg (1883-1970) in Berlin studied red-cell metabolism in 1909, and showed that red cells use little oxygen. Later studies by him and many other investigators elucidated the many enzymes involved in glucose metabolism (p.80).

Hemoglobin (Hgb), the substance that gives the red color to blood, makes up about 96% of the dry content of red cells and about 35% of total content (including water). The name derives from Heme and Globin, reflecting the fact that each subunit of Hgb is a globular protein with an embedded heme group with an iron molecule. In 1825, chemist Johann Engelhart (1797-1837) in Göttingen GE calculated the molecular mass of each Hgb subunit at 16,000 Da. He was ridiculed, because many scientists did not believe that any molecule could be that big. Protein chemist Gilbert Adair (1896-1979) in Cambridge UK, however, confirmed his results in 1925. Friedrich Hünefeld in Greifswald GE discovered that Hgb can carry oxygen in 1840. The binding of oxygen was reversible as demonstrated by Felix Hoppe-Seyler in 1864. He also showed that the blood pigment, which he called

Heme molecule

"*Hämoglobin*" for the first time, can be split into hematin and a protein. The oxygen-binding capacity of hemoglobin was confirmed by French giant Claude Bernard, (1813-1878; in 1870); each Hgb molecule can bind up to 4 oxygen molecules. The total oxygen-binding capacity of blood is 70-fold compared with O_2 dissolved in plasma.

Max Perutz (1914-1992), who initially trained in Vienna AT, but did most of his work in Cambridge UK, determined the molecular structure of Hgb with X-ray crystallography in 1959. He received the Nobel prize in Chemistry in 1962 for this work. In the years that followed, his group documented how Hgb works as a molecular machine, switching between the deoxygenated and oxygenated states. The iron in the heme group stays in the reduced state (Fe^{2+}).

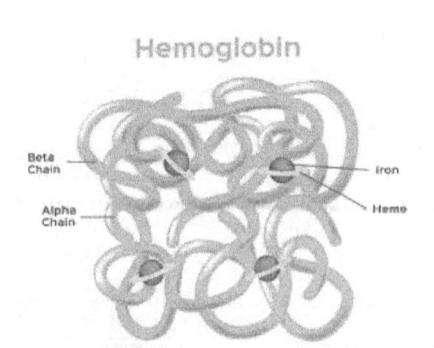

The major Hgb in humans, Hemoglobin A, is a heterotetramer composed of two α-globin and two β-globin polypeptides, encoded by the duplicated *HBA1* and *HBA2* (on chromosome 16) and by the *HBB* (on chromosome 11) genes, respectively. In the human fetus, hemoglobin F (α2γ2) is the main oxygen carrier. HgbF allows the stronger binding of oxygen, to retrieve oxygen from the mother's blood stream through the placenta. After birth, HgbF production decreases and by the first birthday HgbF usually is <1% of total Hgb. Hemoglobin variants, caused by mutations in the genes for the hemoglobin protein, are the basis for many anemias in man.

HEREDITARY ANEMIAS

Thalassemia

Thalassemia is an old disease, although not officially recognized before the early 20th century. Skulls of prehistoric humans found by archeologists sometimes show *porotic hyperostosis*, in which the bones of the cranial vault have localized areas of spongy or porous bone tissue. Although not diagnostic of thalassemia, this abnormality in mummies in Egypt, Incas in Peru, Aztecs in Mexico, and skeletons in Sardinia and Sicily, would fit various thalassemic syndromes. Hippocrates may have referred to children with β-thalassemia, although the *pica* (eating dirt) he described as a symptom, probably fits all types of anemia. The pallor of emperor Constantius Chlorus (*"the green"*) (250-306 CE), the father of Constantine the Great, might be explained by β-thalassemia. He originated from the central Balkan, where the disease was frequent. Clearly, another explanation for his pallor could be pernicious anemia. Early descriptions from medieval Italy can point to many different diseases. The same holds true for the *"anemia infantum pseudoleukemica"*, described by Rudolf von Jaksch (1855-1947) in Prague AT in 1889. He reported children under three years of age with anemia and splenomegaly. On the other hand, thalassemia was/is not frequent in the Czech Republic. Over the next 25 years, "Jaksch anemia" was used for any unusual anemia in infancy.

In 1925, pediatrician Thomas Cooley (1871-1945) in Detroit MI, reported on a "series of cases of splenomegaly in children with anemia and peculiar bone changes". The four children had anemia with hepatosplenomegaly and jaundice, "but no bile in the urine". Similar cases were then reported from other parts of North America and Europe, some still under the name "Jaksch anemia".

Thomas Cooley

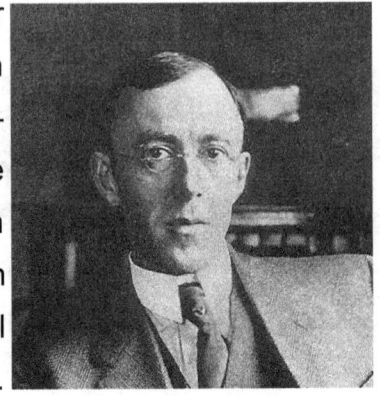

In 1932, pathologist George Whipple (1878-1976) in Rochester NY, described the pathology of the condition and introduced the name thalassemia, from the Greek θαλασσα ("Mediterranean" Sea) and άιμα (blood). Actually, Whipple's classically trained colleague George Corner (1889-1981) probably proposed the name. Corner went on to fame for his early work on oral contraceptives, while Whipple shared in the Nobel Prize in Physiology/Medicine of 1934 for work on "liver therapy in cases of anemia". Fernando Rietti (1890-1954) in Ferrara IT described a mild form of hemolytic jaundice with "increased osmotic resistance of the red cells", clearly different from congenital spherocytosis, in 1925. Other Italian investigators reported similar cases. The condition was called "Rietti-Greppi-Micheli syndrome". It took nearly 2 decades before this syndrome was recognized as the heterozygous form of thalassemia, perhaps partly because their papers were published only in Italian! Both the Greek physician Caminopetros and the Italian Angelini documented that thalassemia was a genetically determined disease in 1936-1938: relatives of patients had red cells with increased osmotic resistance. This was rapidly confirmed by various groups in the US. For example, Max Wintrobe (*p.83*) at Johns Hopkins documented typical changes in the blood of 40 members of three Italian families: some had splenomegaly and/or mild jaundice. Both parents of a child with thalassemia showed these changes. More formal genetic studies after World War II, documented the Mendelian inheritance, with the heterozygous form of thalassemia now called thalassemia minor. Bill Dameshek (*p.188*) pointed out that the blood of patients with thalassemia minor had target cells and he called the disease "target-cell anemia". By 1952, the diseases thalassemia and thalassemia minor were well established, but it already had become clear that it represented probably more than a single genetic disease.

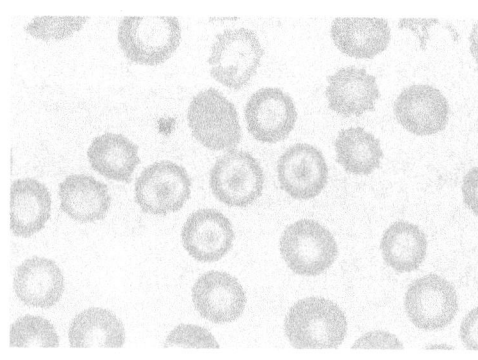

target cells

During the 1940's and 1950's, the knowledge about various hemoglobins rapidly increased. In 1959, Ingram and Stretton presented their theoretical model for the genetic base of thalassemia, based on ideas from multiple sources. Körber in his doctoral thesis for the University of Dorpat (currently Tartu ES) had already shown in 1866 that hemoglobin of human placental blood was more resistant to denaturation with alkali than adult hemoglobin. Many subsequent studies, discussed in the sickle-cell anemia subchapter (*p.65*), provided additional evidence for the structure of hemoglobin. Henry Kunkel (1916-1983) and Gunnar Wallenius in New York demonstrated a minor hemoglobin variant in normal adult red cells: HgbA$_2$. This suggested that a third chromosome locus was involved in the control of human adult hemoglobin. Pauling's group and others found that the globin fractions of hemoglobin A consists of two pairs of identical peptide chains with different terminal amino-acid structures, called α-chains and β-chains. This was in line with Perutz's X-ray crystallographic analysis of horse hemoglobin. Fetal hemoglobin was found to have two α-chains, but also two γ-chains instead of β-chains. The complete amino-acid sequence of the α, β, and γ chains soon followed. Hemoglobin A$_2$ was found to have two δ chains instead of β chains.

Vecchio in Italy concluded in 1946, based on the increased alkali resistance of the red cells of thalassemia, that fetal hemoglobin had persisted . Various combinations of thalassemia, sickle cell anemia, hemoglobin C, hemoglobin H (tetramer of 4 normal β-chains) and hemoglobin Bart's (tetramer of 4 γ-chains) revealed that thalassemia is a rather heterogenous disease. Pauling and Itano suggested in 1954 that the thalassemia gene might be responsible for production of an abnormal hemoglobin of such a nature as to interfere with the inclusion of heme into the molecule. All these facts led Vernon Ingram and Antony Stretton in 1959 to their description of the genetic basis of thalassemia. They suggested the existence of α-thalassemia and β-thalassemia. Hemoglobin H (HgbE) could be explained by a defect to produce α-chains, allowing excess β-chain production.

The genetics of α-thalassemia were clarified in the 1960's, particularly in Thailand. It was found that two types of α-thalassemia genes existed; α-thalassemia was more frequent in the Oriental populations, but also occurred in Arabs and African blacks. Homozygosity for the α-thalassemia-1 gene would lead to hemoglobin Bart's hydrops syndrome with intrauterine death. In Thailand, 20% of the population carry one form or another of α-thalassemia. Many different interactions of α- and β-thalassemia genes have been reported from there and from other parts of the Malaysian peninsula and Indonesia.

The genetic heterogeneity of β-thalassemia was clarified in the same years, mainly based on studies of patients with sickle-cell thalassemia. Some of these patients did not produce any HgbA, but only HgbS and some HgbF. This form of β-thalassemia had completely suppressed β-chain production: the $β^0$-thalassemia. When some production of HgbA was still found, it was called $β^+$-thalassemia. In Mediterranean countries, the carrier state of β-thalassemia was as high as 15-20%. The disease was also common in India and does also occur in Southeast Asia and Africa.

Whereas Cooley originally had described his cases as representing hemolytic anemia, studies in the 1960's stressed ineffective erythropoiesis and premature destruction of the red cells (Fessas in Athens GR;1963). Inclusion bodies in the bone-marrow cells, and in the peripheral-blood cells after splenectomy, represented precipitated α-chains. David Nathan (b.1929) and Robert Gunn in Boston suggested that the precipitated globin chains might interfere with red-cell membrane function. David Weatherall (1933-2018) and colleagues at Johns Hopkins, using radioactive amino-acids *in vitro*, demonstrated in 1964-1965 that thalassemia is characterized by imbalanced globin chain production. Studies showed reduced β-chain mRNA in 1971. The introduction of reverse transcriptase to direct DNA synthesis on RNA templates in 1970, independently by Howard Temin (1934-1994) in Madison WI and David Baltimore (b.1938) at MIT Boston, allowed the copy of complementary DNA from mRNA. Temin and Baltimore shared in the 1975 Nobel prize in Physiology/Medicine. When this technique was applied to the α-chain, it was shown that in HgbBart's hydrops syndrome the α genes were largely deleted. In HgbH disease, three of the four α-genes were deleted.

The molecular basis for the various forms of β thalassemia was more difficult to sort out. Ultimately, it became clear that two major groups of mutations can be distinguished. The "non-deletion" forms had a single-base substitution or small insertion near or upstream of the β globin gene. The "deletion" forms had deletion of different sizes involving the β-globin gene. Mutations are characterized as $β^0$ if they prevent any formation of β chains, or $β^+$ if they allow some β chain formation. Thus, thalassemia minor had $β^+/β$ or $β^0/β$; thalassemia intermedia had $β^+/β^+$ or $β^0/β^+$; thalassemia major had $β^0/β^0$.

Therapy for thalassemia consisted of frequent transfusions, which could easily lead to iron overload. Iron chelation therapy was capable of prolonging life and finally became also available as oral therapy in 2005. The use of "neocyte" (= young red cells, in top layer after centrifugation) transfusions, introduced by Sergio Piomelli (b.1931) in New York in 1979, decreased the required frequency of transfusion. Adequately transfused patients have a lower risk of hypersplenism and less frequently require splenectomy. Hydroxyurea was found to be effective to decrease transfusion need in many children with β-thalassemia, by enhancing fetal hemoglobin production, similar with the situation in sickle-cell anemia. Hydroxyurea worked better in patients with thalassemia intermedia than in thalassemia major. Studies in thalassemia major are ongoing, particularly in countries where stem-cell transplantation is not an economic option. Clearly, these therapies are helpful, but cannot cure the disease.

Allogeneic stem-cell transplantation for homozygous β-thalassemia, with marrow from HLA-identical siblings, was introduced by Guido Lucarelli (b.1934) and his team in Pesaro IT in 1988. Many of the patients came from the island of Sardinia, where no adequate blood-transfusion

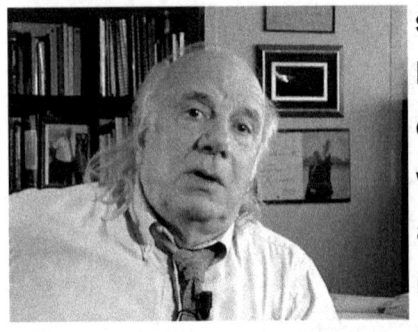

Guido Lucarelli

service was available. Especially in young children and teenagers, the results were impressive with an overall survival of >80% and rejection of only 10%. Mismatched related and matched unrelated donors were also used, but the results were obviously not quite as good. Autologous stem-cell transplantation with lentiviral β-gene transfer of A(T87Q) was performed in 2007 in Paris in an 18-year-old young man with $β^E/β^0$-thalassemia. The patient had already been splenectomized at age 6. He required frequent transfusions, failed hydroxyurea therapy, and did not have an HLA matched donor. After myelo-ablative therapy, he received his transduced bone marrow reinfused and had uneventful hematopoietic reconstitution. His hemoglobin became a combination of HgbF, HgbE ($αβ^E$ dimer) and Hgbβ$^{A(T87Q)}$ ($αβ^{(T87Q)}$ dimer). This treatment received "breakthrough designation" by the FDA in 2015 as betibeglogene autotemcel (Zynteglo®) and was approved in Europe in 2019. Very recently, modification of the transcription factor repressing γ-globin expression, via CRISPR-Cas9 targeting, was successful (2021).

An important approach was preventive treatment by carrier screening and prenatal diagnosis. This was beneficial in some, but not all, societies. Procreation between a β-thalassemia gene carrier and a non-carrier would prevent thalassemia major and would slowly decrease the percentage of carriers.

Sickle Cell Anemia

A recent study at the NIH (Bethesda MD) by Daniel Shriner and Charles Rotimi (b.1957) suggested that the genetic mutation responsible for sickle-cell anemia occurred in a child in the Sahara, then still a green belt of savannas, about 7,200 years ago. Since the mutation occurred in only one copy of the gene, the child remained healthy and passed the mutation down to subsequent generations. As the savanna slowly became desert, the hunters gatherers moved to other parts of Africa and became farmers and cattle-herders. It turned out that the mutated gene protected against one of the main health threats in Africa: malaria. This gave the carriers of the mutated gene a survival, and thus procreation, adventage. The mutated gene spread over wide areas of Africa, but also to southern Europe, the Middle East and India. The problem was, when two carriers of the mutated gene had offspring, two mutated genes might come together, causing fatal sickle-cell anemia. In 1974, Hermann Lehman (1910-1985), a German trained at Heidelberg University but working mainly in Cambridge UK, had suggested in his book *Man's Haemoglobins*

Hermann Lehman

that the sickle-cell gene originated in Neolithic times in Arabia, and then spread to Africa and India. The disease sickle-cell anemia was not reported first in Africa, but in

Blood is Life

Chicago IL by James Herrick (1861-1954) in 1910. A young black dental student from Grenada (West Indies) had presented 6 years earlier with anemia; his blood film showed elongated and sickle-shaped red cells. Herrick suggested that "some change in the composition of the corpuscle itself may be the determining factor". The patient was seen intermittently over the next 3 years. During his long training, Herrick had spent time in the chemistry laboratory of Emil Fisher (1852-1919) in Berlin, where he learned about proteins, polypeptides and amino acids. At the time of this first publication about sickle-cell anemia, a 25-year-old black woman was in the hospital of the University of Virginia. She had suffered for several years from pain episodes, leg ulcers, gall stones, and anemia. The case was also confirmed as sickle-cell anemia. Five years later, Victor Emmel (1878-1928) in St. Louis MO sealed a drop of blood of a patient under a cover slip and observed normal red cells starting to sickle. The patient's father did not have anemia or sickle cells in his blood smear, but the red cells could be forced to start sickling under a sealed cover slip.

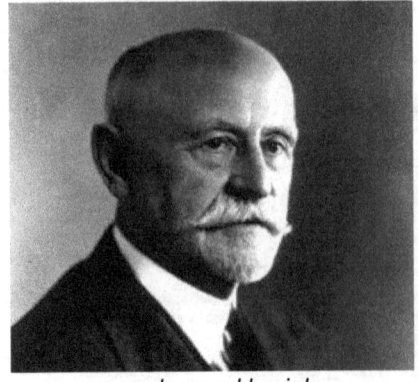

James Herrick

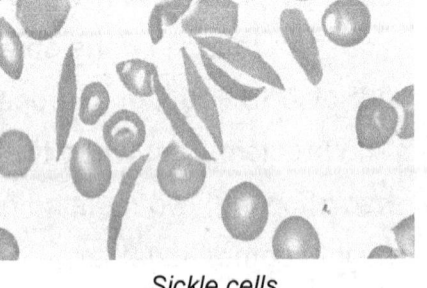

Sickle cells

At Johns Hopkins, the name "sickle-cell anemia" was introduced in 1922, when their first patient was recognized. The next year, at that same hospital, the first genetic study was performed, but it still suggested that the inheritance of a single factor followed Mendelian laws. The term sickle-cell anemia was also used for non-anemic relatives whose cells could be induced to sickle. That same year, Virgil Sydenstricker (1889-1964) and colleagues at the Medical College of Georgia, documented sickle-cell anemia in a patient whose healthy parents could both be induced to sickle. They also described "crisis" for the first time, and suggested that the anemia was hemolytic. Their studies documented "latent sickling"" in 4% of African Americans, but none in Caucasians. Although sickle-cell anemia appeared to be the homozygous state of a gene, it took until 1949 before geneticist James Neel (1915-2000) in Ann Arbor MI, and Colonial Medical Officer Colonel Beet in Northern Rhodesia (now Zambia), independently, concluded that sickle-cell anemia represents homozygosity for the mutant gene.

The first case of sickle-cell anemia in Africa was reported from Khartoum in the Sudan in 1925 . A 10-year-old Arab boy was admitted with a febrile illness. The physicians had not yet heard of sickle-cell anemia, but they reported the case after they learned about the disease in the USA. The first black patient was reported in Ghana in 1932. In a study in West Africa about 20% of the population appeared to have "latent sickling"; in East Africa it was estimated at 13%. The lower incidence of sickle-cell disease in Africa was caused by the enormous infant mortality of children with sickle-cell anemia, as documented by J & C Lambotte-Legrand in the Belgian Congo (later Zaire, now DR of Congo) in the 1950's. Adults with sickle-cell anemia were rare, and the causes of early death were the overall standard of living, the prevalence of infection, nutritional deficiencies, and the level of general health care. As the overall health care improved, so did the chances of patients to survive until adolescence.

The interaction of sickle-cell trait (heterozygosity) and malaria was studied by Colonel Beet in Zambia. He found that 15% of the "non-sicklers" among his hospitalized patients had malaria, but only 10% of the "sicklers". Follow up studies in various countries in East Africa, suggested that "red cells of sicklers (=heterozygotes) offer a less favorable environment for malarial parasites". The investigators suggested that the life cycle of the malaria parasite may be interrupted by sickling and the premature destruction of the parasitized red cell. The South-African geneticist Anthony Allison (1925-2014) noted that the sickle-cell trait in some areas of Kenya was 40%, which would therefore predict a high incidence of sickle-cell anemia. Consequently, the mutated gene would be expected to be rapidly eliminated if there were no advantage to having the trait. He concluded that sickle-cell trait was a true polymorphism, maintained by the selective advantage of the heterozygote.

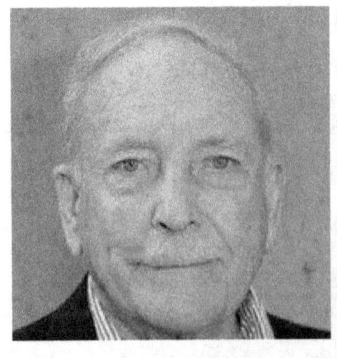

Tony Allison

Red Blood Cells

Why and when do the red cells of sicklers sickle? E. Vernon Hahn (1891-1959; later a neurosurgeon in Indianapolis IN) and Elizabeth Gillespie (later a general practitioner in Cincinnati OH) demonstrated, early in their careers in 1927, that the sickling occurs when the red cells are deoxygenated. Sickling was determined to depend on oxygen tension and pH. Carbon monoxide was as effective is restoring the discoid form as oxygen. It was later shown that prolonged deoxygenation leads to permanently deformed cells. Major work to establish what leads to sickling was done by Lemuel Diggs (1900-1995) in Memphis TN. By studying 3,000 African Americans of whom 8.3% showed sickling, they found In 1932, that sickle-cell trait was compatible with long life, and not associated with leg ulcers or other abnormalities. Irving Sherman (1916-2019) at Johns Hopkins University, who also went on to become a neurosurgeon, showed in 1940 that sickling occurred far more in the venous than in the arterial circulation of patients with sickle-cell anemia. The frequent change in shape should decrease the life span of the red cells. He found that under the polarizing microscope, sickle cells exhibit a definite "birefringence" (optical property to have a refractive index depending on the polarization and propagation direction of light), that disappears when the cells return to their discoid state. This was later interpreted to mean that certain molecules of the cell become orientated when the cells undergo sickling. Linus Pauling (1901-1994), the only person so far to ever receive a Nobel Prize in Chemistry and a Nobel Peace Prize, concluded in 1945 that

Blood is Life

"sicklers" have an abnormal hemoglobin, that when deoxygenated has the power of combining itself into long rigid rods. Pauling put Harvey Itano (1920-2010), who had just been released from incarceration as one of the Nisei during World War II, on the subject at Caltech in Pasadena CA. Itano and his colleagues performed electrophoresis studies and demonstrated in 1948 that the hemoglobin of sicklers was different from normal Hgb. This was caused by a change in the globin, since the heme groups were identical. The Hgb of sicklers had two peaks, whereas sickle-cell anemia Hgb and normal Hgb had each only one (different) peak. This confirmed the heterozygous status of the "sicklers". This was probably the first demonstration of a molecular disease. Two years before, Heinrich Hörlein and Weber had discovered the first abnormal hemoglobin, methemoglobin (now called Hemoglobin M Saskatoon), in four generations of a family in Germany.

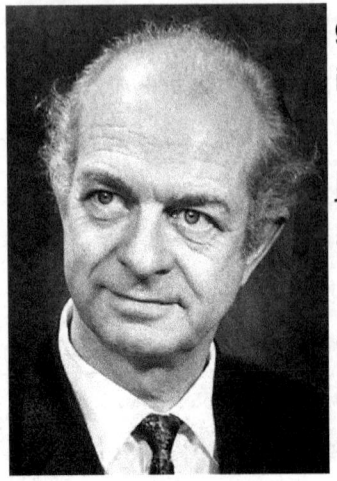

Linus Pauling

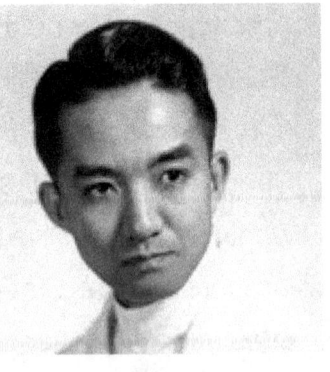

Harvey Itano

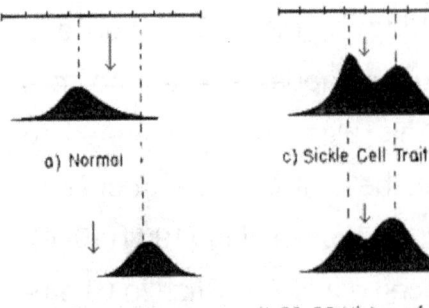

a) Normal
b) Sickle Cell Anemia
c) Sickle Cell Trait
d) 50-50 Mixture of a) and b)

Hemoglobin electrophoresis (Pauling)

Long before that, since 1866, it had been known that fetal hemoglobin differed from adult hemoglobin, and that was also demonstrated with electrophoresis in 1944. Janet Watson (1913-1969) in Brooklyn NY confirmed that red cells of newborns sickled less. Blood samples from her patients ultimately led the group of Perutz to further analyze Hemoglobin S, so named after 1953. In the same year, Itano discovered Hemoglobin C leading to the description of sickle-cell hemoglobin-C disease, which was less severe than sickle cell anemia. Vernon Ingram (1924-2006), originally named Werner Immerwahr, a protein chemist from Breslau GE (now Wroclaw, PO), left for England in 1938. In 1956 at Cambridge, he demonstrated that Hemoglobin S differs from Hemoglobin A in only a single amino acid of the β-chain. To document this, his group used electrophoresis in combination with chromatography.

Vernon Ingram

Therapy for sickle-cell anemia was difficult. Splenectomy had been proposed by Sydenstricker (1922) and performed by Hahn and Gillespie (1927), but did not really take off. Many different therapies were recommended, but all had only ephemeral use. Oxygen administered during crises was tried, but pain was mostly caused by infarction of tissue. Sodium bicarbonate or sodium citrate, by increasing the pH, made sense, but was not shown to help in controlled studies. Anti-sickling agents were also studied. Intravenous urea therapy was highly recommended around 1970, but failed in a double blind trial. Cyanate irreversibly inhibited sickling. Initial studies raised hope, but a severe peripheral neuropathy and cataracts abruptly cancelled the plans for randomized studies. Hydroxyurea was introduced in the early 1980's, and was effective in decreasing pain crises, blood transfusions and hospitalizations. The drug increased the production of Hemoglobin F and made the red cells bigger and more flexible. A multicenter study, starting in 1992, confirmed the value of hydroxyurea and the drug was approved by the FDA for use in sickle-cell disease in 1998. This treatment helps to decrease the clinical problems of sickle-cell anemia, but obviously does not solve the underlying disorder.

Allogeneic stem-cell transplantation from a healthy, or a heterozygous, matched donor might completely cure the disease by eliminating the HgbSS cells. This approach was first attempted by Christiane Vermylen and colleagues in Louvain BE in 1988. Most of their patients were small children and the results were excellent. HLA-matched sibling donors were identified for 49 of 50 patients. Four years earlier, a successful allograft had been performed in a child who had sickle-cell disease but also AML. Several studies showed that a considerable proportion of patients, or their parents, were willing to accept the risks of allografts if the therapy could cure sickle-cell anemia. Unfortunately, in a study only 18% of patients were found to have an HLA-matched related donor. An alternative approach would be autologous stem cell transplantation with a transferred HgbA gene. The gene-transfer science developed during the 1980's, but government approval for clinical use only slowly progressed. The first approved attempt of clinical gene transfer was done by French Anderson (b.1936) and Michael Blaese at NIH in 1990. The 4-year-old girl was suffering from Adenosine Deaminase Deficiency SCID. Repeated infusions of T-cells with a retroviral vector containing the ADA gene, normalized her immune status. I recall that when these results came in, many in the stem-cell transplant community believed that within 5-10 years we would be able to do similar therapy for sickle-cell anemia. Actually, it took more than 25 years, but now studies are ongoing with a lentiviral vector with a modified form of the β-globin gene (LentiGlobin®). The results of stem-cell transplantation for sickle-cell anemia lagged behind thalassemia, undoubtedly connected with the financing of the health-care system, and the limited economic and political power of that particular patient population. Very recently, modification of a transcription factor that represses γ-globin expression (*p.55*) has been successful.

Hereditary spherocytosis

The first descriptions of hemolytic anemia without hemoglobinuria were published in the late 19th century. The distinction between jaundice caused by hemolysis or by liver disease was difficult without laboratory tests. In 1890, Claude Wilson in London described six members of a family with splenomegaly and mild jaundice, suggesting a hereditary condition. Since they also had anemia, it was concluded that the splenomegaly was responsible. The blood smear was initially not described, but in later studies of the same family, Wilson showed microcytosis and anemia. One of the patients died and the autopsy showed the spleen to be engorged with red cells. Active hemolysis of splenic origin was considered the cause of death. In 1871, Constant Vanlair (1839-1914) and Voltaire Masius in Liège BE had described a young woman, who developed icterus, painful splenomegaly and dark stools after a delivery. The peripheral-blood smear showed many microcytes (3-4µm diameter and spherical). Her mother and sister also had jaundice and her sister had splenomegaly. They concluded that this was a clinical entity. William Hunter in London demonstrated in 1888, that all cases of hemolytic anemia had microcytes in their peripheral blood, and that in fact it was an indication that the anemia was hemolytic. Oskar Minkowski (1858-1931) of Strassburg GE studied two families with jaundice, urobilinuria and

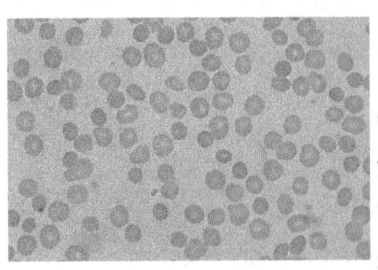

spherocytes

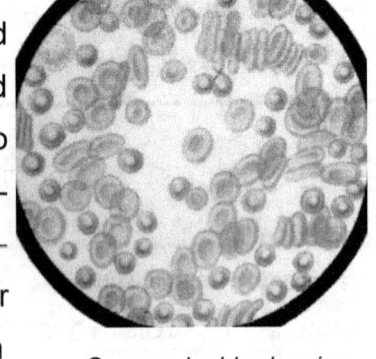

Camera lucida drawing after Vanlair (1871)

Red Blood Cells

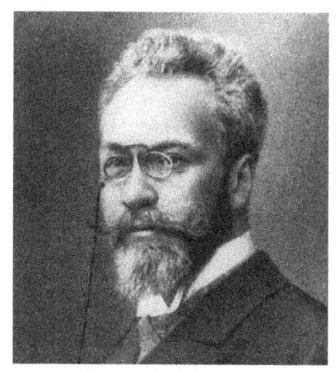

Oskar Minkowski

splenomegaly between 1900 and 1905. The liver of one patient was normal at autopsy. He believed the spleen responsible for the disorder and described the blood as normal! Similar cases were reported from other parts of Germany and from England, but here the patients were anemic (red cells 2.8-3.5 million/mm^3) and polychromasia was noted. Anatole Chauffard (1855-1932) in 1907 in Paris, showed that the red cells of patients with anemia, jaundice and splenomegaly were hemolyzed by hypotonic saline. His osmotic-fragility test became pivotal for the diagnosis of hereditary hemolytic anemia, and the disease became known as the Minkowski-Chauffard disease. Otto Naegeli, in his usual authoritarian way, claimed credit for the name spherocytes ("Sphärozyten";1931), but

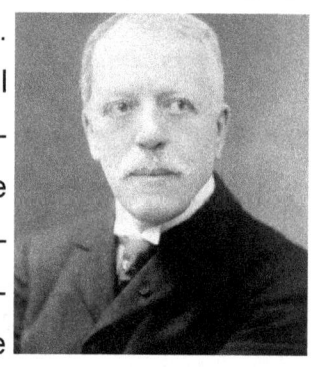

Anatole Chauffard

the term had already been used many years before in studies of malaria: "black water fever". Chauffard also confirmed the existence of polychromasia in these patients, and with the Pappenheim (=May-Grünwald-Giemsa)

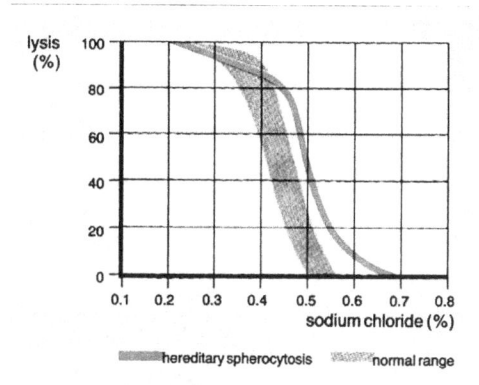

Osmotic fragility study: spherocytes lyse at a lower NaCl concentration than normal red cells.

stain, he rediscovered reticulocytosis. Chauffard measured the red cell as between 3 and 11μm, and concluded that the small cells were the more fragile. He did not know whether the splenic reaction was the cause or an effect of the disease, but believed there was an "active intervention of the splenic parenchyma". This was unlike other cases of hemolysis.

In 1902 in London, Barlow and Shaw found intractable distal leg ulcers in a 10-year-old boy with all the features of hereditary spherocytosis. His mother was also anemic, mildly jaundiced, had splenomegaly and had had a leg ulcer for 27 years. The boy's red-cell count was on average 2.6 million/mm^3. Nucleated red cells were present in his blood smear. The need for increased red blood-cell production often led to extramedullary hematopoiesis involving paraspinal masses. I recall that the only patient with hereditary spherocytosis I saw in 35 years of hematology practice, had large paraspinal masses on X-ray, even many years after splenectomy. Since the spleen appeared to play a major role in the disease, splenectomy was already practiced by Essex Wynter and John Bland-Sutton in England in 1912. The jaundice reportedly disappeared within 12 hours (!), and the anemia had partially corrected after one month. In 1931, Lord Dawson of Penn, the physician-in-ordinary of King George V, reported that a

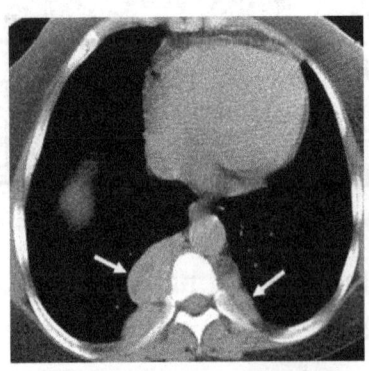

Extramedullary hematopoiesis in a patient with spherocytosis

splenectomy had been performed in 1887 on a 27-year-old woman with recurrent jaundice, who was suspected of fibroids, but was found to have a very large spleen. Forty years later, she was healthy, but still had abnormal osmotic fragility. More recently, partial splenectomy has been recommended, to avoid the increased risk of infection after complete splenectomy.

In 1921 in Copenhagen DE, Elnar Meulengracht (1887-1976) studied seven families and found dominant inheritance of the disease. Newer studies have shown that the disease may be either an autosomal recessive or dominant trait. The disease is particularly frequent in Caucasian populations, with a frequency of up to 1 in 2,000 births.

While the clinical syndrome and therapy of the disease had been well established, its cause was still unclear. From animal studies in rabbits and dogs, it became obvious that red cells coated with antibodies appeared to become smaller and increasingly fragile. Among those who studied this phenomenon was Guido Banti (1852-1925), a pathologist in Florence IT

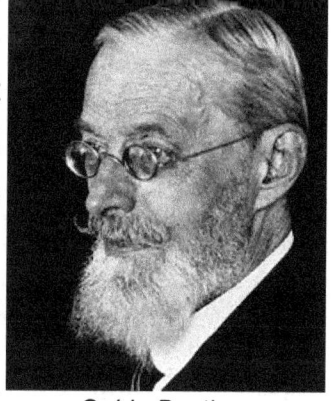

Guido Banti

(1913). Banti also described the syndrome named after him: Banti's syndrome involves anemia, splenomegaly, and ultimately liver cirrhosis with ascites in 1894. He was largely responsible for documenting that the spleen was the principal site of destruction of red blood cells (1895-1912).

It took several decades before the underlying membrane abnormalities of hereditary spherocytosis could be identified. When Ulrich Laemmli in Geneva SU had developed SDS PAGE (sodium dodecyl sulphate-polyacrylamide gel electrophoresis), an improved method to separate proteins, various defects in the membrane proteins spectrin (α and β), ankyrin and others were identified. The membrane proteins in the lipid bilayer are necessary to maintain the normal shape of red cells (biconcave disks). A deficiency of membrane surface area was the primary defect in hereditary spherocytosis leading to spherocytes with decreased deformability. At least 5 gene defects have already been found involving different chromosomes.

G6PD deficiency

Pythagoras (ca.570-ca.495 BCE), the mathematician and philosopher, warned his disciples not to eat beans. It probably was already known that fava beans could cause hemolytic problems in some individuals. Yet very little research happened until treatment for malaria was started with 6-methoxy-8-aminoquinolone drugs (*e.g.* primaquine) in 1926. Wilhelm Cordes, a physician working for the United Fruit Co, reported the next year that acute hemolysis occurred in some workers receiving the drug pamaquine. It took a couple of decades, before this hemolysis was explained. Better understanding of how red cells metabolize sugar, new techniques to study red cell survival, but particularly World War II and the Korean War, were needed to elucidate this problem. The war in tropical and subtropical areas necessitated the development of new synthetic anti-malaria drugs, since quinine supply from Java was cut off by the Japanese. Studies were done mostly on paid prisoner volunteers in the Illinois State Penitentiary in the mid 1950's. These studies were performed by military physicians, under the leadership of Alf Alving of the University of Chicago, and especially by Ernest Beutler (*p.85*). When the prisoners were given a dose of primaquine, some developed acute hemolytic anemia. With ^{51}Cr-labeled red cells, it was shown that red cells from a sensitive subject were rapidly destroyed, when infused into a non-sensitive subject who received primaquine. When labeled red cells from a non-sensitive subject were transfused into a sensitive subject who was taking primaquine, however, no increased red cell destruction occurred. The conclusion was that the defect was inside the red cell itself. The group demonstrated that other drugs, such as sulfonamides, also caused hemolysis in primaquine-sensitive subjects. Small doses of phenylhydrazine destroyed a large part of primaquine-sensitive red cells and led to Heinz bodies, *i.e*, inclusions of denatured hemoglobin. These inclusions were named after Robert Heinz (1865-

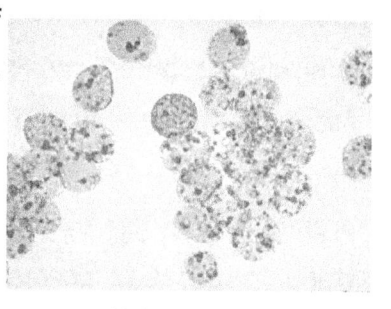

Heinz bodies

1924) from Germany, who had reported them in hemolytic anemia in 1890. The Heinz-body test allowed identification of primaquine-sensitive subjects. The group found that the hemolysis was self-limited. After a nadir, the hemoglobin started to rise again, even when primaquine was continued; young red cells were resistant. To explain these phenomena, earlier work on red-cell metabolism was relevant. Until 1864, when physiologist Felix Hoppe-Seyler in Tübingen GE established that the red pigment of erythrocytes was responsible for oxygen transport, little was known about the role and metabolism of red cells. By the end of the 19th century, it had become clear that red cells increased in size in hypotonic solutions, and that the permeability of the membrane was selective: some molecules entered easily, others did not. The complexity of the red cell was far greater than expected. These cells without nucleus consumed sugar and produced lactic acid. The explanation started with Ottto Warburg, a student of chemist Emil Fischer in Berlin. Warburg showed in 1909 that the human red cells consume some, but not much, oxygen. When 10 years later George Harrop Jr (1880-1945) at Johns Hopkins confirmed the scanty oxygen consumption, but found that it was markedly increased by methylene blue, Warburg restarted his studies another 10 years later. He proposed that methylene blue reacts with hemoglobin to form methemoglobin, which is re-oxidized to hemoglobin in the presence of sugar by molecular oxygen. Although this theory was later proven incorrect, he discovered "Zwischenferment": G6PD (glucose-6-phosphate dehydrogenase) and NADP ("coenzyme II"). Warburg was able to survive in Nazi Germany even though he was half Jewish. Perhaps military officials helped him: Warburg had been decorated in World War I as a member of the elite Uhlanen cavalry regiment. His Nobel Prize in Chemistry in 1931 probably did not hurt either! Gustav Embden (1874-1933) in Frankfurt am Main, and Otto Meyerhof (1884-1951) in Berlin, worked on the pathway that breaks down glucose to lactic acid. Hans Krebs (1900-1981), a pupil of Warburg, moved from Germany to Sheffield UK in 1933. There he documented how cells produce energy from the breakdown of glucose with oxygen consumption: the citric-acid cycle (1937). The Krebs cycle is the only metabolic cycle I learned with an eponym attached, during biochemistry courses in medical school in the late 1960's. Krebs received the Nobel Prize in Physiology/Medicine in 1953 for the discovery of this citric-acid cycle.

Now that much more was known about the metabolism of red blood cells, the formation of Heinz bodies in primaquine-sensitive cells got renewed attention. It was already known that young red cells were metabolically more active than older ones. Ernest Beutler showed that inhibition of glycolysis with fluoride to create Heinz bodies did not work, but inhibition with iodoacetate or arsenite did. Both of these "poisons" act on sulfhydryl groups. This led to the study of the glutathione (GSH) content of the red cells, since GSH is their main sulfhydryl compound. It was shown that primaquine caused an abrupt fall in GSH, when primaquine sensitive red cells were exposed to the drug. Paul Carson

(1925-1985), then working with Alf Alving in the volunteer prisoner project in Illinois, studied the GSH pathway in 1956, and finally showed that the causative problem was G6PD. That same year, William Crosby (*p124*) found that the favism in Sardinia was identical with primaquine-induced hemolytic anemia. G6PD deficiency turned out to be quite widespread in the Mediterranean. Crosby had already delineated hereditary non-spherocytic hemolytic anemia in 1950, and this was found to be a manifestation of G6PD deficiency. The disease was also common in African-American subjects, suggesting a genetic base. It was found in 11% of African Americans and in 50% of the small population of Kurdish Jews. The syndrome proved X-linked (Brown *et al.*, 1957), and Beutler and Susumu Ohno (1928-2000) used this in their studies of the inactivation of one of the X chromosomes in 1966. G6PD deficiency disease was found to be heterogeneous: in the Mediterranean it was more severe than among African Americans. This led the World Health Organization to publish a classification of variants based on severity of the hemolysis. Currently at least 9 variants and mutations are known on X-chromosome band 28. G6PD deficiency appears to protect against Plasmodium falciparum or vivax malaria, which may explain its distribution in malaria-endemic areas. In addition to primaquine and its analogs (chloroquine, hydroxychloroquine), other drugs that

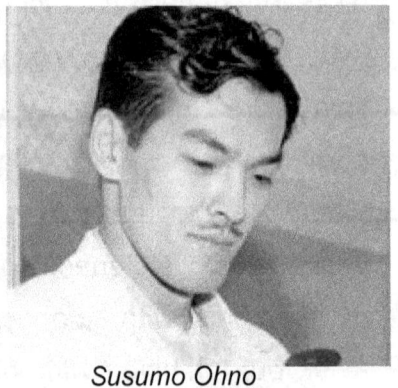

Susumo Ohno

Red Blood Cells

may exacerbate G6PD deficiency include sulfonamides (also cotrimoxazole), nitrofurantoin, isoniazid, dapsone, methylene blue, phenazopyridine, acetanilide, and even high-dose intravenous vitamin C (!) Obviously, fava beans may also cause hemolysis (*favism*), proving Pythagoras right again.

Maxwell Myer Wintrobe *was born in 1901 as Max Weintraub in Sanok, then Austrian-Hungarian empire, now Poland. In his early childhood, his parents and he fled to Canada because of anti-semitism in his homeland. Four of his mother's brothers lived in Halifax CN, and the Weintraubs also ended up there. In 1912, the family moved to Winnipeg, where Max attended St.John's High School. He completed eight years of grade school in six years and was in high school always younger than his classmates. Max entered the University of Manitoba at age 15 and 10 months. During these college years, he changed his name to Maxwell Wintrobe. He majored in political economy and French. In 1920, he entered medical school at the University of Manitoba, and in his sophomore year he took a job in the hospital's blood bank to help finance his studies. He graduated first in his class in 1925. After some more training in Medicine and biochemistry, he moved to Tulane University in New Orleans*

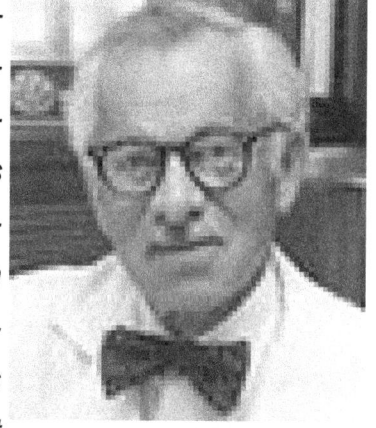

LA. He helped the Chief of Medicine at Tulane to rewrite the section on Diseases of the Blood for the Tice Practice of Medicine. *This set the stage for his later* Clinical Hematology. *At Tulane, he published his work on the microhematocrit, and he introduced the red cell indices MCV, MCH, and MCHC. This led to the three basic forms of anemia: microcytic, normocytic, and macrocytic. In 1929, Max earned a PhD at Tulane on the thesis* The Erythrocyte in Man. *The publication of his studies in the journal* Medicine *led to the invitation to join the Johns Hopkins staff in 1930. Baltimore proved to exhibit blatant antisemitism in contrast to New Orleans. Although socially isolated (even from most of his colleagues), medically and scientifically Hopkins was excellent for Wintrobe. In 1933, he and his wife Becky toured major hematological centers in Europe. On his return, he became Chief of the clinic for nutritional, gastrointestinal and hematologic disorders and his rank was changed in 1935 from instructor to associate (!). In 1943, he was invited to become the first Chairman of Medicine at the newly formed medical school at the University of Utah. He suddenly became a full professor! Arriving in Salt Lake City, the new medical school was located in old military barracks. The dilapidated County Hospital was the clinical facility, without a blood bank and with hardly a laboratory. Nevertheless, he was able to recruit a small first rate faculty. With George Cartwright (1917-1980), he built an outstanding hematology training program. Many of his hematology fellows went on to become faculty at other institutions. His group made major contributions: documenting cryoglobu-*

lins, providing evidence that thalassemia major is a homozygous disease, and studying the effect of nitrogen mustard and antifolates on hematopoiesis (with the Boston group). He wrote more than 400 scientific papers and three books. Clinical Hematology *was first published in 1942, and he remained the sole author until the 7th edition. Then he appointed 5 of his former fellows as co-editors. Wintrobe co-edited* Harrison's Principles of Internal Medicine *from 1951 through 1966, and was its editor-in-chief for the 6th and 7th edition (1970, 1974). He retired as Chairman of Medicine in 1967, but continued to work until 1973. He died from heart failure in 1986. His very important contributions to the history of hematology were made in* Blood, pure and eloquent *(1980; p.2), and* Hematology: blossoming of a science *(1985).*

Ernest Beutler *was born in 1928 at Reichskanzlerplatz, Berlin. The name of this square was changed to Adolf Hitler Platz in 1933 and to Theodor Heuss Platz in 1945. He left with his physician parents and siblings for the USA in 1935, to escape Nazi persecution. He trained in Medicine at the University of Chicago and graduated at the age of 21. He then worked in the laboratory of Leon Jacobson on a humoral radioprotective factor and on iron metabolism. He*

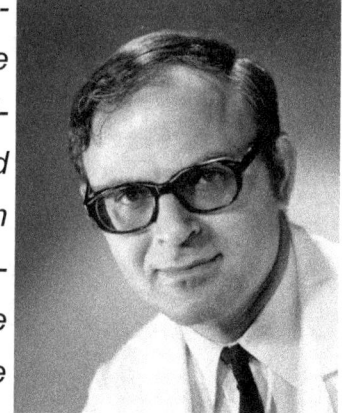

joined the military and was assigned to the Army Malaria Research program. There, he worked on anemia produced by antimalarial drugs and he identified G6PD deficiency, which became part of his life's work. He returned to the University of Chicago in 1955, but In 1959 he became the Chairman of the Department of Medicine of the City of Hope National Medical Center (Duarte, CA). Here he collaborated with Susumu Ohno, a Japanese American geneticist. Ohno had shown that the histological Barr body in female cells was a hyperchromatic X chromosome. Beutler recognized that this might account for the variable expression of X-linked genes in females heterozygous of X-linked mutations. This was found to be the cause of tissue mosaicism in females with G6PD deficiency. Female cells were either normal or completely G6PD deficient; there were no intermediate cells. Around the same time, Mary F Lyon (1925-2014) in Harwell, UK described this X-chromosome silencing in mice. Beutler presented his data first, but Lyon published hers first. It is now mostly referred to as lyonization. *This probably sounded better than* beutlerization? *Beutler continued his work on hemolytic anemias, and he also purified the enzyme that is aberrant in Tay-Sachs disease. His group cloned the gene for Gaucher disease and introduced treatments for this disease. The group designed artificial storage methods for red blood cells and introduced mannitol in this process. He recruited Karl Blume (1937-2013) to the City of Hope, to start their successful bone-marrow transplantation program. In 1979, Beutler assumed the chairmanship of the Depart-*

ment of Clinical Research at the Scripps Clinic and Research Foundation in La Jolla CA. There, his group developed cladribine as a treatment for hairy-cell leukemia. He was the Editor of Williams Hematology for more than 20 years. In 2008 he retired from the Scripps Institute and he died several days later.

ACQUIRED ANEMIAS

Iron-deficiency anemia

Porphyrin compounds are vital for all life on earth. Chlorophyll has magnesium protoporphyrin as important component for photosynthesis, to convert solar energy into chemical energy. Iron protoporphyrin (*i.e.*,"heme") serves in the transport of oxygen to convert chemical energy from food into metabolic energy. Heme is a necessary part of hemoglobin, myoglobin, cytochromes, and many enzymes. The importance of heme makes sufficient supply of iron essential.

Iron preparations were already used in ancient Egypt and Rome for a variety of ailments. On the other hand, Hippocrates recommended bleeding as a method to restore harmony of the four humors and hence health. This was especially recommended in case of fever, to reduce body heat. This therapy persisted for 2,000 years and may well have been the immediate cause of death of George Washington. The enthusiasm of Benjamin Rush "MD" (1745-1813), one of the signers of the Declaration of Independence, for bleeding may have contributed to the high mortality during the 1793 Philadelphia yellow-fever epidemic. Galen, though, had recommended removing only a small volume of blood!

Our supply of iron comes under normal conditions from food. In areas with insufficient iron in the diet from childhood on, the iron deficiency may lead to attempts by the body to increase marrow production. This may lead to *porotic hyperostosis* (*p.57*). Examples of archeological findings in that respect are the Native Americans living in the canyons of New Mexico, who lived mainly on corn (maize) with little iron, as compared with those who lived on the plains, where meat was more easily obtained.

In the 16th century, "chlorosis" was described as a medical condition in Western Europe. Shakespeare described it as "green sickness" in *Fallstaf* (1597). The disease was especially frequent in young women, was painted as "lovesickness", and some thought it hysterical in nature. German physician Johannes Lange (1485-1566) described severe anemia in 1554. The young girl was pale, but he did not mention "green". She had shortness of breath on

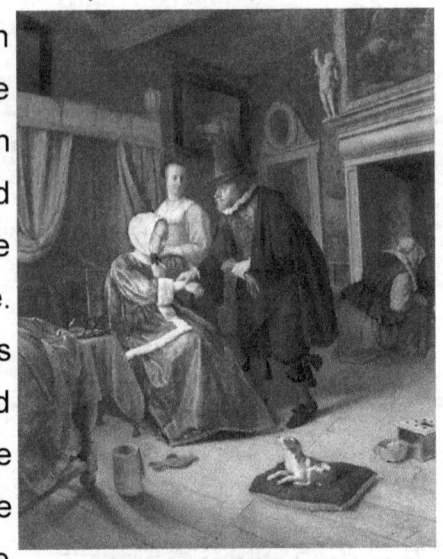

Jan Steen: The Sick Girl (1666) (Mauritshuis, Den Haag)

exertion and palpitations. She disliked meat and had anorexia. He suspected retention of menstrual blood (!) and recommended marriage and pregnancy. Thomas Sydenham (1624-1689), by many considered the father of English Medicine, saw chlorosis as a manifestation of hysteria, but in 1681 advocated its treatment with iron preparations! He saw good effect of his therapy already after 30 days. This was 32 years before iron was found in the ash of blood (Lemery and Geoffrey; 1713), and a century-and-a half before iron deficiency was documented in chlorotic blood (Faedisch; 1832). Pierre Blaud in France recommended pills that contained 64 mg of elemental iron in 1832. Then in 1889, George Hayem in Paris saw that the red cells in chlorosis were smaller (6 instead of 7.5µm) and had less hemoglobin per cell. Still, it took several years before the mechanism of action of iron became known. Gustav von Bunge (1844-1920) in Basel SU demonstrated the presence of iron in hemoglobin in 1885, but he refused to believe that iron was absorbed from the gastrointestinal tract. Similarly, in 1912, Von Noorden in Germany argued that iron stimulated hematopoiesis, but that this effect was unrelated to its presence in the hemoglobin molecule. On the other hand, Ralph Stockman (1861-1946) in Scotland demonstrated, in 1893, that oral or parenteral iron resulted in a significant increase in hemoglobin in chlorotic women. George Whipple (1878-

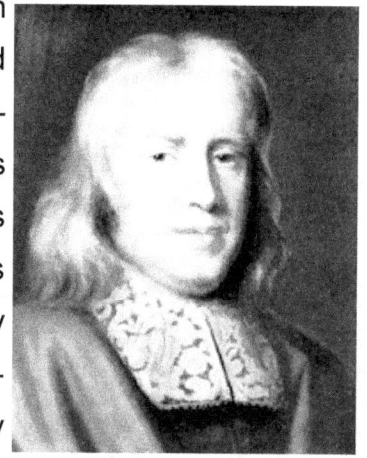

Thomas Sydenham

1976) and his group in Rochester NY studied various food products and, in 1925, found raw liver to be particularly effective to favor hemoglobin production. For this he shared in the 1934 Nobel Prize in Physiology/Medicine. Since their studies included patients with various types of anemia, they initially believed that iron pills were not effective, unless the patient had anemia from chronic blood loss. It became clear later, that the effect of liver probably was caused by its iron content! In the early 1930's, Heath, William Castle(1897-1990) and George Minot(1885-1950) in Boston provided evidence of a close correlation between the amount of parenteral iron and the amount of iron gained in the hemoglobin. They found that only a small fraction of oral iron was absorbed: from 1 to 50%, depending on the presence of iron-deficiency anemia (Reimann, 1936).

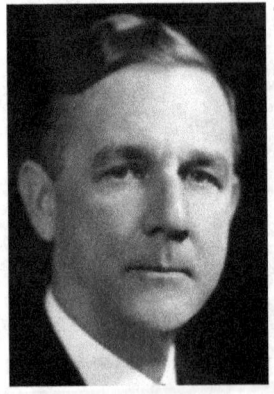

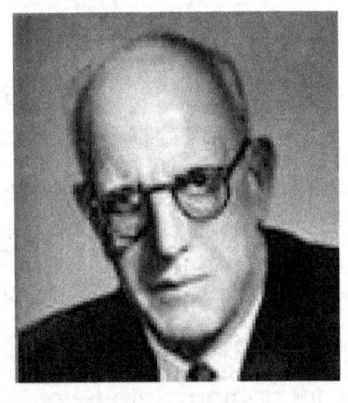

George Whipple

William Castle   *George Minot*

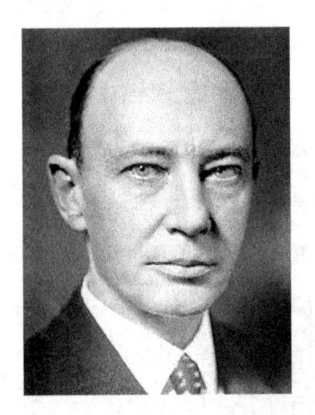

With radioactive iron, the fate of iron metabolism could be much more precisely studied (1939).

Iron-deficiency anemia is still very widespread (1.48 billion worldwide), with 54,000 fatal cases in 2015. The most frequent cause is parasitic disease, particularly hookworms (*Ancylostoma, Necator*). Overt blood loss (gastrointestinal bleeding, menorrhagia) and insufficient intake or absorption (achlorhydria, celiac disease, bariatric surgery) are also common. The estimated average requirement for men is about 6 mg/day, for women (with monthly periods) about 8 mg/day. The daily dietary allowance is obviously definitely higher (8 mg for healthy men to 27 mg for pregnant women).

Pernicious Anemia

In the early 20th century, a form of fatal anemia was increasingly seen in hospitals in Europe and North America. The patients were mostly middle-aged, and survival was only 1-3 years, as reported by Richard Cabot (1868-1939) in Boston MA in 1908. This poor outlook led to the name "pernicious" anemia. In 1926, also in Boston, George Minot and William Murphy (1892-1987) announced that they had abolished the anemia with a diet of half a pound of liver per day for some months. They shared in the 1934 Nobel Prize in Physiology/Medicine with George Whipple. Thomas Addison (1793-1860) at Guy's Hospital in London had described this type

Blood is Life

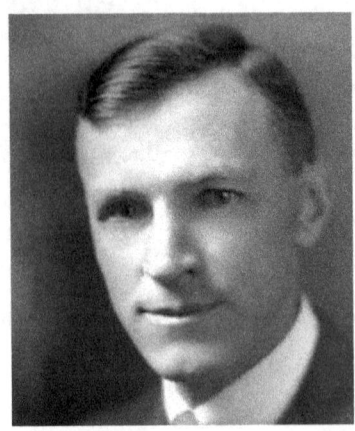

William Murphy

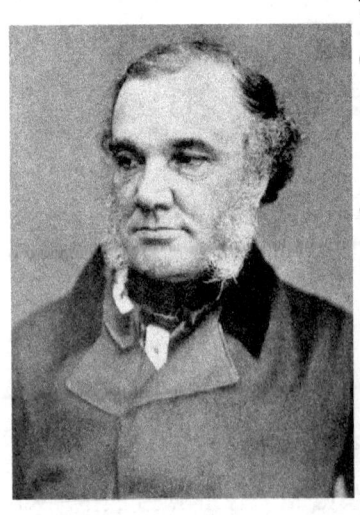

Thomas Addison

of anemia for the first time in 1855. He did not do microscopy of the blood and called it "idiopathic". He also did not mention any specific symptoms of mouth, fingers/toes, or jaundice. The prevalence of sore tongue was emphasized by William Hunter in London in 1897, but he believed the disease to represent oral sepsis. Cabot stressed the sore tongue, jaundice and spinal-cord damage in 1908. The spinal-cord lesions had been documented in the 1870-1880's, both clinically and through autopsies. In those same years, the macrocytic red cells, and poikilocytosis were reported from several countries, but perhaps first by Sörensen in Denmark in 1874. Paul Ehrlich reported large nucleated red cells in the blood of patients with pernicious anemia in 1880: *megaloblasts*. In the following years, he observed bluish particles in some of the red cells. He believed that these were degenerating red cells, whereas in fact they were reticulocytes, as shown by Theobald Smith (1859-1934) in Washington DC in 1891.

The disease pernicious anemia was also seen in continental Europe in the 1870's, particularly in poor women after childbirth. Samuel Wilks in London, who also gave Thomas Hodgkin his dues for describing Hodgkin's disease (*p.192*), claimed Addison's priority for the first report of pernicious anemia. This discussion in 1874 about priority gave additional attention to pernicious anemia.

When Ernst Neumann and Giulio Bizzozero had established the bone marrow as the source of red-blood-cell production in 1868, it became difficult to explain the increased immature red-cell production seen at autopsy of patients with pernicious anemia. For many years opposing explanations for Ehrlich's megaloblasts were coined. In 1875, William Pepper (1843-1899) in Philadelphia PA, who had just returned from working in Germany, believed that the cellularity of the bone marrow at autopsy represented a form of "pseudoleukemia". Two years later, Ernst Neumann explained that the immature red-cell precursors in pernicious anemia were similar to those in patients with chronic hemorrhage. Some investigators believed a red-cell toxin was responsible for the anemia. On the other hand, when after 1926, the use of liver was found to dramatically improve the anemia, a factor in liver promoting red-cell development and differentiation was suspected. Not until radioactive ferrokinetics became available, did Clement Finch (1915-2010) and his colleagues in Seattle WA show in 1956, that ineffective red-cell production in the bone marrow led to decreased release of reticulocytes into the blood stream and premature release of hemoglobin. The released red cells also had a shorter life span. Ineffective hematopoiesis could also explain leukopenia and thrombocytopenia, seen in many patients with pernicious anemia.

The toxin theory did fit well into the late 19th century, when bacterial toxins were widely studied and published, particularly in Germany (Koch, von Behring, Ehrlich) and France (Pasteur). That a factor might be "lacking", received its first evidence in 1897 when Christiaan Eijkman (1858-1930), a Dutch physician working on Java (Dutch East Indies, now Indonesia), demonstrated that the use of polished rice led to beriberi, a debilitating disease. Unpolished rice did not result in beriberi, and Eijkman thought that the "silver skin" contained an antidote to the nerve poison of the disease. Five years later, his colleague Gerrit Grijns (1865-1944) showed that beriberi was actually caused by the lack of a certain factor. In 1926, it was finally isolated as thiamine (vitamin B1). The Polish biochemist Casimir Funk (1884-1967) had tried to isolate the factor preventing beriberi in 1912, and since it had an amine group he called it "vitamin". He claimed four vitamins at that time: "anti-beriberi, anti scorbutic, anti-pellagric and anti-rachitic". He believed that rickets, pellagra, scurvy and coeliac disease could also be cured with vitamins.

That pernicious anemia was due to a missing factor in insufficient nutrition had been suggested by several clinicians in the late 19th century (*e.g.*, Anton Biermer; 1871). The work of Minot and Murphy in Boston in 1925, however, with liver therapy finally proved the point. Their 45 patients at first had a hard time getting down 120-240 grams of lightly cooked beef liver each day. The rapid rise in reticulocytes after 7-10 days, followed by a rise in hemoglobin level, persuaded the patients to persevere. Many other groups confirmed their results. Minot believed that the high protein content of their diet was responsible for the improvement. Subsequent studies by his group, however, revealed that the liver proteins were inert, but the water-soluble alcohol-insoluble precipitate (liver fraction G) was active. This liver fraction was soon (1928) commercially available to the medical profession through Eli Lilly and Company (George Clowes; 1877-1958) in Indianapolis IN. Now only 12.7 grams were sufficient, instead of 300 grams of beef liver. The patent was given to the public. In 1930 in Tübingen GE, Gässlen produced a protein-free injectable form made from only 5 grams of liver. That drug became available in 1935.

While the nutritional anemia of pregnancy could be successfully treated with liver, Lucy Wills (1888-1964) and Barbara Evans, working in Bombay (now Mumbai) India in 1938, found the purified liver extract to be ineffective. Working with a monkey model, they showed that a defective diet led to a macrocytic anemia different from pernicious anemia. The missing factor, initially called the "Wills factor", received many different names (*e.g.*, vitamin M, factor U, pure L. Casei factor) until the vitamin was isolated from yeast and liver, in fierce competition between Lederle Laboratories and Parke-Davis Laboratory in 1943. Then the folic acid was rapidly synthesized as pteroylglutamic (or pteroylheptaglutamic) acid.

After World War II the study of the active factor in liver (extracts) was resumed. When it was shown in 1947, that a certain lactobacillus needed an essential growth factor present in purified liver extract, isolation of the necessary factor became possible with chromatography. It was identified in 1948 as crystalline cyanocobalamin, and chemist Karl Folkers (1906-1997) and colleagues at Merck and Co in Rahway NJ called it vitamin B12.

The flesh or milk of ruminant animals is the ultimate source of vitamin B12. The daily bacterial production of vitamin B12 in the colon is sufficient to prevent pernicious anemia. The total synthesis of vitamin B12 was not accomplished until 1973, by organic chemist Robert Woodward (1917-1979) at Harvard University. Woodward had already earned the Nobel Prize in Chemistry in 1965 for his earlier work on the synthesis of complex organic molecules.

How did vitamin B12 and folic acid interact in causing macrocytic anemia? In the early 1960's, an increased level of the usual form of folic acid (methyl tetrahydrofolate or methyl THF) was found in patients with pernicious anemia with a low vitamin B12 level. This accumulation of methyl THF was due to its failure to be converted into (methylene) THF, a molecule essential for production of the double-helix DNA. Thus, vitamin B12 deficiency causes a secondary defect in the metabolism of folic acid, whereas folic acid deficiency more directly causes insufficient methylene THF. The Danish hematologist Sven-Aage Killmann confirmed this with ^{3}H-thymidine studies in 1964. Vitamin B12 proved essential to form THF out of methyl THF. Rapidly dividing tissues, such as bone marrow, tongue and small intestine, feel the scarcity of vitamin B12 or folate the earliest. Massive doses of folic acid would restore the bone-marrow production, but at the expense of neurological symptoms, as documented by Richard Vilter (1911-2006) and colleagues in Cincinnati OH in 1947. This discrepancy was caused by the lack of the adenosyl-cobalamine coenzyme, essential for the final step of the fatty acid sequence responsible for the integrity of the lipoid myelin sheaths of the nerves of the spinal cord.

In 1860, only 5 years after Addison's description of pernicious anemia in England, Austin Flint (1812-1886) in Buffalo NY suspected the stomach to be involved. He remarked in a lecture about anemia that the stomach might "undergo degenerative disease not apparent to the naked eye". He attributed this form of anemia to a reduction of the amount of gastric juice, "so that assimilation of food is rendered inadequate". This phenomenon was later called *achylia gastrica*. His thoughts were confirmed a decade later by Samuel Fenwick (1821-1902) in London, who examined at autopsy the mucosal lining of the stomach of a patient who had died from pernicious anemia. Cahn and Von Mering in Germany documented that hydrochloric acid was lacking in the stomach of a patient with pernicious anemia in 1886. . Four years later, Faber and Bloch in Copenhagen DE found this to be true in a series of patients, and in 1921, Samuel Levine (1891-1966) and William Ladd in Boston MA, confirmed this in an even larger series. Shortly after Minot and Murphy had shown that treatment with liver could overcome pernicious anemia, William Castle in Boston, while still a resident physician in 1927, came up with the idea that the stomach of a healthy person could derive something from ordinary food that was equivalent to liver for patients. He showed that daily lean steak did not produce a reticulocyte rise in a patient with pernicious anemia. When a healthy person ate the steak and his gastric contents were collected one hour after eating, the liquefied healthy contents given daily to the patient, resulted in a reticulocyte rise after 6 days. Healthy gastric juice by itself was ineffective; only the combination of gastric juice and beef worked. The beef was the extrinsic factor, but an "intrinsic factor" was also essential. Over the next 20 years, the intrinsic factor was found to be secreted only by the human stomach. In 1948, Castle's associate Lionel Berk found that oral liver extract or vitamin B12 was only effective when given with gastric juice. Ralph Gräsbeck (1930-2016) in Helsinki FI identified intrinsic factor with electrophoresis in 1956, and in 1966 his group isolated the intrinsic factor from human gastric juice; it proved a glycoprotein. Forty liters of gastric juice yielded only 8 mg of intrinsic factor. Philip Hoedemaker in Groningen NL demonstrated that the factor was produced by the parietal lining cells of the stomach in 1964. Parenteral vitamin B12 proved far more active than oral vitamin B12 with gastric juice. Radioactive vitamin B12 given with gastric juice to a patient with pernicious anemia, decreased its excretion in the feces, but increased it in the urine. The latter, studied by Robert

Schilling (1919-2014) in Madison WI in 1953, became the basis of the Schilling test. At the University of Minnesota in 1957, Alfred Doscherholmen and Paul Hagen found that for the uptake of a small dose of vitamin B12, intrinsic factor was helpful, but for the uptake of more massive doses of vitamin B12, intrinsic factor was not needed. This explained why the massive doses of liver given by Minot and Murphy had been effective.

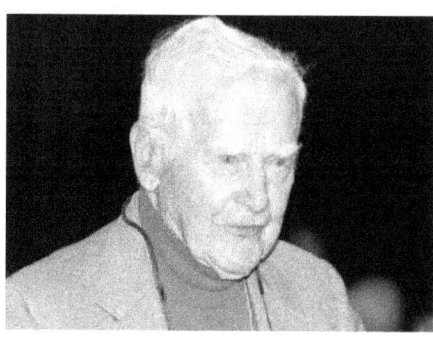

Robert Schilling

As far as the cause of atrophic gastritis was concerned, Michael Schwartz in Copenhagen DE reported in 1958, that the serum of some patients with pernicious anemia who had become refractory to treatment with a refined preparation of hog stomach, prevented the uptake of radioactive vitamin B12 together with hog intrinsic factor. This was confirmed by Keith Taylor at Oxford University UK for patients who had never received hog stomach, and he ascribed it to an antibody against human intrinsic factor. It was then shown that these autoantibodies either blocked the binding of vitamin B12 by intrinsic factor *in vitro*, or the binding of the vitamin B12-intrinsic factor complex to the surface of the mucosal cells of small intestine. The frequent association of anti-intrinsic-factor autoantibodies and anti-thyroid auto-antibodies (*Hashimoto's disease*) was reported in 1963 by Deborah Doniach and colleagues in London.

Treatment of megaloblastic anemia became standardized to 1 mg/day of parenteral (i.m.) cyanocobalamin and oral folic acid 1-5mg/day for severely ill patients. Therapy for vitamin B12 deficiency became 1 mg/day im x 7, followed by twice weekly for 1 week, then 1 mg/week for 4 weeks, and then 1 mg/month indefinitely. For patients refusing parenteral therapy, 1 mg/day by mouth should be effective.

Acquired hemolytic anemia

Galen of Pergamom (130-200 CE) in Rome reported on a slave of emperor Marcus Aurelius (121-180 CE) who was bitten by a snake. The slave developed jaundice, but Galen cured him by prescribing *theriac,* a supposedly homeopathic concoction. This may have been the first report of acquired hemolytic anemia. Galen suggested a relationship between the jaundice and the spleen; it took about 1,600 years for that connection to be confirmed! More than a millennium later, Johannes Actuarius (1275-1328) in Constantinople (now Istanbul TU) reported some cases of cold hemoglobinuria with azure, livid or black urine after exposure to the cold. Pathologist Gabriel Andral (1797-1876) in Paris described a spontaneous anemia, arising without any prior blood loss in 1843. He proposed that the anemia was caused by destruction of red cells.

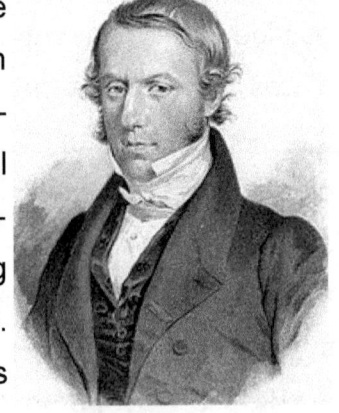

Gabriel Andral

Julius Vogel (1814-1880) in Germany found that the color of the urine was caused by the same substance in the blood and came from "decomposition of blood discs" in 1853. The degree of "blood decomposition" could be measured by the color of the urine. In the late 19th century, cases of familial or congenital hemolysis were found as reported in the previous subchapters. In 1898, Georges Hayem (*p.48*) described cases of acquired hemolytic jaundice. He entitled his paper "Sur un variété particulaire d'ictère chronique". He noticed that the patients became jaundiced, but had no biliary pigment in their urine. Their blood did show bilirubin, as detected with the Gmelin test. This test had been developed in 1844 by Leopold Gmelin (1788-1853) in Heidelberg GE, and was a non-quantitative colorimetric test involving nitric acid. The patients also had splenomegaly and anemia, but Hayem considered the disease to start in the liver. About ten years later, also in Paris, Georges Widal (1862-1929) reported on cases of hemolytic jaundice that could start suddenly or gradually. The adult patients were mostly seriously ill, unlike Chauffard's cases of congenital spherocytosis who were jaundiced but not really ill ("ictèrique plutôt que vraiement malade"). Auto-agglutination of red cells was often observed. Since Widal's cases were similar to those of Hayem, the disorder was now called "Hayem-Widal disease". Further developments were interrupted by World War I, but in 1925 and 1930, Max Lederer (1885-1952), a pathologist in New York, reported six cases presenting with acute onset, fever, jaundice, splenomegaly, severe anemia and leukocytosis.

Not being aware of the French and German contributions, the name "Lederer's anemia" was coined, or even "Lederer-Brill disease" when in 1926, Nathan Brill (1860-1925) in New York, reported an additional case. The blood smear showed reticulocytosis, poikilocytosis and microcytosis. Brill's patient recovered promptly after transfusion.

In 1940, Bill Dameshek (p.184) and Steven Schwartz in Boston summarized the world literature on acute hemolytic anemia in a 96-page (!) review in the journal *Medicine*. They proposed that all cases of acute hemolytic anemia were caused by "hemolysins". The presentation would depend on the concentration of hemolysin, as they showed in the figure.

At the start of World War II, acquired hemolytic anemia was well recognized. The anticipated enormous need for blood transfusions led to increased attention for anemia. In England, the Medical Research Council (MRC) moved the Galton Laboratory Serum Unit from London to a supposedly safer place in Cambridge. Their task was to select suitable donors, and to produce the blood-group typing sera.

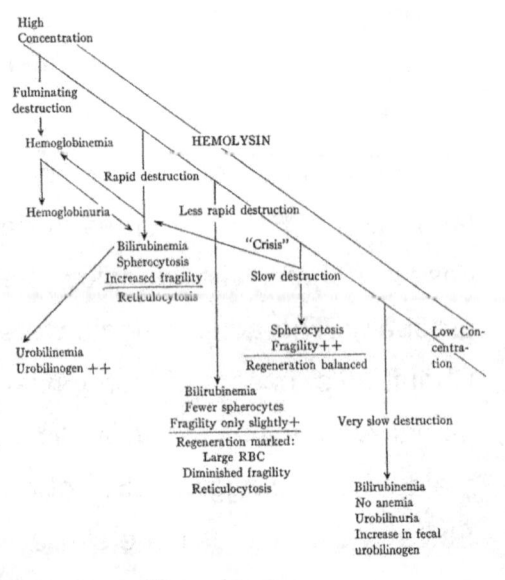

Concentration of hemolysins and hemolysis according to Dameshek & Schwartz

Red Blood Cells

Robert Race (1907-1984) was investigating the newly discovered Rhesus blood-group system (*p.299*) there. Some of his anti-D antisera directly agglutinated D-positive cells ("complete"), but others did not ("incomplete"). When the D-positive cells were first incubated with the incomplete antiserum, the complete ones did not agglutinate cells any longer. The young veterinarian Robin Coombs (1921-2006) joined the group and he conceived the principle of the anti-globulin reaction. He came up with the idea by remembering Paul Ehrlich's (*p.49*) side-chain theory. His technique became known as the Coombs test. When he published his paper in 1945, he learned from a colleague that Carlo Moreschi (1876-1921) in Pavia IT had reported this phenomenon already in 1908 in a German journal; Coombs added this to his galley proofs. The protein fraction responsible for sensitization of red cells was shown to be gamma globulin. With the Cambridge results, John Loutit's group in London with Barbara Dodd (1917-2000) and Kathleen Boorman (1918-2000) rapidly showed that their 5 patients with acquired hemolytic anemia all had a positive direct anti-globulin reaction, whereas their patients with familial hemolytic anemia did not (1946).

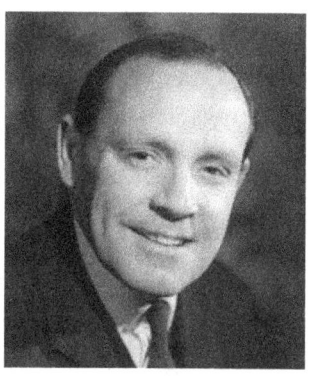

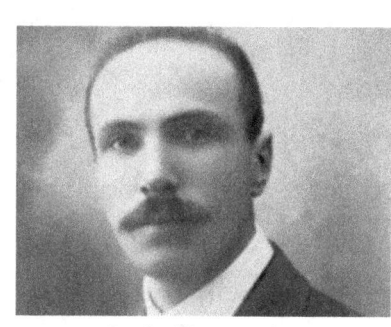

Robin Coombs

Carlo Moreschi

In 1951, the term "auto-immune hemolytic anemia" (AIHA) was first coined, and although several diseases were associated with AIHA, the majority were idiopathic.

John Dacie (*p.120*) reported on the variation in temperature range and pH amplitude of the agglutinating and hemolysing properties of patient sera in 1962. Then in 1971, he summarized the existing hypotheses of autoantibody formation: response to modified red cell antigens, not true autoantibodies but a cross-reactivity to viruses, followed by the development of a "forbidden" clone of antibody-forming cells.

The pediatrician and immunologist Michael Frank (1937-2019) at NIH (Bethesda MD) elucidated in the 1970's the significance of red-cell-bound complement and its involvement in both intravascular and extravascular hemolysis. His group showed that in AIHA red cells coated with complement are sequestered in the liver, whereas those coated with IgG only are taken up by the spleen. Studies in the 1980's started to investigate the immunological mechanisms of autoimmunity, and the role of HLA glycoproteins in the presentation of antigens by macrophages to T lymphocytes.

Lucas Dressler (1815-1896) of Würzburg GE had described a 10-year-old boy who developed cold hemoglobinuria (PCH) in 1854; perhaps the boy had congenital syphilis. In the next decade, several cases were reported from England, all with red urine but no hematuria. In 1879, Kuessner in Halle GE found that "cupping" (= putting heated cups on the skin to create suction and hyperemia) a patient with PCH during an attack, resulted in red-tinged serum. This was the first evidence that hemoglobin in the urine originated from hemoglobin in the serum. Paul Ehrlich (*p.49*) showed that the finger of a patient with PCH, cooled with ice after a ligature had been applied, resulted in red-tinged serum. Around this time, the association of PCH and syphilis was recognized. In a series of papers starting in 1904, Julius Donath (1870-1950) and Karl Landsteiner (*p.321*) in Vienna AT established that hemolysis was due to an autolysin that bound to the patient's red cells at low temperature, and that labile serum factors ("alexin" = complement) caused lysis of the sensitized cells. Ehrlich had casually suggested something like that in 1899. This Donath-Landsteiner antibody was in 1963 determined to be an anti-P antibody. Syphilis fortunately has become much more rare after Salversan and penicillin. Other cold autoantibodies are anti-I associated with cold hemagglutinin disease (CHAD), a disorder possibly related to Waldenström's disease. Warm autoantibodies, which react best at 37^0C, are the most typical of AIHA. Warm AIHA antibodies of IgG1 and IgG3 subclasses predominate, but IgG2 or IgA are not rare. Therapy of AIHA obviously consisted of immunosuppression.

Aplastic anemia

In 1888, Paul Ehrlich probably reported the first case of severe acquired aplastic anemia (SAA), although he did not use this terminology. He reported on a 21-year old woman admitted for menorrhagia of 18 days duration; she died after 7 days with fever from the complications of pancytopenia. Subcutaneous injections of blood had failed to benefit her (!). The autopsy showed the femoral bone marrow to be yellow (fatty), instead of reddish. Ehrlich inferred that bone-marrow failure was the cause of the pancytopenia. The name "aplastic anemia", derived from the Greek α (not, un-), πλάσσειν (to make, to create) and άιμα (blood), was first used by Louis Vaquez and Charles Aubertin in France in 1904 ("*aplasique*"). Over the next 50[+] years, several more cases and some small series were published, but these included even cases with hyperplastic bone marrow! Many different names were introduced for this type of anemia: bone-marrow failure, aleukia hemorrhagica, aregenerative anemia, panmyelophtisis, progessive hypocythemia, refractory anemia, and adynamic anemia. In 1950, a nomen-

Ehrlich's 1888 paper

clature committee came up with "hypoplastic normocytic or macrocytic anemia, due to unknown cause". The objection against the name "aplastic anemia" was that in part of the cases the bone marrow was normocellular or hypercellular, and several cases did not have **pan**cytopenia. Nevertheless, the name "aplastic anemia" persisted. In 1959, Wintrobe's group in Salt Lake City UT required for the diagnosis that 1) pancytopenia is present in combination with definite evidence of decreased marrow production of all the formed elements of the peripheral blood, and that 2) primary diseases of the bone marrow with infiltration or replacement of active hemopoietic tissue are absent. Thus, leukemia would be excluded, but Fanconi's congenital anemia would be included. Normocellularity caused by benign lymphocytes would also qualify.

Joseph Smadel (1907-1963) at the Armed Forces Epidemiological Board, Washington DC, while reporting on the use of chloramphenicol in the treatment of typhoid fever, suggested in 1949 that this drug might cause blood dyscrasias, based on the presence of the nitrobenzene ring in the formulation. This was already confirmed over the next couple of years by cases of aplastic anemia associated with the use of chloramphenicol. The first case was reported by Rich *et al.* in 1950. In series in the 1950's, chloramphenicol was listed as a cause of aplastic anemia in 2-12% of cases. Adel Yunis in Miami FL presented evidence in the 1960's that chloramphenicol could cause dose-related reversible bone-marrow suppression (mainly of erythropoiesis), in addition to the rare devastating bone-marrow aplasia. In 1991, the sale of oral chloramphenicol was halted in the USA. It is interesting, though, that the incidence of aplastic anemia in Hong Kong was not higher than in the "Western countries and Australia", but the use of chloramphenicol was 11-442-fold higher. Additional drugs associated with dose-independent aplastic anemia were sulfonamides, gold salts, phenylbutazone, and diphenylhydantoin. Chronic exposure to benzene (benzol) vapor had already been shown to be myelotoxic in 1897 by Carl Santesson (1862-1939) in Stockholm SW, and was confirmed many times as a cause of aplasia. Benzene was also associated with various forms of leukemia, as shown clearly by Muzaffer Aksoy (1915-2001) for cobblers in Istanbul TU (1985). With the increased use of chemotherapy agents and radiation, dose-dependent aplastic anemia became more common. Mary Sklodowska Curie (1867-1934), who discovered the elements Radium and Polonium, and who introduced the term "radioactivity", died from aplastic anemia; this was possibly caused by her careless handling of radioactive products. Some drugs, *e.g.*, busulfan, have even been used as an animal model for "idiopathic" aplastic anemia.

Starting already in the 1950's, viral infections became associated with cases of acquired aplastic anemia. Thus, viral hepatitis was linked to the disease in the 1950's and 1960's, Epstein-Barr virus in the late 1970's, parvovirus B19 in the late 1980's, and Human Herpesvirus 8 in 2000. With increasing causes of aplastic anemia being recognized, the proportion of cases without established causes ("idiopathic") decreased; yet, idiopathic cases still constitute the vast majority! Since various agents and mechanisms can lead to aplastic anemia, it made sense that therapeutic options would also vary. Basically, the two possible explanations of aplastic anemia are: 1) Absence of hematopoietic stem cells or 2) presence of stem cells, but suppression of their growth by other factors. Radiation and chemotherapy would be examples of immediate destruction of stem cells. In these cases resupplying stem cells (autologous or allogeneic) should be curative. Such an approach was taken in 1937 by Edwin Osgood (1888-1969) in Oregon for a girl with aplastic anemia. She received 18 ml of sternal bone marrow from her ABO-compatible brother infused; she died 5 days later. The first successful infusion of identical-twin bone marrow was performed by Moreno Robins and Noyes in Seattle in 1960. The 7-year-old patient with epilepsy had developed severe aplastic anemia, perhaps drug-induced. Twenty-four days after the onset of illness, she received a bone-marrow infusion, obtained with 44 aspirations from her identical twin (5-6 x10^9 nucleated cells). Within 5 days, the patient started to improve and 2 days later her white-cell count was already 2,900 (AGC>500/mm^3). The rapid recovery after bone marrow infusion makes it impossible to ascertain that the hematologic recovery was not spontaneous. When more patients with aplastic anemia received bone marrow infused from their identical twin, about one third improved. The others required a conditioning regimen. The results of allogeneic stem-cell transplants are covered in that chapter (*p.236*).

Treatments to stimulate remaining stem cells included anabolic steroids. The first reports of the beneficial effect of testosterone in children with aplastic anemia came in 1959 from Louis Diamond (1902-1999)'s group at Children's Hospital in Boston. Nevertheless, the mortality for children treated with testosterone remained over 50%. Sanchez Medal and colleagues in Mexico City and Monterrey ME introduced oxymetholone, a synthetic derivative of testosterone in 1964, and reported that it had a greater erythropoietic stimulating activity than testosterone. Dameshek's group in Boston saw positive results in 5 children with aplastic anemia that was resistant to testosterone in 1967. A study in Sweden from 1970-1975 of 53 patients showed that about half the patients with hypoplastic bone marrows had a remission on oxymetholone and a 2-year survival of 75%. Patients with hypercellular bone marrows, who may have had preleukemic states, responded poorly and 63% died of acute leukemia. A collaborative study in France (1971-1977) of 352 patients treated with one of four forms of androgen therapy for 10 months, showed that after 20 months half the patients had died, primarily during the first 3 months. Patients who survived at least 3 months appeared to benefit from the therapy. When patients survived at least 2 years on androgen therapy, their mortality markedly decreased, with a low risk of acute leukemia, but a slightly higher risk of paroxysmal nocturnal hematuria (PNH). When more active therapies (allogeneic stem-cell transplantation, immunosuppressive therapy) became available, the interest in androgen therapy decreased, even though the therapy remained popular in Japan and Mexico.

When hematopoietic growth factors became available in the 1980's, they obviously were also tested in aplastic anemia to stimulate remaining stem cells. GM-CSF (sargramostim) did stimulate the production of white cells 2-10-fold, mainly neutrophils and eosinophils, but had little effect on platelets and red cells. Colony-forming cells in the bone marrow also failed to increase. Studies with G-CSF (filgrastim), IL-1, IL-3, IL-6, and stem-cell factor (SCF) were equally disappointing. Occasional patients responded to these therapies. Prolonged administration of these growth factors potentially led to clonal disease, especially the proportion of any pre-existing monosomy-7 cells (2006).

To address the possibility that aplastic anemia was caused by suppression of the hematopoietic stem cell, immunosuppressive therapy would be tried. As with nearly all serious diseases, corticosteroids were tried in aplastic anemia. Allan Erslev (1919-2003) and his group at Yale (New Haven CT) reported in 1951 that cortisone and ACTH improved peripheral blood values in patients with hypoplastic anemia. As with corticosteroid therapy for many other poorly defined diseases, this therapy did not catch on. In addition, it could not be considered truly immunosuppressive therapy. Eleanor Roosevelt died in 1962, after receiving steroids for her aplastic anemia, which caused her dormant tuberculosis to flare.

Then in the late 1960's, the group of Georges Mathé (1922-2010) (p.123) in Villejuif (suburb of Paris) performed unsuccessful allografts in aplastic anemia. The group used only antilymphocyte globulin (ALG) as conditioning regimen. Surprisingly, two of the four patients (chloramphenicol and virus-associated aplastic anemias) had autologous recovery. This observation led to acrimony between European investigators, who believed the data, and American investigators, who did not, and who demanded randomized studies. Bruno Speck (1934-1998), a young Swiss investigator who had just moved to Leiden University NL, followed up on the Mathé results, both in the laboratory (animal experiments) and in the clinic. In 1973, he published the combined positive results in 41 patients of Basel SU, where he had relocated, Paris (Hôpital St.Louis) and Leiden. Part of the patients had received haplo-identical bone marrow, in addition to the ALG or antithymocyte globulin (ATG). Speck believed the haploidentical graft to be of importance, but later studies did not confirm that. ALG became first-line therapy for severe aplastic anemia for patients without an HLA-matched sibling donor, and for patients considered to be poor candidates for allografts. Alberto Marmont (1918-2014)'s group in Genova IT showed that massive doses of methylprednisolone (the "Genova bomb") gave results similar to ALG. Starting in 1979,

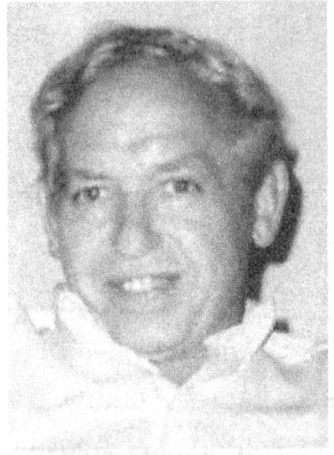

Bruno Speck

American groups did randomized studies that confirmed the beneficial effect of ALG in aplastic anemia. When cyclosporine became available in 1983, this immunosuppressive drug gave results similar with ALG. The first studies with cyclosporine came from Japan, where ALG was not readily available. Studies in France/Belgium/Switzerland and in Germany demonstrated that the combination of ALG and cyclosporine was superior. Moderate doses of corticosteroids were used only to prevent serum sickness induced by ALG.

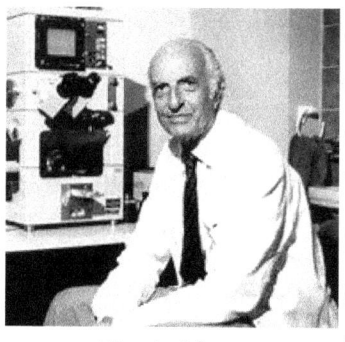

Alberto Marmont

In 2007, eltrombopag, a small orally bioavailable thrombopoietin receptor agonist, was introduced by Glaxo-SmithKline (GSK). It was shown to be effective in chronic idiopathic thrombocytopenic purpura (ITP), but in 2012 also in a proportion of patients with refractory aplastic anemia. Given in combination with ALG and cyclosporin at the NIH, it appeared also to increase the response rate to immunosuppression. It was added to standard therapy shortly after that.

A few patients treated with moderate dose cyclophosphamide responded, but the Johns Hopkins group in the 1990's treated patients with aplastic anemia, who did not have an HLA-matched donor, with cyclophosphamide doses similar to the conditioning regimen for allografts. More than half the patients had a durable remission, but the prolonged pancytopenia resulted in considerable early toxicity.

How could ALG or cyclophosphamide be effective?

Blood is Life

Although American clinicians did not yet want to entertain immunosuppressive therapy for aplastic anemia in the 1970's, their laboratory researchers did. The first studies came from Malcolm Moore's group at Sloan-Kettering in New York in 1975. The studies showed that aplastic-anemia bone marrow contains lymphocytes that suppress myelopoiesis. These results were rapidly confirmed on both sides of the Atlantic. Neal Young (b.1947)'s group at the NIH (Bethesda, MD) found activated suppressor T-cells in the peripheral blood of patients with aplastic anemia.

Response to immunosuppressive therapy was often incomplete, and relapses of the aplasia were frequent (up to 20%), requiring additional therapy. Acquired aplastic anemia likely was a chronic disease.

Important subtypes of aplastic anemia are Fanconi anemia (FA) and Paroxysmal Nocturnal Hemoglobinuria (PNH). Fanconi anemia was first reported by Guido Fanconi (1892-1979), the Swiss pediatrician who became the Head of the Kinderspital in Zürich. In 1927, he described a hereditary panmyelopathy with short stature and hyperpigmentation. This rare disease had impaired response to DNA damage, due to an autosomal recessive genetic defect in a cluster of proteins responsible for DNA repair via homologous recombination. At least 22 FA or FA-like genes have been identified.

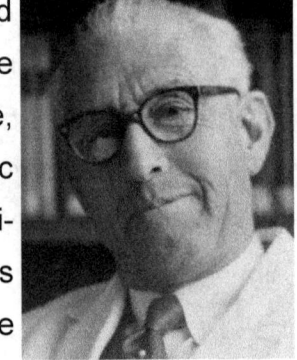

Guido Fanconi

Red Blood Cells

A majority of patients develop aplastic anemia, and a minority acute myeloid leukemia. Allogeneic bone-marrow transplantation was the treatment of choice, but in 1980 Éliane Gluckman (b.1940) in Paris showed that the conditioning regimen should be far less aggressive than for other transplants for aplastic anemia. She was also the clinician responsible for the first ever umbilical cord-blood-cell transplant, with cells collected in North Carolina and processed in Indianapolis IN by Hal Broxmeyer (b.1944) in 1988. The 5 year-old boy with Fanconi anemia received umbilical cord blood cells from his HLA-identical sister, who did not have the genetic defect, and he fully recovered.

Paroxysmal Nocturnal Hemoglobinuria, mostly abbreviated to PNH, was first reported in 1882 by Paul Strübing (1852-1915) of Greifswald GE as paroxysmal hemoglobinuria. Strübing had followed a 29-year-old cartwright since 1880. The patient had attacks of hemoglobinuria, especially in the morning when the urine was more concentrated. More than two centuries before him, the Dutch physician Johannes Schmitz (1621-1652) had described a disease in "an elderman whose urine turned black when he had attacks of abdominal pain". During severe attacks, the plasma was also red, proving that hemolysis did not occur in the kidney, as suggested by Ettore Marchiafava (1845-1935) in Rome as late as 1911. Nevertheless, PNH was called Marchiafava Micheli disease until the 1960's. Ferdinando Micheli (1872-1937) in Turin IT had also described hemolytic anemia with hemoglobinuria in 1931. Actually, the name Paroxysmal Nocturnal Hemoglobinuria was first coined by Dutch physician Jules Enneking in 1928. Strübing had demonstrated with spectroscopy that the red color of the urine was hemoglobin. Leonard Landois, his colleague at Greifswald, suggested that the more acidic conditions during sleep favored hemolysis of the abnormal cells. Attempts to cause hemolysis by giving the patient oral acid were unsuccessful.

Fifty-five years later, Thomas Ham (1905-1987) in Boston MA was able to increase the acidity of serum by giving the patient a single dose of ammonium chloride, and he did observe increased hemoglobinemia and hemoglobinuria (1937). This led to the *acidified serum test of Ham* in 1939. Ham also discovered that complement played an important role in the lysis of PNH red cells. John Dacie, then still in Manchester with John Wilkinson (1897-1998), confirmed this the next year. Interestingly, Abraham Hijmans van den Bergh (1869-1943) (of *"Hijmans van den Bergh reaction"* for bilirubin fame) in Rotterdam (later Utrecht) NL had already in 1911 studied the role of complement, the heat-labile cytotoxic factors of the serum proposed by Paul Ehrlich in 1899. Hijmans van den Bergh heated the serum for 30 min at 50°C and did not observe the hemolysis of PNH cells anymore when he added diluted fresh serum; he concluded that complement was not responsible for the hemolysis. Forty-three years later (1954), it was shown by Louis Pillemer (1908-1957) in Cleveland OH that the alternative pathway of complement (properdin) requires more fresh serum than Hijmans van den Bergh had used. The lysis of PNH cells was complement dependent, but antibody independent. The classic description of PNH came in 1953 from William Crosby (1914-2005) (*p.124*), who at that time was still at Walter Reed Army Hospital in Bethesda MD. His review occupied 43 pages in *Blood*! He concluded that PNH was an acquired disease of the hematopoietic system, in which abnormal red cells, white cells, and platelets are produced. The lesion of the cells involves the stromal proteins, which makes them susceptible to the proteolytic effect of plasma enzymes. Chronic leukopenia leads to susceptibility to infection. Inhibition of the hemolytic factors is easily destroyed by thrombin, allowing increased hemolysis. This interaction and the platelet abnormality which leads to agglutination, explain the increased risk of thrombosis. Thrombosis was the cause of death of 24/53 patients in Crosby's study. Coumadin may protect patients from thrombotic accidents and sometimes even relieve the hemolysis. Heparin, on the other hand, actually increased hemolysis. John Dacie in London postulated in 1963 that the occasional myelofibrosis in PNH resulted from an attempt at regeneration by a damaged bone marrow, leading to a somatic mutation with production of a new clone of abnormal stem cells, with an unusual biological advantage that enabled them to crowd out and replace the normal stem cells, producing red cells with the PNH defect. Lucio Luzzato (b.1936)'s group in Ibadan NI, concluded from studies of two patients who were heterozygotes for G6PD, that the PNH cells came from one clone. Wendell Rosse (b.1933), working at the time in London with John Dacie, developed a PNH

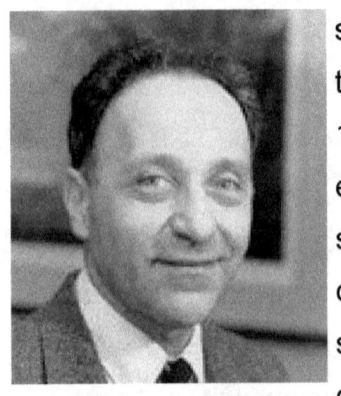

Lucio Luzzato

specific complement lysis sensitivity test using a lytic "anti-I" as antibody in 1966. This test also showed the existence of a distinct clone of complement sensitive cells. The percentage of PNH cells varied between 4 and 80%. By separating the cell populations, Rosse documented the importance of acetylcholinesterase deficiency in PNH (1969). His group at Duke University (Durham, NC) also reported, in 1973, that PNH red cells bind more C3 than normal red cells, and are more easily lysed at a certain level of C3. This was caused by an aberrant regulation of the C3 convertase and aberrant regulation of the membrane attack complex (MAC) of complement. MAC is inhibited by Membrane Inhibitor of Reactive Lysis (MIRL), also known as CD59. Edward Hoffmann showed in 1969 that an extract, prepared from human erythrocyte stroma, contained a factor that inhibited complement mediated hemolysis. He called the factor(s) decay accelerating factor (DAF). Anne Nicholson-Weller and colleagues in Boston in 1982 purified DAF (CD55) and found it to be deficient in PNH cells. Victor Nussenzweig's lab at New York University reported four years later that DAF was released from the cell membrane by phosphatidylinositol-specific phospholipase C (PI-PLC). All proteins of the hematopoietic cells *(i.e.*, acetylcholinesterase, leucocyte alkaline phosphatase) that are deficient in PNH, are GPI-anchored (glycosyl phosphatidylinositol anchor). The next year the structure of the GPI anchor had been elucidated and in 1993, Taroh Kinoshita and his group in Osaka JA cloned the gene, which they named *PIG-A*. This gene is X-linked, but since all hematopoietic cells express only one X chromosome, the mutant *PIG-A* can occur in both men and women.

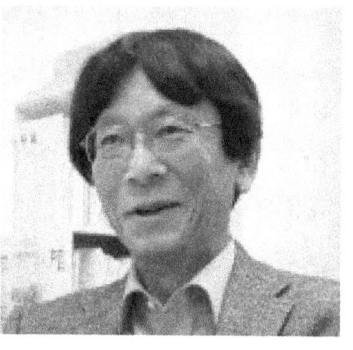

Taroh Kinoshita

In 2004, a humanized monoclonal antibody against complement component C5 was produced and called eculizumab. It blocked the proinflammatory and cytolytic effects of terminal complement activation in PNH. It was marketed as *Soliris*® by Alexion Pharmaceuticals. Its staggering price ($500,000 per year) created major discussion, even though a randomized study, published in 2006, had shown eculizumab to be effective in reducing hemolysis. Subsequent complement-pathway inhibitors have been approved for use, *e.g.*, ravulizumab and pegcefacoplan.. For the few patients with debilitating PNH who have an identical twin, bone-marrow transplantation would be a more permanent and definitely cheaper option. The infusion of the syngeneic stem cells must be preceded by a myeloablative preparative regimen, because the mutant stem cells have a survival advantage. Lucio Luzzato, now in Dar-es-Salaam TA, postulated in 2018 that the *PIG-A* mutant clone of PNH expands by Darwinian selection, exerted by a glycosyl-phosphatidyl-inositol specific auto-immune attack. He hypothesized that a similar process may operate when the auto-immune attack is a clone missing that molecule. Other mutant clones frequently found in aplastic anemia, due to a combination of genetic drift and selection, may emerge and lead to myelodysplasia or acute leukemia. In contrast to the PNH clone, they would not be able to effectively reconstitute hematopoiesis. This theory would nicely tie aplastic anemia and hypoplastic myeloid malignancies together, and explain the transition from aplastic anemia to myeloid malignancy.

John Vivian Dacie was born in Putney, London, in 1912. He graduated from King's College Hospital Medical School in 1935. He trained in clinical pathology and spent six months in Janet Vaughan's department at Hammersmith Hospital, which stimulated his interests in anemia, and especially hemolytic anemia. He finished his training at the Manchester Royal Infirmary, where he saw a patient with paroxysmal nocturnal hemoglobinuria (PNH). During the war he was in the army and involved with blood transfusions. After the war, he went back to Postgraduate Medical School (Hammersmith Hospital), and in 1957 he was appointed to the first Chair of Hematology in the United Kingdom at the University of Lon-

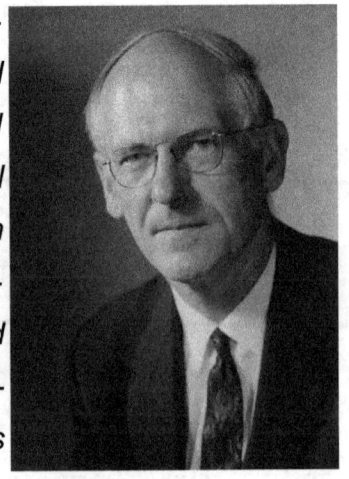

don. Hematologists in England were primarily clinical pathologists, although they also saw patients, mainly in the outpatient clinic. They were often boarded both in Pathology and Medicine. Dacie collected a very talented group of investigators/clinicians around him, including David A G Galton (1922-2006) and Daniel Catovsky (b.1937) in leukemia morphology, A Victor Hoffbrand (b.1935) in anemia and folate/vitamin B12 metabolism, Edward C "Ted" Gordon Smith in aplastic anemia, Alexander S "Sandy" D Spiers (1936-2014) and John M Goldman (1938-2013) in leukemia, Patrick Mollison (1914-2011) and Sheila Worlledge (1928-1980) in blood transfusion, and S Mitchell Lewis (1924-2018) in laboratory hematology. He became the first editor of the British Journal of Haematology *(1955) and remained in the position until 1962. Then he became Chairman of the Editorial Board. His team organized excellent postgraduate courses* "Advances in Haematology", *which I attended several times in the 1970's. I remember "Sandy" Spiers once asking: "Sir John, may I make a point?" Answer: "Yes, but one minute and no slides!" In 1960, Dacie founded the* Leukaemia Research Fund, *and in 1969 he established a Leukemia Research Unit at Hammersmith Hospital under David Galton. This unit also performed the first bone-marrow transplants in the United Kingdom (Ted Gordon-Smith, John Goldman). John Dacie became a fellow of the Royal Society in 1967 and he was knighted in 1976. He retired in1977, and after an interregnum of 4 years was succeeded by Lucio Luzzato, who rekindled the interest in red blood cells with his studies in G6PD* (glucose-6-phosphate dehydrogenase) and PNH. John Dacie died in 2005.

John Dacie's scientific contributions were extensive. In the field of hemolytic anemia, he studied the osmotic fragility test and autohemolysis after incubation for 24h at 37°C. They were able to distinguish hereditary spherocytosis from other forms of hemolytic anemia with glucose addition. These studies led to his book Practical Haematology in 1968; later editions were authored by Dacie and Mitchell Lewis. An unstable hemoglobin (Hemoglobin Hammersmith) was diagnosed with a globin-chain mutation.

He published The Haemolytic Anaemias, in 4 volumes between 1960 and 1967; these volumes covered congenital and autoimmune hemolytic anemia, cold hemagglutinin disease, microangiopathic hemolytic anemia, and paroxysmal nocturnal hemoglobinuria.

Although coagulation was not a major interest of the Hammersmith group, they did describe Christmas disease, named after the patient Stephen Christmas. Now it is known as Factor IX deficiency (Hemophilia B). The paper was published on 27/12/1952, as close to Christmas as possible! Outside the medical field, Sir John Dacie collected and classified butterflies and moths, and he published three papers in the Entomologists' Record.

Red Blood Cells

Georges Mathé was born in 1922. During World War II, while in medical school in Paris, he was part of the resistance. He was captured and sent to a concentration camp in Poland; the war ended soon thereafter. He finished medical school and then worked with Jean Hamburger (1909-1992) and Baruj Benacerraf (1920-2011). This was followed in 1951 by a fellowship with Joseph H Burchenal (1916-2006) and David Karnofsky (1914-1969) in New York.

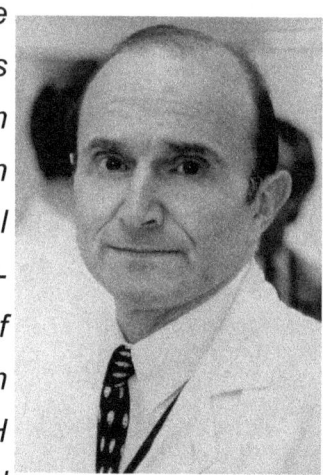

Georges Mathé

Upon his return to France, he joined Jean Bernard's group in Paris to study immunological approaches to leukemia therapy. He showed that in the mouse, allogeneic bone marrow/spleen cells after total body irradiation could cure leukemia L_{1210}, whereas syngeneic cells could not. This approach was attempted in humans, and even though most of the patients did not benefit, a 26-year-old physician with refractory ALL was cured after a bone-marrow transplant from six of his relatives. The patient died after one year from a viral infection, while still in remission. This constituted the first successful allogeneic bone-marrow transplant in man (1963). In 1958, Mathé joined the group of the Curie Institute in Paris to help treat the 6 physicists of the Vinca Nuclear reactor accident in Serbia. Five of the six patients received a bone marrow transplant from ABO-compatible volunteers, but none had permanent engraftment. Four had autologous bone marrow *recovery. With funding from his work for the Vinca Reactor victims, Mathé moved his program to the Institute Gustave Roussy in Villejuif and he built the first state-of the-art isolation unit at Hôpital Paul Brousse. By 1965, he had introduced the term "adoptive immunotherapy" for the transfer of allogeneic lymphocytes/stem cells, with the primary goal of immunological therapy of cancer. The non-myeloablative stem-cell transplants that became popular in the 1990's basically were grounded on this concept. Mathé left the field of bone marrow transplantation to utilize more general immunological leukemia therapies, i.e., irradiated allogeneic leukemia cells and BCG. In 1962, he became the founding president of EORTC (European Organization for Research on Treatment for Cancer). EORTC now has cancer centers in 40 countries as participating members. After his retirement he focused on immunological therapy of HIV/AIDS, and he introduced several unorthodox therapies. He died in 2010 in Villejuif.*

William Holmes Crosby *was born in 1914 in Wheeling WV. He studied Medicine at the University of Pennsylvania, interrupted by a bout of tuberculosis. He graduated in 1940 and enlisted in the army, starting a 25-year career there. After World War II, he did his internal medicine at*

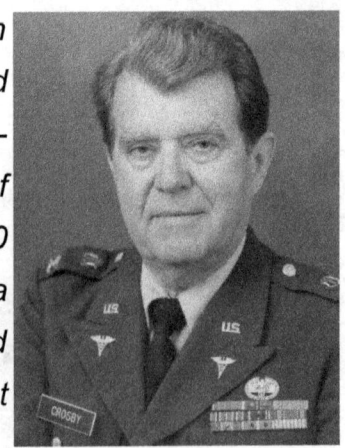

Red Blood Cells

Brooke General Hospital in Texas. Since no hematology support existed in that state, he did self study in the field. William Dameshek was so impressed, that he requested formal hematology training for him; Crosby was transferred to Boston. After a year in London, he established a hematology and oncology service at Walter Reed Hospital in Bethesda MD in 1951. He started research there and studied iron deficiency anemia, interrupted by assignment to a MASH unit in Korea. He published about the hemostatic response to injury in 1955. Then, after his return to Walter Reed Hospital, he studied coeliac disease among soldiers and invented the Crosby capsule to obtain intestinal tissue biopsies (1957). He also studied non-hereditary spherocytic hemolytic anemia ("Crosby's syndrome"; G6PD deficiency) and its risk of iron overload. He wrote a 43-page review of that syndrome for Blood *in 1950. Crosby recommended energetic phlebotomy for hemochromatosis and protested against iron supplements of bread. He retired from the military in 1965 and succeeded William Dameshek in Boston. Seven years later, he moved to the Scripps Clinic in San Diego CA to establish a hematology-oncology training program. Then in 1979, he was recalled to active duty and spent another four years at Walter Reed Hospital. At age 69, he finally retired to private practice in Joplin MO, where he died in 2005 at age 90. In addition to his medical work, he was active in translating poetry. He translated Charles Baudelaire (1821-1867) from French into* Flowers of Evil *and* Paris Spleen.

Blood is Life

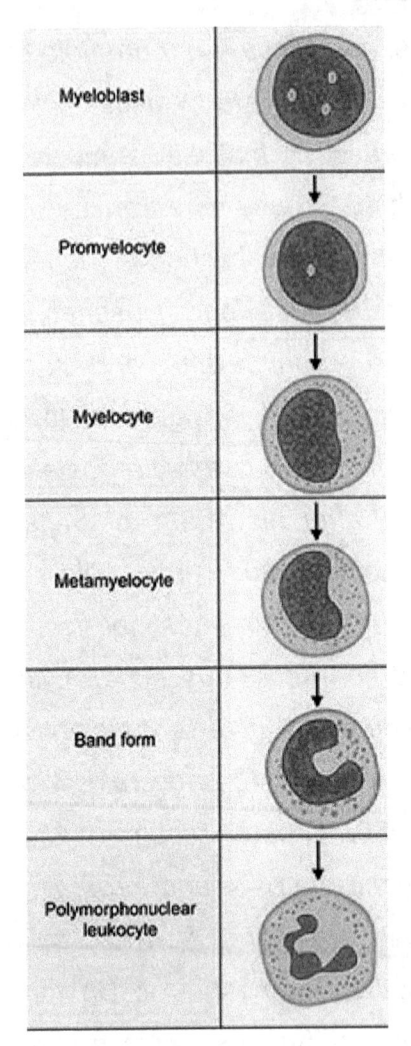

Otto Naegeli, 1900 (p.8)

Paul Ehrlich, 1880 (p.26)

Rudolf Virchow, 1845 (p.130)
Paul Ehrlich, 1880 (p.130)

Stages of myelopoiesis

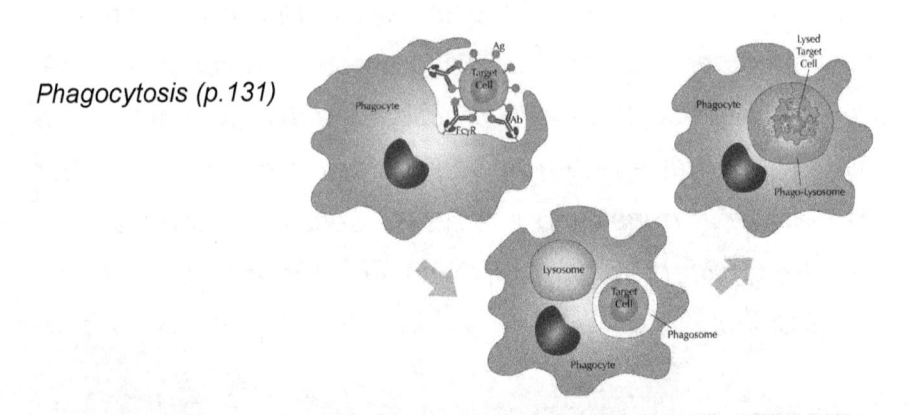

Phagocytosis (p.131)

WHITE BLOOD CELLS

Joseph Lieutaud in Paris (*p.25*) probably was the first to see white blood cells ("globuli albicantes") in unstained blood smears around 1759. He reported that in his book *Précis de la Médicine Pratique*. Slightly later, William Hewson (*p.25*) in London also reported them, together with the entire lymphatic system. He discovered that leukocytes had nuclei ("central particles") and assumed that these cells were formed in lymph nodes and transported to the blood via the thoracic duct. He did not assign a specific function to the white blood cells and he did not recognize different varieties. Before them, Jean-Baptiste de Sénac (1693-1770), who studied in Leiden NL (under Boerhaave) and London but practiced in Paris, had recognized these "globules blancs" in pus in his book on cardiology *Traité de la structure du Coeur, de son action, et de ses maladies* of 1749. He believed that these globules derived from chyle.

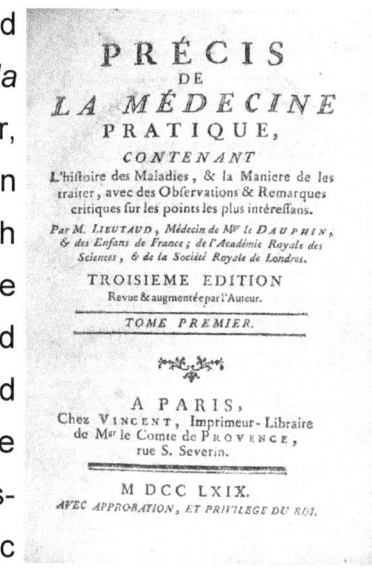

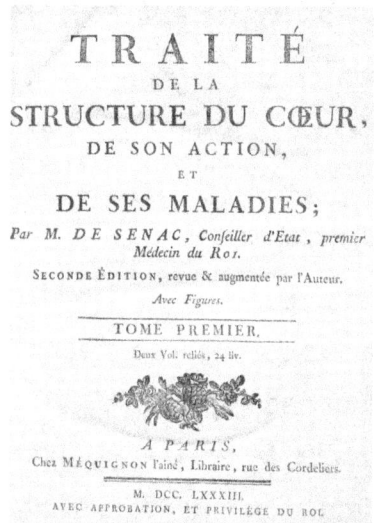

Blood is LIfe

The defensive nature of inflammation started to get recognized in the first half of the 19th century. Before that, and basically since Hippocrates, inflammation was approached based on attempts to modify the body's imbalance of humors. Infections, such as smallpox and cholera, were thought to try to correct themselves by vesicles and diarrhea, respectively. Various concoctions were made to restore the balance and named "galenicals" after Galen of Pergamom. Bloodletting was also recommended. As an example, the Salerno School of Medicine on the Amalfi coast in Italy, which started in the early 9th Century, taught "Bleeding soothes rage, bringing joy to the sad, and saves all lovesick swains from going mad". Although some physicians objected to the practice, *e.g.*, Paracelsus (1493-1541) and Thomas Sydenham *(p.89)*, this approach survived until the first half of the 19th century. Pierre Louis (1787-1872) in Paris, perhaps the first epidemiologist, showed in 1836 that bloodletting was not only not helpful, but even harmful.

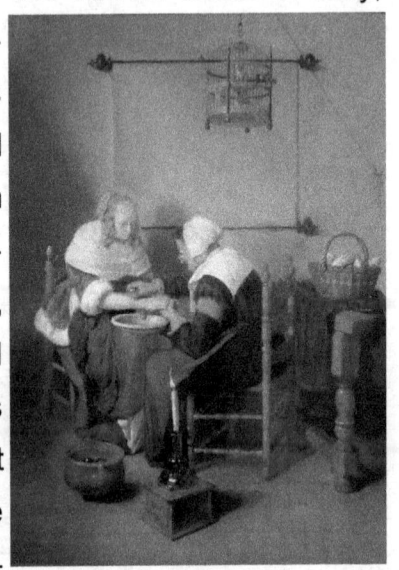

Q van Brekelenkam, The Bloodletting (1660; Mauritshuis, Den Haag)

Slowly more attention was paid to the defense mechanisms of the body. Part of the problem had been that William Harvey (1578-1657), in his book *De Motu Cordis*, had described the arterial and venous circulation, but not capillaries! The microcirculation and the origin of pus cells from the circulation was not entertained until William Addison (1802-1881) in Malvern UK (*not Thomas Addison of London!*) insisted that the colorless corpuscles of blood were identical with those of pus in 1843. Even the great Rudolf Virchow (*p.168*) believed for the longest time that pus arose from precursor cells in the mesenchyme of various connective tissues (1847). Addison's concept of leukocyte diapedesis was not easily accepted, since capillaries were supposed to be completely enclosed structures. Augustus Volney Waller (1816-1870) in London studied diapedesis in the microcirculation of the frog tongue in 1846. He saw that, over 44 hours of observation, leukocytes migrated through small pores between endothelial cells on their own power, but his work was ignored. Two of Virchow's assistants, Friedrich von Recklinghausen (1833-1910) and Julius Cohnheim (1839-1884), observed migration of leukocytes through vascular walls and the "wandering" of leukocytes in the blood in 1863 and 1867-1873, respectively. Cohnheim did not yet believe that the leukocytes moved towards bacteria, but two years later Joseph Richardson (1836-1886) in Philadelphia PA likely did.

Then came Ilya Mechnikov (1845-1916), a zoologist from Odessa RU (*p.135*). He studied the amoeboid cells in the marine sponge. He designated these cells showing digestive activities as "phagocytes" (Greek φαγειν = to eat) in 1882. He subsequently studied larval starfish and observed that these phagocytes moved towards intruders. Virchow visited him in Messina, Sicily in 1883 and was skeptical, but published Mechnikov's data in his own journal (*Archiv Pathol Anat,* now called *Virchows Archiv*) anyway. Virchow reminded him of the opinion of Robert Koch (1843-1910), who still believed in 1878 that certain bacteria multiplied in white blood cells and spread this way through the body. Mechnikov spent the next 25 years proving his own concept.

Virchow had already documented that not all leukocytes looked the same. Many were granular and had irregular nuclear shapes; others were agranular and mostly had rounded nuclei. Paul Ehrlich (*p.49*) introduced his triacid stain of blood smears in 1877, and was able to differentiate various granulocytes based on their granules: neutrophils, basophils, and acidophils (now called eosinophils) in 1880. He also distinguished non-granular cells: lymphocytes, large lymphocytes (both with round nuclei), and large mononuclear cells with idented nuclei (monocytes). Neutrophils increased markedly in many types of infection. Eosinophilia was seen with bronchial asthma, dermatitis, worm infections and in cancer. He assumed that specific bone-marrow production responded to "special chemotactic stimuli". He doubted the importance of phagocytosis, and believed that antibodies were the keystone of body defense. Ehrlich also recognized the myelocyte in the bone marrow as the precursor of granulocytes.

In the first half of the 20th century, new non-surgical therapies for infections became available. In 1928, Alexander Fleming (1881-1955) in London discovered penicillin, while studying bactericidal enzymes such as lysozyme. The drug became clinically available in 1940. Around the same time, agranulocytosis started to appear, leading to rapid death of patients following acute pharyngitis. It was first reported by Philip Brown in San Francisco CA in 1902, but was seen more regularly in the 1920's. In the mid 1930's, an association of agranulocytosis with aminopyrine use was found. This compound had become part of several analgesic and anti inflammatory drugs. Similar effects were later found with other drugs, *e.g.*, phenylbutazone.

The production of neutrophils was studied in the 1950's. Incorporation of radioactive ^{32}P-orthophosphate into the DNA of precursor cells showed that neutrophils appeared in the peripheral blood after 5-6 days and circulated less than one day, as shown by Jens Ottesen in Copenhagen DE in 1954. The production of neutrophil granulocytes was regulated by growth factors, colony-stimulating activity (*p.16*). Each day about $5\text{-}10 \times 10^{10}$ neutrophils were produced. The amoeboid activity of neutrophils was regulated by chemotactic factors, including components of complement (*e.g.*, C5a). The actual killing of bacteria in the neutrophils was accomplished by granules containing acid phosphatase, nucleases, cathepsin and β-glucuronidase. These granules were called "lysosomes", as described by the group of Christian de Duve (1917-2013) in Louvain BE in rat liver tissue in 1955.

Christian de Duve

The phagosome would fuse with the lysosome. This also happened in neutrophils, as reported by Rochelle Hirschhorn and Gerald Weismann (1930-2019) in New York in 1965 (*p.126*). During phagocytosis, neutrophils consumed far more oxygen (1911) and glucose (1959).

As far as macrophages are concerned, Ludwig Aschoff (*p.9*) had developed the concept of the Reticulo-Endothelial System (RES) between 1913 and 1923. The word "Reticulo" derived from the tendency of large phagocytic cells in various organs to form a lattice or reticulum; "Endothelial" referred to the proximity of the cells to vascular endothelial cells. As discussed on pages 9-10, disagreements existed about the relationship of the RES and hematopoietic stem cells. Studies in the 1960's made clear that neutrophils and macrophages (via monocytes) derive from the same progenitor cells that can be cultured *in-vitro* as CFU-GM. In 1968, the Mononuclear Phagocyte System (MPS) replaced the RES; the MPS was described by Zanvil Cohn (1926-1993) in New York with Ralph van Furth (1929-2018) in Leiden NL.

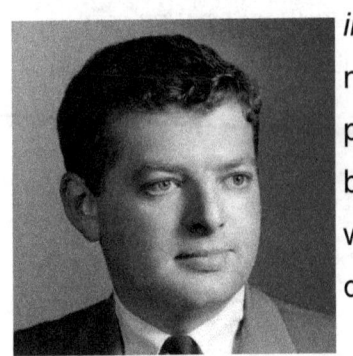

Zanvil Cohn

Lymphocytes belong more to the discipline of immunology than of hematology. They will be briefly discussed here, since they are important for the discussion of leukemia and malignant lymphoma. These diseases definitely belong to the field of hematology.

William Hewson (*p.25*) in England was the first to study the lymphatic system. He suggested that all white blood cells ("globuli albicantes") came from the lymphoid organs. When staining of blood smears became possible, Paul Ehrlich (*p.49*) did not assign any function to the lymphocytes, because they did not have stainable features. Around the same time, the histologist Louis-Antoine Ranvier (1835-1922) in Paris described the structure of lymph nodes in great detail, and tried to study the function of lymphocytes. He found that between 30° and 37°C lymphocytes were motile, but they died above 40°C. They did not move in suspension, but only on a solid surface. Because Paul Ehrlich did not agree with these findings, the discussion in the literature lasted 40 years. Ultimately, Ranvier's opinion prevailed, but lymphocytes move far more slowly than phagocytes. Paul Ehrlich, who introduced the name "lymphocyte" (before him they were called *lymph corpuscles* or *lymphatic elements*), believed that they represented a separate class of leukocyte and were produced in lymph nodes and spleen. This dualism lasted for 80 years, before Neumann's monophyletic theory was confirmed! Ehrlich studied the formation of antibodies, which had been discovered by Behring and Kitasato in 1890. In studies between 1899 and 1900, Ehrlich suggested that the cellular machinery for making an antibody was present before the first exposure to the particular antigen. Antibodies were stimulated when the antigen selected the appropriate receptor (his "side chain theory"). He also claimed that one cell may express many or all antibody specificities. Interestingly, Ehrlich never associated lymphocytes with antibody production: he believed that all cells had this capacity! Since colored antigens were taken up by macrophages, during the first half of the 20th century, macrophages were suspected as the production site of antibodies.

In the late 1930's, evidence started to accrue that antibody production might occur in the lymph node draining the antigen, after injection into the skin. In 1939, Arnold Rich (1893-1968), Lewis, and Maxwell Wintrobe (*p.83*) at Johns Hopkins studied the spleen after injection of foreign protein. They observed a marked increase in large lymphocytes, and suggested that lymphocytes might play a role in antibody production. Ehrich and Harris in Philadelphia PA confirmed the production of antibody in the draining lymph node in 1945-1946. Around the same time, in Copenhagen DE and Stockholm SW, investigators focused on the bone-marrow plasma cell as the main source of antibody, until that was finally established by Astrid Fagraeus (1913-1997) in 1947.

Meanwhile, developments in cell-mediated immunology had established that lymphocytes were involved with rejection of transplanted tumors. The work of James Murphy (1884-1950) in New York, between 1912 and 1921, was of particular importance here. This was the start of transplantation immunology (*p.39*).

The modern understanding of the immune system dates to the early 1960's. The role of the thymus was established by Robert Good (1922—2003)'s group in Minneapolis MN. In 1956, Bruce Glick in Columbus OH had discovered that the Bursa of Fabricius (1533-1619) was pivotal for antibody formation in birds. Then in 1970, markers were found for the human thymus-dependent T lymphocytes and the Bursa-equivalent B lymphocytes (*p.144*).

Ilya Ilyich Mechnikov *was born in a village near Kharkov RU in 1845. He studied biology, first in Kharkov and then in various cities in Germany. In Giessen GE, he discovered intracellular digestion in flatworms in 1865. He planned to do his PhD in Naples IT, but went back to Germany when a cholera epidemic hit Naples. He then went to St.Petersburg RU to get his doctorate. When he was only 21, he became a docent at the new university in Odessa RU. His life was complicated by depression, partly caused by illnesses of his two spouses. The first died from tuberculosis (1873) and the second suffered from severe typhoid. Mechnikov attempted suicide twice, the second time (1882) by injecting himself with Borrelia of relapsing fever. He got severely ill but survived. In 1882, he resigned because of political turmoil after the assassination of the czar. He moved to Messina IT. Ultimately, he ended up in Paris in the Pasteur Institute. He was the father of natural immunity. His research was mostly with minute animals: flatworms and larvae of starfish.*

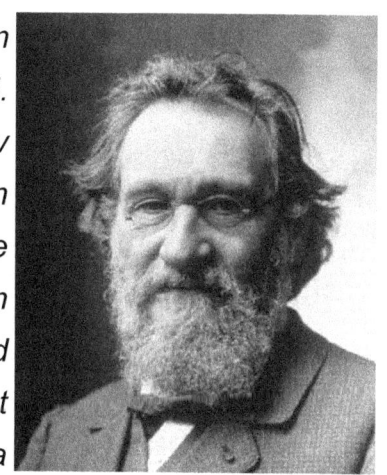

In 1882, he observed that when he inserted small citrus thorns in the larvae, unusual cells surrounded the thorns. He deduced that in animals that have blood, the white blood cells gather at the site of inflammation, and he hypothesized that this could be the way bacteria were attacked and killed. In 1887, he observed that leukocytes from various animals were attracted towards certain bacteria. With Ehrlich's stains, he distinguished microphages (polymorphonuclear leukocytes; neutrophils) from macrophages (motile and fixed) in organs such as the liver (Kupffer cells), spleen, lung (alveolar dust cells), lymph node and intestine. He noted different kinetics and contributions in clearance, uptake, and killing of micro-organisms during chronic and acute inflammation. He noticed amoeboid nature, directed migration and pseudopod extensions during different types of phagocytosis, by envelopment or sinking into the cytoplasm. He shared the 1908 Nobel Prize in Physiology/Medicine with Paul Ehrlich. Mechnikov also developed the theory that aging was caused by toxic bacteria in the gut. He introduced the term gerontology. *He believed that lactic acid could prolong life and advocated the use of lactic acid bacteria, i.e., soured milk. He died in 1916 in Paris. His second wife Olga outlived him for 28 years, but she did die from typhoid.*

Leukemia

No cases of leukemia were documented until the mid 19th century. Even though we know that leukemia must have occurred throughout human (and animal) history, the diagnosis required study of the peripheral blood and/or bone marrow. As discussed before (*p.23*), this required advanced microscopy. Compound microscopes were not invented until the 17th century, but improved dramatically in the 19th century. Alfred F Donné (1801-1878) taught microscopy classes in Paris and "photographed" blood smears with daguerreotypes. Perhaps the first cases of leukemia (1839-1844) were documented by him. Before that, in 1829, Alfred Velpeau (1795-1867) in Paris had reported on a 63-year-old florist with massive hepatosplenomegaly, and blood "like porridge or yeast of red wine". Most medical historians accept that the first well documented cases were reported in 1845, almost simultaneously from Scotland and Germany. John Hughes Bennett (1812-1875) studied medicine in Edinburgh, Paris and Berlin. He returned to Edinburgh and taught classes in polyclinical medicine. He ultimately became Professor of Medicine of the Institute of Medicine there. His case concerned a 29-year-old man in Edinburgh with splenomegaly and the presence of many leukocytes in the peripheral blood. The patient survived for about 3 months. Bennett proposed the name *leucocythaemia,* for what probably was chronic myelogenous leukemia (CML). Later that same year,

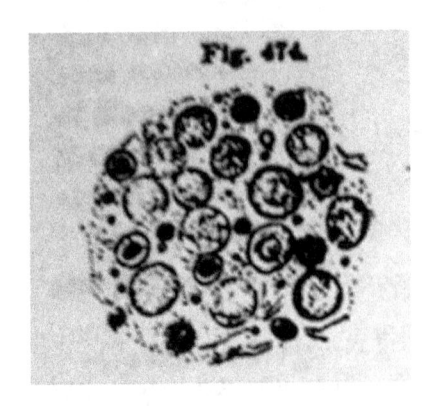

Drawing of blood smear seen by John Bennett (1845)

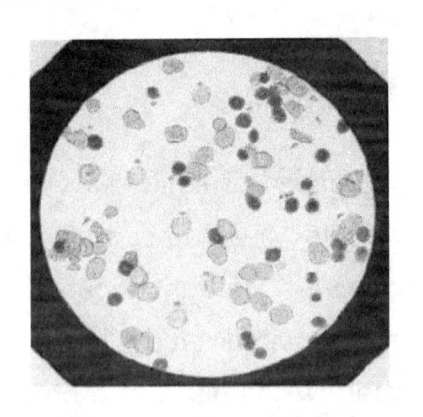

Daguerreotype of leukemia cells by Alfred Donné

Rudolf Virchow (*p.168*) reported from Berlin the case of a 50 year-old woman with a 4-year history of ill health and abdominal swelling. She died 4 months later and was found to have enormous numbers of white ("pus") cells everywhere in her body. He proposed the name *Leukämie* (leukemia) as the Greek translation (λευκος = white; αιμα = blood) of the German "Weisses Blut" for his case that was either CML or, more likely, chronic lymphocytic leukemia (CLL). His name stuck! He also observed that not all white blood cells ("lymph particles") were the same. Many were granular and had irregular nuclear shapes; others were agranular and had mostly rounded nuclei. In 1856, he proposed to subdivide leukemia into two types: "splenic" or "lienal" (*lien = spleen in Latin*) leukemia, and "lymphatic" leukemia. This was accepted, but 14 years later Ernst Neumann (1834-1918), who had co-discovered the function of bone marrow 2 years earlier, reported that the splenic leukemia originated in the bone marrow. The terminology now changed to "spleno-medullary" leukemia, but several authors still considered the spleen as more important. Many leading physicians of the second half of the 19th century, were suspicious about the existence of a separate entity "leukemia" and they also mocked those who saw the potential of the microscope. That started to change, when Paul Ehrlich (1854-1915) introduced the staining of peripheral blood smears with aniline dyes, his "triacid" stain. Artur Pappenheim (1870-1916), and his friend and colleague Hans Hirschfeld (1873-1944) in Berlin, did important work in the dissection of the cells of the peripheral blood, and the latter identified that cells giving rise to granulocytes were non granular cells in the bone marrow. In 1900, Otto Naegeli, the Swiss hematologist, called these non-granular cells "myeloblasts". In 1913, Reschad and Schilling-Torgau reported on a "new" form of acute leukemia with "splenocytes" (= monocytes) in the peripheral blood. They believed these cells derived from the histiocytes of the reticulo-endothelial system (RES). Naegeli never accepted that form of leukemia as separate from acute myelogenous leukemia (AML), but for several decades AML was now divided into 3 subtypes: Myeloblastic, Naegeli-type (myelomonocytic) and Schilling-type (monocytic). Since clinical studies had already separated acute from chronic leukemia in the 1880-1890's, four main types were now recognized: acute lymphocytic leukemia (ALL), AML, CML and CLL. Because the clinical features and therapy of these four subtypes are so different, they will be discussed consecutively.

Blood is LIfe

In 1938, Claude Forkner (1900-1992) of Cornell University, New York, wrote in his book *Leukemias and Allied Disorders:* "Although leukemia is a fatal disease, much can be done to add to the comfort, and promote the general health of sufferers from the chronic forms of the disease. Unfortunately, acute leukemia does not respond satisfactorily to any form of therapy". Forkner later became the personal physician of the shah of Iran, Mohamed Reza Pahlavi. His depressing statement about acute leukemia was correct, even though a single patient with AML had been cured in 1927. A 49-year old businessman from New York consulted dr. Gloor in Otto Naegeli's clinic in Zürich SU with AML (WBC >100,000/mm^3 with 92% myeloblasts). He was treated with splenic irradiation, arsenic, radioactive radium, and sibling blood transfusions. He attained complete remission and remained disease free for 50^+ years. Was this the effect of the arsenic, radiation or an early example of immunotherapy induced by sibling blood transfusion? When dr. Gloor published his case in 1930, he expected academic credit, but instead he was fired and spent the rest of his career in a small canton.

Arsenic trioxide had been introduced in 1786, by Thomas Fowler (1736-1801) of York UK as an 1% potassium arsenite solution. Fowler's solution was recommended for the "cure of agues, remittent fevers, and periodic headaches", and became a popular tonic. In 1865, Abraham Lissauer (1832-1908) of Danzig (now Gdansk PO) used it in a woman with CML, and he was surprised when she markedly improved; the improvement lasted for several months.

Others also used it with success in CML. William Osler recommended it in his *The Principles and Practice of Medicine* (1892). In fact, Forkner himself also studied it in CML. Arsenic continued to be used at times for CML until, in the mid 1950's, busulfan (Alkeran®) arrived. Arsenic regained popularity for the treatment of acute promyelocytic leukemia after successful studies in China in 1992 and 1997 (*p.152*).

Acute Lymphocytic Leukemia (ALL).

ALL may occur at any age, but the vast majority of cases occur in children. Paul Ehrlich just about ignored lymphocytes, since the cells did not have any stainable features. Consequently, the disease was defined as a disease of very immature cells without granules. The lymphoblasts tended to have only 1-2 nucleoli, a high nuclear/cytoplasmic ratio, and nuclei that were not indented. This was the morphological picture, especially in children. Cases in older patients had more heterogeneous cells, with irregular nuclear shape and more abundant, quite basophilic, cytoplasm. For many years, the diagnosis was made just based on the morphology of cells in the peripheral blood and/or bone marrow. No therapy was available, except for blood transfusions and antibiotics, until the 1940's. Alkylating agents started to be studied in 1943. Nitrogen mustard, the first alkylating agent studied (with the sulfur of mustard gas changed to nitrogen), produced temporary partial remissions in ALL, but with considerable toxicity. Analogs of nitrogen mustard, and other alkylators, were synthesized that had less acute toxicity.

More effective agents in ALL proved to be the antifolates aminopterin and amethopterin -better known as methotrexate-, which emerged from nutrition research into folate. When folate was given to patients with ALL, it appeared to stimulate the leukemia. The antifolates produced clinical and hematological remissions in children with ALL, as shown by Sidney Farber (1903-1973) and colleagues in Boston in 1947. This was followed by reports of the efficacy of corticosteroids at the Mayo clinic (Rochester MN) in 1950 and of the antipurine 6-mercaptopurine by Joseph Burchenal (1912-2006) and colleagues at Memorial Sloan-Kettering in New York in 1953. When a combination of chemotherapy agents, *e.g.*, corticosteroid plus antifolate or antipurine was used, survival became more prolonged, but nearly all patients still died from relapse. The group of Emil "Tom" Frei III (1924-2013) at the NCI introduced the periwinkle alkaloid vincristine (Oncovin®). This led to the combination VAMP (vincristine, amethopterin (MTX), mercaptopurine, and prednisone) in 1961. The combination chemotherapy produced a high remission rate, but no cures. The next important step was made by Donald Pinkel (1926-2022) at St. Jude Children's Research Hospi-

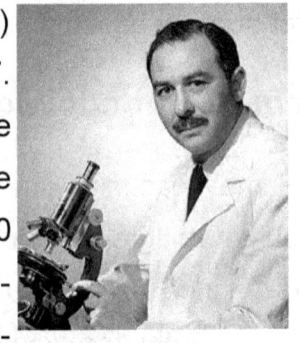

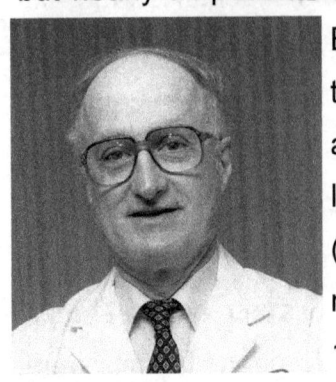

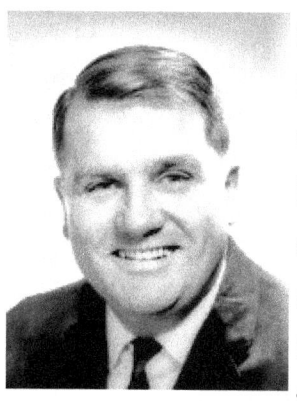

Donald Pinkel

tal in Memphis TN in 1961. Pinkel had trained with Sidney Farber in Boston and was recruited to St. Jude's by the entertainer Danny Thomas (1912-1991), who spearheaded the founding of the hospital named after the patron saint of the hopeless and despaired. The St. Jude's "total therapy" program for childhood ALL consisted of remission induction, consolidation, pre-emptive meningeal treatment (radiation and intrathecal chemotherapy) and continuation of treatment for 2-3 years. Subsequent studies slowly improved the results, and by 1967 a 50% cure rate was obtained. These cures with combination chemotherapy have lasted for 25$^+$ years! When L-asparaginase was shown in 1966 by veterinarian William Dolowy to be effective against Gardner 6C3HED lymphosarcoma xenografts, and by physician Joseph M Hill and colleagues at the Wadley Institute in Dallas TX against human acute leukemia (1967), it rapidly became part of the combination chemotherapy. Asparaginase had already been discovered in 1953 by John Kidd (1908-1992) of Cornell University, who showed that guinea pig serum regressed 6C3HED lymphosarcoma xenografts in mice. John Broome (b.1939), a pathologist at Cornell, showed in the early 1960's that this anti-lymphoma effect was due to L-asparaginase. Consecutive combination chemotherapy studies by the Children's Cancer Group (CCG), which included asparaginase and improved supportive care, pushed the cure rate to 90%

by 2010. Per study 1,300-3,700 children were enrolled! Among the features important at the time of diagnosis were morphology of the leukemic cells, white blood-cell count, age, and immunophenotype of the blast cells. In the early 1970's, immunological phenotyping became available. First, Victor Nussenzweig (b.1928)'s group at New York University found that T-lymphocytes form rosettes with sheep erythrocytes. Around the same time, Ellen Vitetta (b.1942) in Dallas TX was able to isolate surface immunoglobulin from mouse splenic B-lymphocytes.

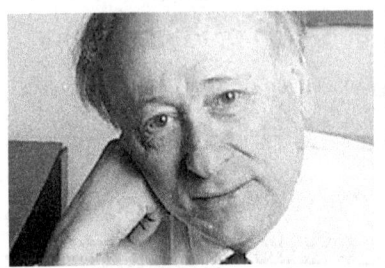

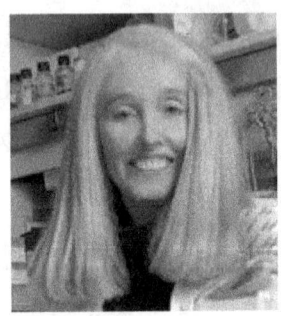

Victor Nussenzweig

Ellen Vitetta

Melvyn Greaves (b.1941)'s group in London produced polyclonal antisera against a frequent antigen on ALL cells, called CALLA (*common ALL antigen*) in 1975. The same year, Georges Köhler (1946-1995) and César Milstein (1927-2002) in Cambridge UK, published their method to create monoclonal antibodies by fusing antibody-producing cells with myeloma cells. This accomplishment earned them the Nobel Prize in Physiology/Medicine in 1984. Monoclonal antibodies against CALLA were made by several laboratories (*e.g.,* J5

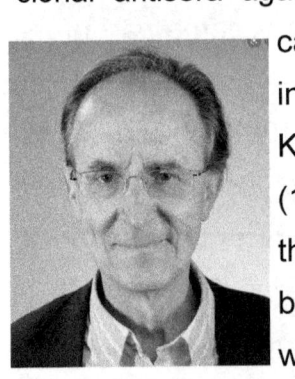

Melvyn Greaves

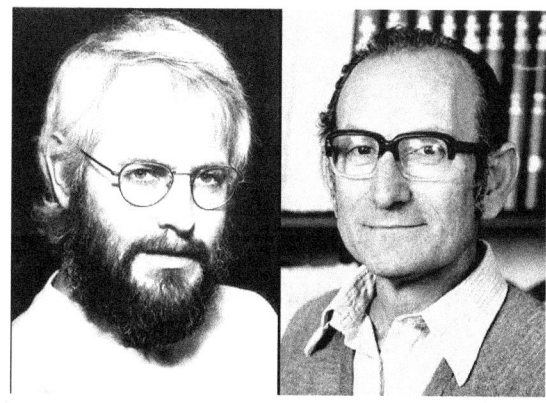

Georges Köhler   *César Milstein*

in Boston) and when the HLDA (International Workshop and Conference of Human Leukocyte Differentiation Antigens) was held in Paris (1982), CALLA became CD10. Many additional monoclonal antibodies were made against differentiation antigens of the lymphoid lineage. Among the more important for early B-cells were CD19, CD20, CD9, and CD24. For early T-cells were important CD7, CD5, CD2 (E-rosette receptor), CD1, CD3, CD4, and CD8. It became clear that T-cell ALL and mature B cell ALL were more difficult to cure than pre-B ALL. Thus, the immunophenotype proved an important prognostic factor. Cytogenetic findings also proved of importance: t(8;14) associated with Burkitt's lymphoma, t(9;22) associated with the Philadelphia chromosome, and t(4;11)(q21;q23) associated with congenital ALL, predicted worse than average outcome, whereas t(1;19)(q23;p13) was associated with pre-B ALL and suggested a better than average outcome.

In 1976, the FAB (**F**rench-**A**merican-**B**ritish) group came out with a classification of acute leukemia, especially to distinguish ALL from AML. The group consisted of Marie Thérèse Daniel and Georges Flandrin of Hôpital St.Louis in Paris and Claude Sultan (1936-2008; Hôpital Henri Mondor, Créteil); John Bennett (b.1933; University of Rochester) and

Harvey Gralnick (1937-2020; NIH); and Daniel Catovsky and David Galton of Royal Postgraduate Medical School, London. They divided ALL into three types: L1 (small cells, mostly in children), L2 (larger cells) and L3 (Burkitt type). The FAB group based their diagnosis on morphology and, if necessary, cytochemistry. When immunological and genetic markers became available, the WHO (World Health Organization) classification of 2009 subdivided ALL into 9 categories, to a large degree based on gene arrangements. Examples were B-ALL with t(9;22) *BCR-ABL1*, or t(1;19)*TCF3-PBX1,* and T ALL.

In adult ALL, which is less frequent than childhood ALL, the cure rate has been substantially lower, partly because of the high frequency of unfavorable prognostic features. The induction chemotherapy for adults with ALL was initially similar with that for children, but soon started to include chemotherapy drugs that had shown activity in AML. In 1965, the group at NCI introduced POMP (**P**redniso(ne)(olone), vincristine (**O**ncovin), **M**ethotrexate, and **P**urinethol (6-mercaptopurine)) for both ALL and AML. In 1968, the group at MD Anderson Hospital, led by Emil ("Jay") Freireich (1927-2021), reported COAP (**C**yclophosphamide, **O**ncovin, **A**ra-C, **P**rednisolone) for both types of acute leukemia. With the introduction of L-asparaginase and anthracyclines, the complete

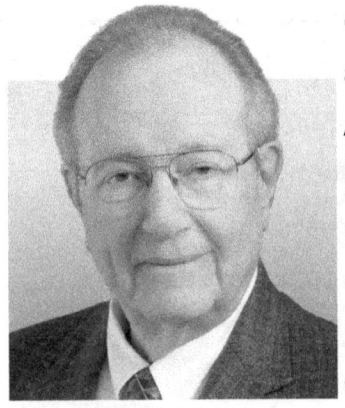

Emil Freireich

remission rate in adult ALL increased from 36-67% with vincristine/prednisone to 72-89% with vincristine/prednisone/anthracycline or vincristine/dexamethasone/asparaginase/methotrexate. Many different regimens were introduced in the 1980's, resulting in 64-82% complete remissions, and 30-40% continuing remissions after 3-10 years. Consolidation and maintenance therapy, often with Ara-C (cytarabine), and CNS intrathecal treatment were important components of successful therapy. For patients who did not enter complete remission, the outlook was much poorer. Allogeneic stem cell transplantation was capable of salvaging a few, but allografting was more successful for high-risk patients in first or second complete remission (p.237).

Immunotherapy is being used increasingly in adult ALL: rituximab for CD-20$^+$ ALL, blinatumomab for residual disease after remission induction, inotuzumab-ozogamycin (antibody-toxin combination) that targets CD-22, imatinib (p.155) for Ph' ALL, and CAR-T cells (p.209).

Acute Myelogenous Leukemia

The efforts of Ernst Neumann (1870), Otto Naegeli (1900) and Victor Schilling-Torgau (1912) had established AML as a separate form of leukemia. This leukemia occurred at all ages, but mostly in adults with increasing incidence with increasing age.

The most immature form of AML is represented by leukemic cells with a primitive nucleus (with prominent nucleoli) and cytoplasm with few or any granules. More frequently, though, the cytoplasmic granules are more prominent, and sometimes many cells even have the morphology of abnormal promyelocytes. In 1947, Cazal showed that azurophilic granules stain with peroxidase, but the neutrophilic granules do not. Peroxidase-positive blasts were, by definition, myeloid and not lymphoid. Similar conclusions could be drawn when the blast cells showed Sudan black B positivity. This lipophilic stain was originally introduced by George Wislocki and Edward Dempsey of Harvard (1946), but the clinical use of this stain was shown in 1964 by Frank Hayhoe (1920-2009)'s group in Cambridge UK. Leukocytes contain many esterases. The non-specific esterases (*e.g.*, α-naphthyl acetate esterase) are positive in cells of monocytic lineage (and sensitive to inhibition by sodium fluoride) as shown between 1968 and 1971. The specific esterases (*e.g.*, naphthol-AS-D-chloroacetate esterase) are negative in monocytes, but positive in granulocytes.

The FAB group convened in Paris in 1974 at the suggestion of David Galton (1922-2006), and proposed their classification in 1976. The main goal was to distinguish myeloid from lymphoid acute leukemia, because of the important implications for therapy. They subdivided AML into 8 (by 1980: 9) types. M1 was myeloblastic without maturation, M2 myeloblastic with maturation, M3 hypergranular promyelocytic, M4 myelomonocytic (the old Naegeli type), M5A monoblastic, M5B differentiated monoblastic (the old Schilling type), M6 erythroleukemia and M7 megakaryoblastic leukemia. Again, only light microscopy and cytochemistry were used for the classification.

White Blood Cells

When immunological techniques, cytogenetics, and FISH (**F**luorescence **I**n **S**itu **H**ybridization) and RT-PCR (**R**everse **T**ranscriptase **P**olymerase **C**hain **R**eaction) techniques became available and were used since the 1970-1990's, new classifications became important. Some of the new subtypes had important therapeutic and prognostic implications. Thus, AML with inv(16)(p13;q22) or t(16;16)(p13;q22) had a better than average prognosis, as did acute promyelocytic leukemia with t(15;17)(q22;q12). AML with 11q23 abnormalities, on the other hand, had a high risk of relapse and worse than average survival. These subtypes were part of the WHO classification of 2002, updated in 2008 and again in 2016.

The therapy for AML initially was similar to that for adult ALL, *e.g.*, POMP. When the pyrimidine antagonist cytosine arabinoside (cytarabine, Ara-C) was introduced in 1961 by the Upjohn Company, it proved active against leukemia. Ara-C is a synthetic nucleoside that differs from cytidine and deoxycytidine by having arabinoside instead of ribose or deoxyribose as the sugar moiety. This leads to a strong inhibition of DNA synthesis. The drug proved effective both against ALL and AML, as reported by several groups in 1968. It was also part of the COAP regimen, reported by the MD Anderson group in Houston. Since Ara-C by itself gave a relatively low percentage of complete remissions, it was rapidly combined with an antipurine or a DNA-intercalating natural anthracycline (daunorubicin or adriamycin). Mercaptopurine had the disadvantage that, in combination with allopurinol to prevent excessive uric acid production, the elimination of mercaptopurine was retarded, leading to excessive bone-marrow suppression. Therefore, 6-thioguanine (6-TG) became the antipurine of choice to combine with Ara-C. The combination Ara-C/6-TG became standard as published by Timothy Gee (1935-1999) and Bayard Clarkson (b.1926) of Memorial Sloan Kettering in 1969. The next studies often used Ara-C/ 6-TG in combination with daunorubicin. This latter drug, developed simultaneously in Italy (daunomycin) and France (rubidomycin) around 1967, proved to be very active, but had to be given intravenously with often serious side effects, including cardiotoxicity. The combination was known as DAT, as used by the Medical Research Council in England, or – in combination with prednisolone – as TRAP used at Hammersmith Hospital in London. By 1973, the complete remission rate was about 60% for patients with AML and the cure rate 20%. Consolidation therapy proved also important in the treatment of AML. Various anthracyclines were compared with daunorubicin. In the early 1990's, idarubicin was found to be superior in three randomized studies and not more toxic. Joseph Bertino (1930-2021)'s group at Yale (New Haven, CT) showed in 1979 that high-dose Ara-C (HDAC) could induce remis-

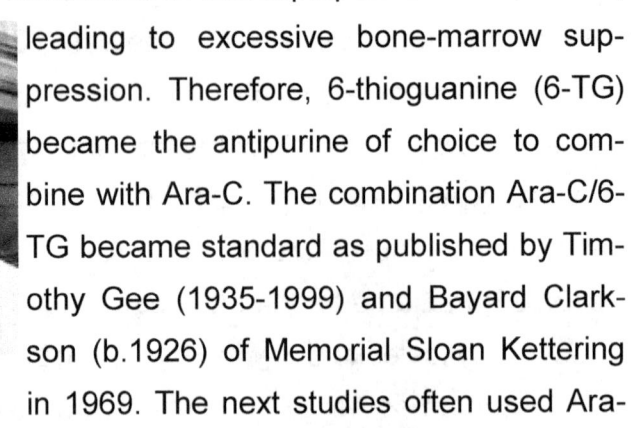

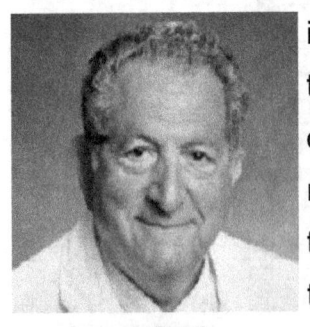

Bayard Clarkson

Joseph Bertino

sion in refractory AML. In 1991, a study from Vancouver CN and the Cleveland Clinic OH reported a 90% complete remission rate and a 27% long-term disease-free survival for 70 patients <60 years of age after HDAC and daunorubicin. Randomized studies could not prove superiority of HDAC, but did show increased toxicity to the CNS. HDAC became a drug typically used for consolidation therapy for patients who did not go on to autologous or allogeneic stem-cell transplantation (p.237). For patients whose leukemia cells express CD33, gemtuzumab ozogamicin (Mylotarg®) was an option for induction therapy, in particular for older patients. This humanized monoclonal antibody-drug conjugate was first studied in 1991. Recently, drugs against molecular targets (e.g., *FLT3* and *IDH1* and/or *IDH2*) have been introduced.

As mentioned before, acute promyelocytic leukemia (APL, M3) required a completely different approach. The leukemic cells with many azurophilic granules, which may cause the increased hemorrhagic diathesis (DIC) seen with this disease, have the retinoic acid receptor-A (RAR-α) rearrangement. This rearrangement represents the translocation between the long arms of chromosomes 15 (*PML* gene) and chromosome 17 (*RAR-α* gene). The first report on APL came in 1957 from Leif Hillestad in Oslo NO, who called it the "most malignant form of acute leukemia", because his three patients died within a few weeks from bleeding. In 1973, Jean Bernard's group in Paris showed that the disease was relatively sensitive to daunorubicin with a complete remission rate of 55%. After that, the combination of daunorubicin and Ara-C, resulted in 80% complete remissions, but only if the DIC bleeding tendency could be controlled with platelet and clotting factor support. Discussions about the use of heparin were frequent. I recall Misha Brozovic during the "*Advances in Hematology*" course at Royal Postgraduate Medical School in London (mid 1970's) stating: "Heparin in DIC stops the DIC, but kills the patient"! In 1985, treatment with ATRA (*all-trans retinoic acid*) was started by Zhenyi Wang (b.1924) and Zhu Chen in Shanghai CH. A five-year-old girl with APL, who had failed induction chemotherapy, was given ATRA by mouth for one year and achieved a complete remission that lasted 20^+ years! Follow-up studies in Shanghai, Europe, USA, and other countries in the 1990's and early 2000's, confirmed that ATRA alone, or in combination with daunorubicin/Ara-C, resulted in 90^+% complete remissions and 60-80% disease-free survival. ATRA appeared to work through differentiation of the APL cells. The same group in Shanghai also published on arsenic trioxide (ATO; As_2O_3) in the therapy of APL. This drug had been studied in the early 1970's in northeastern China as a general anti-cancer drug. Sun and colleagues reported, in 1992, that intravenous treatment with 1% ATO induced complete remission in 65% of patients with APL, with 30% survival after 10 years. Studies at Harbin Medical University and in Shanghai in 1996-1997, confirmed the high remission rate

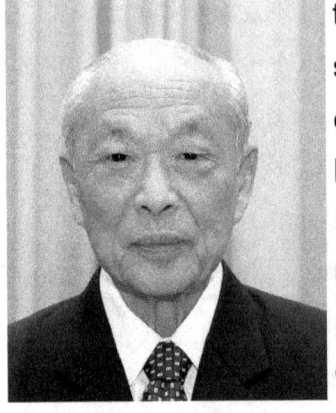

Zhen-Yi Wang

using pure ATO. Similar results were also obtained with As_4S_4, an oral formula. Since APL cells strongly express CD33, treatment with gemtuzumab ozogamicin also was a viable option. With the contributions of the Chinese investigators, based on traditional Chinese medicine, APL had become a curable disease.

Chronic Myelogenous Leukemia (CML)

Nearly all the early cases of leukemia reported in the mid 19th century were CML. That was logical, since the extreme splenomegaly and leukocytosis, in addition to the more prolonged course of the disease, were typical of that diagnosis. After the introduction of staining techniques for peripheral blood and bone marrow, the distribution of the granulocytic series in CML was found to be quite different from that in severe bacterial infections. Whereas in the latter, a progressive left-shifted distribution was found, in the former myelocytes and granulocytes were overrepresented. In addition, in CML the morphology of the myeloid cells was often aberrant. Absolute basophilia and eosinophilia were almost ubiquitous. Max Wachstein (1905-1965) in Passaic NJ reported, in 1945, that the segmented neutrophils in CML had a marked decrease in their alkaline phosphatase (NAP or LAP), in contrast to bacterial infections where the NAP was elevated. The disease occurred at any adolescent/adult age, but was most frequent between the ages of 40 and 70. The chronic phase with slow progression may last several years, but then a majority of patients enter an accelerated phase. In that phase, the disease stops responding to previously effective therapy ("*metamorphosis*") with clinical and hematological deterioration. Ultimately, a sudden fulminating clinical deterioration may occur with death within weeks.

In 1959, Bernard's group in Paris showed that patients may also suddenly transform into a kind of *de novo* acute leukemia ("blast crisis").

The first consistent treatment of CML consisted of splenic irradiation. A total dose of 1,000-1,500 rads over 9-15 days was effective in reducing spleen size and high leukocyte count, as shown by Edwin Osgood (1899-1969) in Portland OR in 1952. Chemotherapy consisted initially of arsenic, but was less popular than splenic radiation, despite Forkner's support for arsenic. That changed when David Galton in London reported that oral busulfan (Alkeran®), an alkylating agent, was effective in the chronic phase of CML in 1953. This remained the standard treatment of CML for many years. In 1975, George Canellos' group, then still at the NCI, showed that hydroxyurea, either intravenously or by mouth, was effective in patients with CML, who had either accelerated phase or excessive myelosuppression from busulfan. In the early 1980's, Moshe Talpaz's group at MD Anderson introduced α-interferon therapy, which proved a major improvement, often leading to cytogenetic remissions.

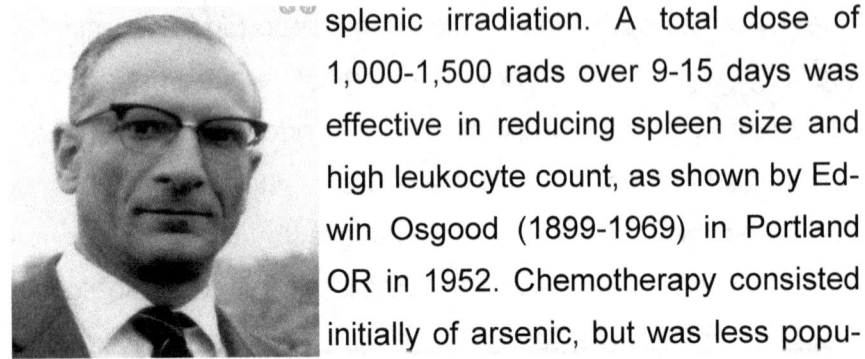

David Galton

A major development had occurred in 1960, when Peter Nowell (1928-2016) and David Hungerford (1927-

White Blood Cells

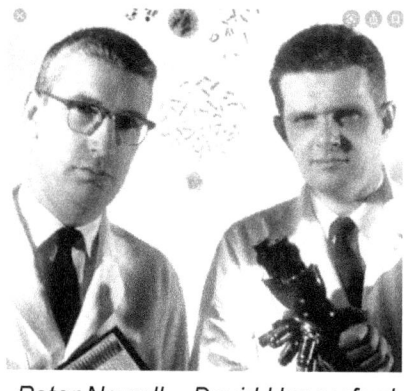

1993), working in Philadelphia PA, reported on an abnormally small acrocentric chromosome in the leukemic cells of CML. Their observation was rapidly confirmed by other groups, but was initially thought to involve chromosome 21. In 1971, it was shown to involve chromosome 22 instead, and in 1973 Janet Rowley (1925-2013) at the University of Chicago used quinacrine fluorescence and Giemsa banding to prove that the Philadelphia chromosome was the 22q- of t(9;22). This translocation resulted in the juxtaposition of the sequences in the breakpoint cluster region *(bcr)* of chromosome 22 with the cellular oncogene *c-abl* of chromosome 9 to form a hybrid gene *(bcr-abl1)* (1982-1985), as the causative event in CML. A collaboration between university laboratories and pharmaceutical company Ciba-Geigy (now Novartis) led to the development of a *BCR-ABL* kinase inhibitor, imatinib mesylate (Gleevec®), by Brian Druker (b.1955) at the University of Oregon and Nicholas Lydon (b.1957) at Novartis, Basel SU in 1996. Once it was

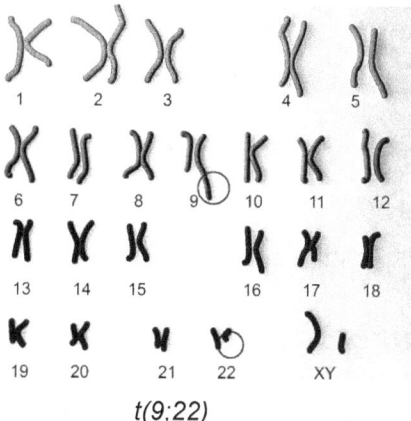

Peter Nowell   David Hungerford

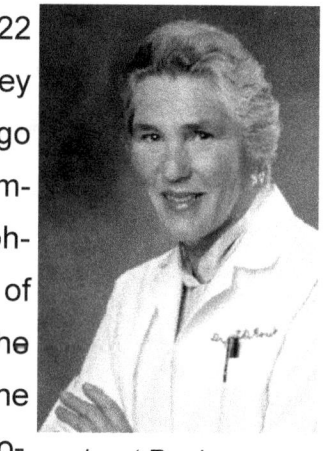

Janet Rowley

t(9;22)

approved by government agencies, this drug and several of its successors, completely changed the treatment of CML. It even replaced allogeneic stem cell transplantation (*p.238*) as first line therapy. Imatinib proved also more effective than α-interferon. The majority of patients have deep and durable responses to *BCR/ABL1* inhibitors and appear to have survival similar to their non-leukemic peers. Part of these deep-response patients may be able to withhold all treatment after 2 years without signs of progression, for prolonged treatment-free remissions.

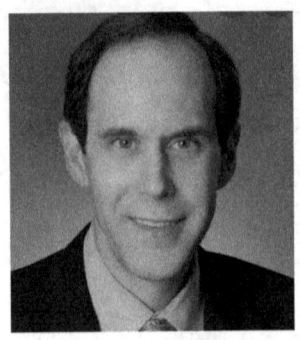

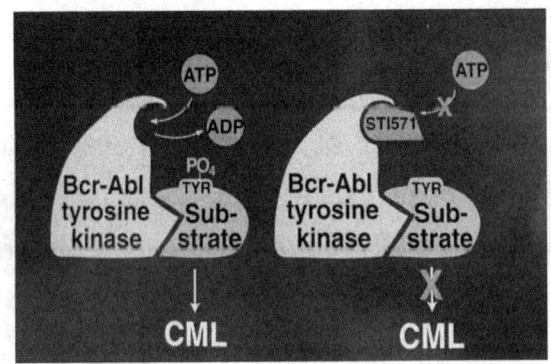

Brian Druker

Mode of action of imatinib (=ST1751)

The few patients with CML (5%), who do not have t(9;22)(q23;q11.2) or *BCR-ABL1* by FISH technique, are obviously not candidates for tyrosine-kinase inhibitors.

Chronic Lymphocytic Leukemia(s)

Joseph Lieutaud (1703-1780), who became the personal physician of Louis XVI, probably was the first to see white blood cells ("globuli albicantes"), but William Hewson first identified them and described the lymphatic system. Rudolf Virchow documented in 1845 the first case of chronic lymphocytic leukemia. In 1856, he summarized his studies of leukemia by documenting not only an increase in "colorless corpuscles", but also a decrease in red blood cells. He distinguished between splenic leukemia with splenomegaly and lymphatic leukemia with swelling of the lymph nodes and presence of lymph-node cells in the peripheral blood. His concept of leukemia was not easily accepted, because many physicians believed that "there are already enough diseases without inventing any new ones". Quite a chaos ensued in the classification of lymphatic diseases. William Gowers in 1879 correctly attributed the leukemic cells in the blood stream to an "overflow" of cells produced in the hematopoietic tissue, but he also equated lymphatic disease with Hodgkin's disease! New names were introduced: lymphosarcoma (Kundrat;1893), leukosarcoma, myelosis, pseudoleukemia (Ebstein;1888), *etc*. The introduction of staining techniques by Ehrlich in 1877-1880 helped to define various lymphatic cells. In 1901, Felix Pinkus (1868-1947) gave a comprehensive description of CLL. He defined the neoplastic lymphocytes as "small cells", sometimes even smaller than red blood cells. He also suggested that sometimes an absolute increase in the number of lymphocytes was the first detectable sign of the disease (*Pinkus' sign*). The cells were monotonously uniform small cells with heavily clumped chromatin (*grumuleé*), a narrow rim of cytoplasm and many smudge cells ("*Gumprechtse Schollen*"; 1896). Not all lymphatic cells

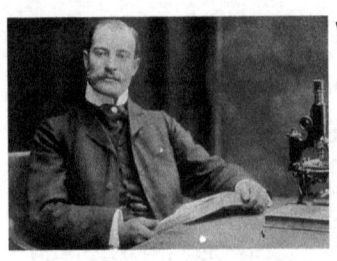

Artur Pappenheim

were small, though. In his 1905 *Atlas der menschlichen Blutzellen* (Atlas of human blood cells), Artur Pappenheim (1870-1916) in Berlin tried to determine the various development stages of lymphocytes, but he was not truly successful, according to current knowledge. Pappenheim believed that the myeloblast of Naegeli also could give rise to "lymphocytes". He subdivided the lymphocytes into small lymphocytes, lymphoidocytes (=larger lymphocytes), and "lympho-leukocytes" with more cytoplasm and an often not round nucleus. CLL mostly showed the small lymphocytes, but could have components of all three. Wilhelm Türk (1871-1916) in Vienna AT established the close relationship between CLL and malignant lymphoma (1903). The next year, Carl Sternberg (1872-1935) in Vienna (*of Reed-Sternberg cell fame*) separated CLL with infiltration of small lymphocytes from leukosarcoma with infiltration of non-lymphatic organs. The situation remained confused, but in 1929 Flashman and Leopold, reporting on a case of retroperitoneal lymphoma that ended in leukemia, went back to the description of CLL by Türk. This definition of CLL was now well established and little changed until the early 1970's, when immunological methods to study lymphocytes became available. Rosette techniques, immunoglobulin analysis, and most importantly monoclonal antibodies, were then used to dissect the leukemic lymphocytes. The resulting separate entities will be discussed consecutively.

CLL is the most common form of chronic leukemia in Caucasians, accounting for 25% of all leukemias. The disease is far less frequent in Asia. Before 1950, radiation therapy to spleen and/or enlarged lymph-node groups was the standard of care for CLL. This therapy was less effective than in CML. William Dameshek tried corticosteroids, sometimes with good success. `In the early 1950's, chlorambucil (Leukeran®) was developed by Everett and colleagues at the Chester Beatty Research Institute (now Royal Marsden Hospital) in London. This oral alkylating agent, by itself or in combination with prednisone, became the standard therapy of CLL for many years. Chlorambucil may have controlled the symptoms and leukocyte count, but it probably did not have a true effect on survival. Survival ranged from weeks to 25^+ years. Kanti Rai (b.1932) at Brookhaven NY in Eugene Cronkite's group, developed a

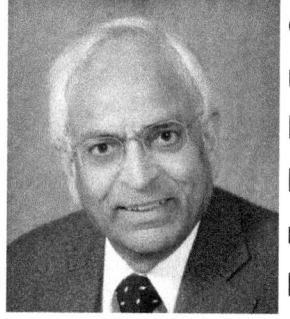

Kanti Rai

staging system for CLL in 1975. This staging system, with stages 0-IV, was based upon lymphadenopathy (stage I), hepato- and/or splenomegaly (Stage II), anemia (stage III) and thrombocytopenia (stage IV). The staging system was a reasonable predictor of median survival. Therapy was indicated for patients with constitutional symptoms, painful lymphadenopathy or splenomegaly, rapidly increasing organomegaly, auto-immune cytopenia, or progressive bone marrow impairment. When the disease became therapy resistant, *e.g.*, by the occurrence of a more malignant clone (Richter's syndrome, 1928) or progressive bone-marrow failure or constitutional symptoms, therapy became difficult. Fludarabine (Fludara®), developed in 1968, proved extremely lympholytic. The drug was used intravenously as a single agent in CLL with success by Michael Grever (b.1945) and colleagues at Ohio State University, Columbus OH (1985) and at MD Anderson Hospital in Houston TX by Michael Keating (b.1942) and colleagues. In previously untreated patients, fludarabine proved effective. Addition of prednisone did not appear to improve survival. At the same time, studies with intravenous 2-chlorodeoxyadenosine (cladribine; Leustatin®) by Ernest Beutler's group (*p.85*) at the Scripps Clinic (San Diego CA) gave results quite similar to fludarabine. In 1987, Rai revised his staging system to the Rai-Sawitsky system with only 3 stages: low risk (formerly stage 0), intermediate risk (formerly stages I and II), and high risk (formerly stages III and IV). This staging is now still used in the USA. In Europe, most clinicians continue to use the 1977 Binet system, named after Jacques Louis Binet (b.1932) of Paris. Stage A: <3 lymph-nodes areas involved and no anemia or thrombocytopenia;

Jacques-Louis Binet

stage B: more than 3 lymph-nodes groups involved; and stage C: anemia and/or thrombocytopenia. Both systems predict median survival rather well. The immunological and genetic techniques introduced since the 1970's have led to delineation of entities that originally were included among CLL.

White Blood Cells

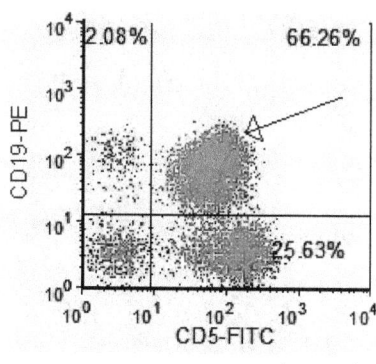

CLL cells are CD19⁺ CD5⁺ (2 color fluorescence)

The cases of CLL "proper" have cells with weak surface immunoglobulin, mostly of μ or μ+δ class, strong CD5 (as determined by Ivor Royston (b.1945)'s group in San Diego CA in 1981) and CD19; they lack FMC7. Many cases have translocations of chromosomes with a breakpoint at 14q32. Cases with del(17p), involving the mutation of the *TP53* gene involved with apoptosis, have more therapy-resistant disease. Since 2010, several monoclonal antibodies and kinase inhibitors have been introduced to the treatment of CLL. Thus, rituximab and obinutuzumab, which both are humanized anti-CD20 monoclonal antibodies, have shown clinical activity against CLL and are often used in combination with chlorambucil. Similarly, the Bruton's tyrosine kinase (BTK) inhibitors ibrutinib and zanubutrinib have shown activity and perhaps keep patients in remission longer than the monoclonal antibodies. The *bcl-2* inhibitor venetoclax alone, or in combination with other modalities, has resulted in deep responses, that may be durable even without indefinite treatment. Over the most recent 20 years, the therapeutic options for CLL have dramatically improved, to a large extent based on the molecular changes in the leukemic cells and their pathways.

Several distinct entities have been separated from CLL. These entities will be discussed sequentially; first the T-cell and then the B-cell diseases.

Blood is LIfe

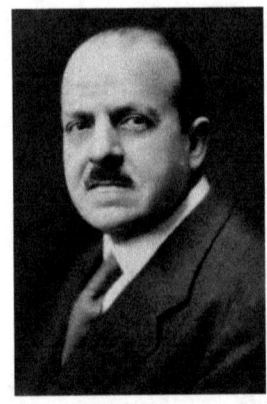

Albert Sézary (1880-1956), a dermatologist and syphilologist at Hôpital St. Louis in Paris, described a case of exfoliative erythroderma with "monstrous" cells in the skin and the peripheral blood in 1938. Their cerebriform nucleus could be observed much better with electron microscopy than with light microscopy. In 1973, several groups reported that these cells were T lymphocytes with a T-helper cell phenotype (CD2, CD3, CD5, CD4 positive). The T-cell receptor is clonally rearranged. In addition to leukapheresis and PUVA phototherapy, many chemotherapy drugs have been used with monoclonal antibodies (*e.g.*, alemtuzumab) and BTK inhibitors among the more recent.

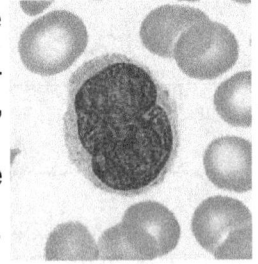

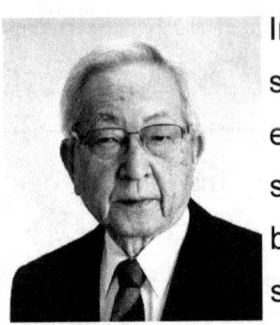

Albert Sézary

Sézary cell

In 1974, an unusual syndrome was reported in some adults in south-western Japan by the group of Kiyoshi Takatsuki (b.1930) in Kyoto. The peripheral blood of these patients had many lymphoid cells with "clover-leafed" or "flower-like" nuclei. Similar cases were then reported from the Caribbean, including immigrants into the USA and England. The cells were shown to be activated T-helper cells (CD2, CD3, CD4, CD5, and CD25 positive). The disease was called

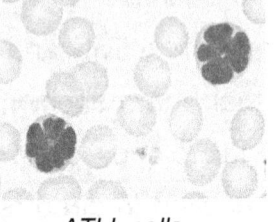

Kiyoshi Takatsuki

ATLL cells

T-cell Leukemia/Lymphoma (ATLL). Then in 1980, Robert Gallo (b.1937)'s group at NIH (Bethesda MD) found the causative agent: HTLVI, a human type-C retrovirus. Combination chemotherapy as for other aggressive malignant lymphomas has been used: CHOP, hyper-CVAD. Antibodies and kinase inhibitors have also been used.

Tom Loughran, Jr (b.1953) and colleagues at the Fred Hutchinson Cancer Research Center in Seattle WA reported on a leukemia of large granular lymphocytes (LGL) in 1985. These cells had T-cell/NK (natural-killer) cell characteristics. The large cells with abundant cytoplasm and azurophiliic granules looked like reactive lymphocytes. Their cell markers were CD2, CD3, CD8, CD57 (HNK-1) positive for T-LGL, or CD2, CD8, CD56 (neural cell adhesion molecule) for the NK-LGL. T-LGL was shown to be clonal for the T-cell receptor, but for NK-LGL clonality was difficult to prove. Before 1985, these diseases had been classified under many different names, *e.g.*, T-CLL by Jean Claude Brouet and colleagues in Paris in 1975. Since neutropenia is often a clinical feature of LGL, low-dose chemotherapy (methotrexate, cyclophosphamide) or even cyclosporine have been used.

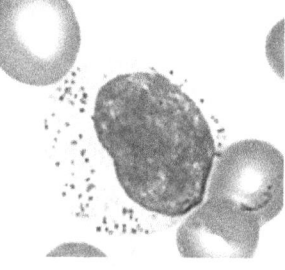

LGL cell

Most cases of CLL proved to be of B-cell origin, but other B cell entities were identified, although initially under other names. In 1958, Bertha Bouroncle (1919-2013) and colleagues at Ohio State University reported on 26, mostly

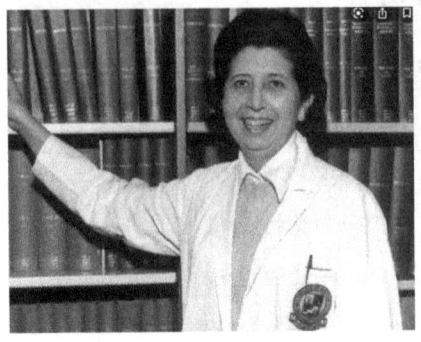

Bertha Bouroncle

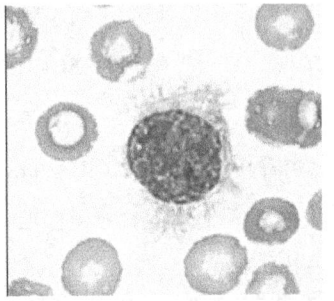

hairy cell

male, patients with splenomegaly and in the peripheral-blood smear cells with a serrated border. The authors considered them to be free "reticulum cells", which they thought to be very immature cells following Ewald's concept from 1923. Similar cases had already been reported by Hal Downey (1877-1959) in 1938 in Minneapolis MN, and Nathan Rosenthal and Stanley Lee in New York in 1951. The paper by Bouroncle on "leukemic reticuloendotheliosis" received a lot of attention. Even though some initial studies still reported the cells as "reticulum cells", their similarity to lymphocytes and monocytes was obvious. They were now described as "hairy cells" of leukemic reticuloendotheliosis (Schrek & Donnelly, 1966). The bone-marrow biopsy showed loose infiltration by neoplastic cells with increased reticulin, leading in France to the name "myélofibrose lymphoide" (George Duhamel, Paris, 1966). In 1971, Lung Yam (1936-2013) and colleagues in Boston reported that the acid-phosphatase activity in these "reticulum cells" was not inhibited by preincubation with tartaric acid (TRAP). In the early 1970's, the name "hairy cell leukemia" (HCL; French: Leucémie à Tricholeukocytes; German: Haarzellenleukämie) became more popular. In the same years, the concept of reticulum cells as stem cells had become outdated. The discussion was now between lymphocyte and monocyte. I recall asking the French hematologist Felix Reyes, at a conference in Paris in 1978, about his opinion. Following French diplomatic tradition, he called himself an "agnostic". Arguments for a monocytic origin were severe monocytopenia (Rama Seshadri, Hamilton CN; 1976), phagocytosis (as seen by several groups in 1974) and cytochemistry. The phagocytosis, however, appeared to be mainly "virtual", as demonstrated by our group in Leiden NL in 1979 with several techniques. Then, when monoclonal surface immunoglobulin was detected on the hairy cells by several groups in the mid-1970's (*e.g.*, Daniel Catovsky and colleagues in London; 1974) and reactivity with monoclonal antibodies specific for B lymphocytes in the early 1980's (our group; 1981), it had become clear that HCL was definitely a B-cell leukemia. Among the antibodies most important to determine the maturation stage were CD19, CD20, FMC7, CD25 and CD103; CD5 was absent. The cells often had multiple heavy chains on their surface (*e.g.*, Hayhoe's group in Cambridge UK; 1978) and reacted weakly with OKM1 (CD11b; our group), but strongly with Leu-M5 (CD11c; Kiel group; 1985).

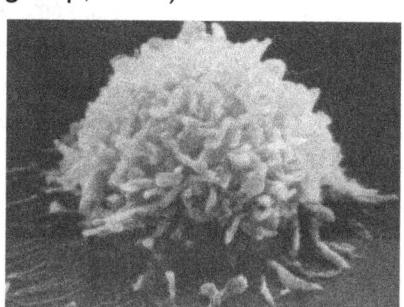

Scan EM picture of hairy cell

Brunangelo Falini *et al.* identified point mutation *BRAF*^{V600E} *as the* causing genetic event in hairy-cell leukemia in 2011. This mutation causes the constitutive activation of the *RAS-RAF-MEK-ERK* signaling pathway.

The therapy of HCL went through as many changes as the name of the disease. The splenomegaly, in combination with pancytopenia, made splenectomy more attractive than chemotherapy. In the 1970's, splenectomy was found to be beneficial for patients (*e.g.*, Harvey Golomb (b.1942)'s group in Chicago IL, 1978; our group for a collaborative study, 1981). Based on the collaborative-group material, our team developed a staging system in 1982. By that time, however, alternative therapy had become available. Jordan Gutterman (b.1938)'s group at MD Anderson (Houston TX) started treating patients with recombinant α-interferon. Several patients attained complete remission. This therapy rapidly spread around the globe, and was used even without splenectomy. In 1995, an NCI-sponsored multicenter study showed that the purine analog pentostatin (2'-deoxycoformycin; Nipent®) produced higher responses and relapse-free survival than α-interferon. During the same period (1991), Ernest Beutler's group in San Diego CA had studied 2-CDA (cladribine, Leustatin®), which they showed to be strongly immunosuppressive and active in HCL. This drug could also be administered subcutaneously, which had practical advantage over intravenous pentostatin.

For relapsed or therapy-refractory patients, cladribine in combination with rituximab was used. Now that the point mutation BRAF^{V600E} had been identified in nearly all cases of "true" HCL, BRAF inhibitors (*e.g.*, vemurafenib) became a logical approach. The cases of HCL that are *BRAF^{V600E}* negative had already been recognized as different from typical HCL in 1980 by Frank Hayhoe's group as HCL, type II. The FAB group in 1989 renamed it HCLv (HCLvariant), partly because Daniel Catovsky (b.1937) considered it to be an intermediate form between HCL and Prolymphocytic Leukemia. The latter disease was first described by David Galton at Royal Postgraduate Medical School in London in 1974.

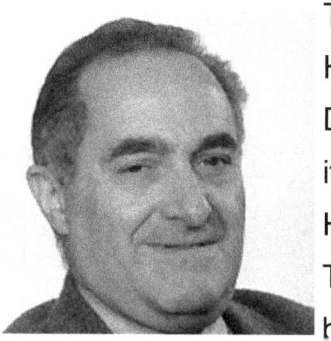

Daniel Catosvky

Patients often presented with massive splenomegaly, high white cell counts, cells with a large vesicular nucleolus, and rapidly progressive disease. The cells could have either a B-cell or a T-cell phenotype. B-cell Prolymphocytic Leukemia cells were positive for CD19, CD20, FMC7, but negative for CD5 and CD25. Therapy is similar to other mature lymphocytic leukemias with increasing attention to treatment with antibodies or B-cell receptor inhibitors.

The current era promises to be as interesting for the treatment of the chronic lymphocytic leukemias, as the 1970's were for their differential diagnosis.

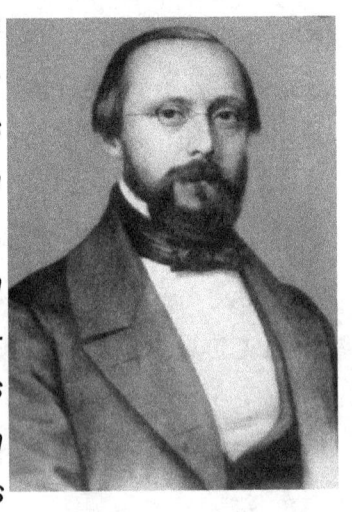

Rudolf Ludwig Carl Virchow *was born in 1821 in Schivelbein, Pomerania, now Swidwin PO. He did his medical training in Berlin and was a polymath (or an Uomo Universale, as the Italians express it so much more poetically). His field was pathology, but he is also known for his political activities, public health efforts, and forensic work. As far as his political work is concerned, he participated in the Revolution of 1848, which led to his dismissal from the Charité Hospital in Berlin. He founded a new political party (Deutsche Fortschrittspartei) and was elected to the Reichstag. He opposed Otto von Bismarck and almost had to fight a duel with the latter (Sausage Duel). His public-health efforts were wide ranging and he coined the aphorism "Medicine is a social science and politics is nothing else but medicine on a large scale". After 5 years, he returned to the Charité Hospital as the Chair of the new Pathology Department. His contributions to pathology were even more important. When he was only 24 years of age, he introduced the term "leukemia" after seeing one of the first patients in whom the diagnosis was made. His book* Cellular Pathology *(1858) was the basis of modern pathology. He postulated that all cells come from pre-existing cells ("Omnis cellula e cellula"), Virchow also founded a number of scientific journals in pathology. He named several new phenomena, such as "thrombosis",*

"chordoma", "embolism" and Virchow node (*left supraclavicular lymph node in cases of intestinal cancer*). *In cellular pathology, he introduced the names "chromatin", neuroglia", "osteoid" and "parenchyma". Even Virchow was not always correct: he called Charles Darwin an "ignoramus", believed that the Neanderthal man was just a deformed human, and he did not believe Ignaz Semmelweis' idea of disinfection or Louis Pasteur and Robert Koch's germ theory. Later in life, he was active in anti-racist activism and called the Aryan race a "Nordic Mysticism". He had studied nearly 7 million children and concluded that Jews and Germans could not be differentiated based on hair, skin or eye color. Virchow died in 1902 from hearth failure, and he received a state funeral.*

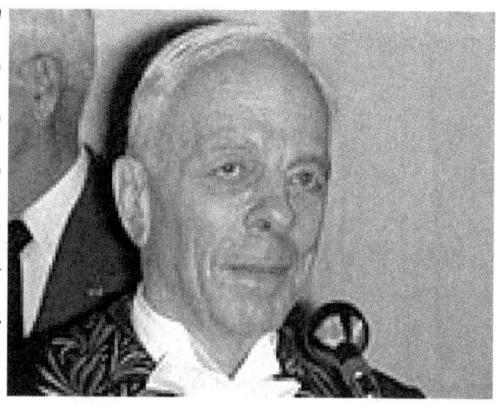

Jean Bernard was born in 1907 in Paris. He became an extern at Salpêtrière Hospital in Paris 1927. He failed his first exam for internship and started to work as a temporary intern at Beaujon hospital in Levallois-Perret (NW Paris) with Paul Chevallier (1884-1960), a hematologist. This profoundly influenced him to become a hematologist. In 1932, he started his doctorate thesis on an experimental model of leukemia; he also became secretary of the French Hematology Society, the first one of its kind in the world. He reported on high-dose radiation therapy for Hodgkin's disease the same year and obtained his doctorate in 1936. He was in the French army in 1939, and after the defeat of France, he became one of the first 500 members of the French Résistance in 1940. He was responsible for collecting weapons parachuted into the Vaucluse. He was arrested by the Germans in 1943, and spent 6 months in captivity. After the war, he became an associate professor in 1949 and Professor of Oncology at the Pasteur Institute in 1956. His Professorship in Hematology happened in 1961 and the next year he also became director of the Georges Hayem Institute of the University of Paris (Hôpital St.Louis). He retired in 1970 but remained active: 1982 President of the Academy of Sciences and from 1983-1992 President of the National Consultative Committee on Ethics. He died in 2006 at age 98.

His scientific interests were wide. He studied childhood leukemia, and in 1947 he and Marcel Bessis treated a 6-year old child with acute leukemia with exchange blood transfusions. The child improved and the second exchange transfusion normalized the blood smear. The remission lasted 2 months. With the introduction of new chemotherapy agents (e.g., daunorubicin) for ALL, the remission rate increased and several patients survived at least 5 years after the introduction of reinduction (=consolidation) therapy in 1965. He was able to organize national studies in 1974, based on prognostic factors that he had described in 1972. Based on these studies, they were able to decrease the duration of therapy from 5 to 3 years.

In 1950, while at the Pasteur Institute, he described the first chemically induced leukemia in industrial workers. Then he showed that tar invariably caused leukemia in rats when injected into the bone marrow.

In acute promyelocytic leukemia (M3), he made major contributions. In 1957-1959, he described the coagulation problems in M3 leukemia. In 1973, his group reported on the high remission rates and the first cures. In chronic myelogenous leukemia he obtained in 1956 a complete cure of a 3-year-old patient. He studied the impact of acute leukemia and its therapy on the psyche of children. Psychologists and psychiatrists were part of his team before anywhere else (1950's).

He and his pupil Georges Flandrin were responsible in Tehran for the diagnosis of the Shah of Iran, Mohammad Reza Pahlavi, with Waldenström's macroglobulinemia in 1974. Until the shah's deposition in 1978, most of the therapy was secretly arranged. George Flandrin told me once that his wife was afraid that he had an affair, because about every month he disappeared for a weekend without giving her information about where he went.

In addition to his extensive work in hematology, Bernard was a published poet (3 volumes) and a philosopher and ethicist (20 books). He was considered the "pope of hematology", being distant and intellectually dominating. But he was also reported to be gentle and to interact well on a one-on-one basis.

Blood is Life

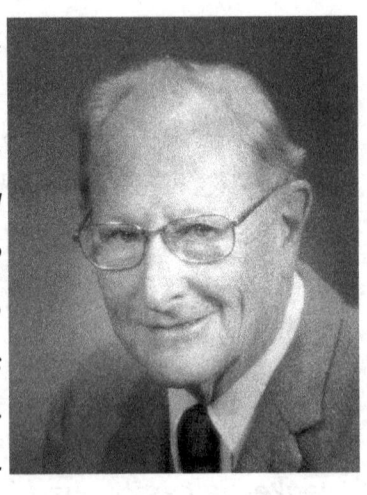

Eugene P Cronkite was born in Los Angeles in 1914. He graduated from Stanford University's Medical School in 1940. He then enlisted in the Medical Corps U S Navy and served from 1942 until 1954, after which he joined the Brookhaven National Laboratory as senior physician and Head of the Division of Experimental Pathology. He became Chairman of the Medical Department (1967-1979), but then returned to research. He retired in 1993 as Rear Admiral, USNR. During his years in the Navy, he was first assigned to the Naval Operating Hospital in Norfolk VA, since his training in Medicine only, made him unfit for ship's doctor. His research there started with skin grafting on heavily burned German submarine survivors. Later in the war, he was involved with mooring the first target ships for the nuclear bomb test at Bikini in the Marshall Islands. He did a medical survey of the local population, before they were evacuated from the island. Then, he was appointed to be the "hematologist" for "Operation Crossroad", the nuclear bomb tests. The Navy put a series of animals – goats, pigs, rats, guinea pigs, etc. – on the island to study the effect of the 23 nuclear bombs between 1946 and 1958. He and George Brecher (1913-2004) researched the effect of radiation on bleeding and thrombocytopenia by transfusing platelets from healthy fox hounds into fox hounds that had been exposed to 600 cGy. It worked well to prevent death from bleeding, but now the recipients died from neutropenic infections. Granulocyte *transfusions helped for a while, but the hounds developed antibodies and still died. Their work with platelet transfusions corrected the concept of "heparinemia' as the cause of bleeding after radiation, as had been suggested by Leon Jacobson.*

In 1954, the winds around the Marshall Islands changed direction, and many Marshallese were exposed to radioactive fall out. They often developed skin burns or bone-marrow failure. Cronkite directed the studies of the effect of this radiation on the increased risk of cancer, similar with the observations made after the Hiroshima/Nagasaki bombs. He worked extensively in the field of radiation biology, and he also studied the formation and life span of neutrophils. He pioneered extracorporeal radiation for leukemic cells (especially chronic lymphocytic leukemia; 1965) and studied bone-marrow growth in diffusion chambers (1970's). After his clinical retirement, he worked again on leukemia, but also on the drug AZT (zidovudine; Retrovir®). Many young investigators, from all over the world, spent time in his laboratory and clinical services. He died in 2001, when he was 86.

Myelodysplastic syndromes (MDS)

Many cases of AML were preceded by abnormalities of bone marrow function that could last up to a couple of years before overt AML was diagnosed. The first report of that stage of *preleukemia* came in 1953 from Mathew Block and colleagues at the University of Chicago. They observed 12 patients for up to 27 months prior to development of acute leukemia. Three years later, Sven-Erik Björkman in Lund SW described 4 cases of refractory anemia with increased free iron in the erythroblasts: a*cquired refractory sideroblastic anemia*. One case was followed for over 18 years. Even earlier, in 1938, Cornelius Roads (1898-1959) in New York had already reported on a series of patients with refractory anemia. Jack Rheingold and colleagues in Washington DC confirmed the existence of a preleukemic stage of acute (myeloid) leukemia in 1963, but some patients died from other problems before the acute leukemia was obvious, mostly from infections. They used the term *smoldering leukemia*. In 1973, James Linman (b.1921) and his medical resident Matti Saarni at the Mayo Clinic (Rochester MN) published on 34 patients with a preleukemic syndrome before the onset of AML. This was a follow-up to their 1971 report on myelomonocytic leukemia (*Naegeli*-type AML). In that earlier report, 31% of their patients had a preleukemic phase. One of their patients lived for 5 years after diagnosis. They used the name *preleukemic syndromes*. Cytopenias dominated the picture. The syndrome was further delineated by James Linman, now in Portland OR, and Grover Bagby (b.1942).

Presenting symptoms of the mostly elderly patients were pancytopenia (44%), anemia with thrombocytopenia (20%), or anemia (15%). The bone marrow was normocellular or hypercellular, with maturation defects in all blood-cell lineages: the white-cell series often had monocytoid features, the red cell series had megaloblastic changes. At a conference on the diseases in 1976, the name *hemopoietic dysplasias* was chosen. Guido Tricot (b.1950) in Louvain BE stressed the importance of the bone-marrow biopsy in 1984, documenting that patients with abnormally localized immature precursors (*ALIP*) had a higher risk of developing AML earlier.

When the FAB group (*p.143,146*) proposed their classification of acute leukemias in 1976, they included two *dysmyelopoietic syndromes* (DMPS): refractory anemia with excess of blasts (RAEB) and chronic myelomonocytic leukemia (CMML). The first group would include preleukemia, smoldering leukemia, and "subacute leukemia". In the hypercellular bone marrow, myeloblasts + promyelocytes were between 10 and 30% with abnormal maturation. The second group had a peripheral blood monocyte count of >1,000/mm^3 with atypical monocytes. The bone marrow was often quite similar with RAEB. In their update from 1982, they now had 5

The 1982 French-American-British (FAB) Cooperative Group classification of the myelodysplastic syndromes

Subtype	Myeloblasts in peripheral blood (%)	Myeloblasts in bone marrow (%)	Ringed sideroblasts (%)	Absolute monocytes in peripheral blood	Auer rods present in bone marrow?
Refractory anemia (RA)	<1	<5	<15	–	No
Refractory anemia with ringed sideroblasts	<1	<5	>15	–	No
Refractory anemia with excess blasts	>5	21-30	–	–	No
Refractory anemia with excess blasts in transformation	<5	20-30	–	–	Yes or no
Chronic myelomonocytic leukemia	<5	<20	–	>1 × 10^9/L	No

subcategories of what they called *myelodysplastic syndromes* (MDS): refractory anemia (RA), refractory anemia with ringed sideroblasts (RARS), RAEB, RAEB in transformation (RAEB-t) and CMML. This remained the standard for two decades, even though CMML was considered probably more a myeloproliferative than a myelodysplastic syndrome.

Then in 2002, the World Health Organization (WHO) committee changed everything around, and introduced 3 additional subcategories: refractory anemia with multilineage dysplasia (RCMD), two variants of RAEB, and the 5q⁻ syndrome. The latter syndrome, with deletion of part of the long arm of chromosome 5, had been described by Herman van den Berghe of Louvain BE in 1974. In the same year 2002, a review by David Steensma (b.1970) and Ayalew Tefferi (b.1956?) of the Mayo Clinic listed 21 names for the syndromes used between 1907 (*Anemia pseudo-aplastica* in Italy) and 1982 (*MDS*).

Another type of disease that was difficult to classify was the *Di Guglielmo disease*. Giovanni Di Guglielmo (1886-1961) was a Brazilian-born Italian hematologist who, between 1917 and 1961, extensively studied neoplastic proliferations of erythroid cells. The first publication probably involved a case of erythroid leukemia, which he published while he was a physician at the war front in Alto Adige (South Tyrol). A follow-up on this paper also showed involvement of myeloblasts and platelet-producing megakaryocytes in the circulation. In 1923, he reported a case of *eritremia acute*. During these years, he followed his mentor Adolfo Ferrata (1890-1946), the father of Italian hematology, to his various

White Blood Cells

Giovanni Di Guglielmo

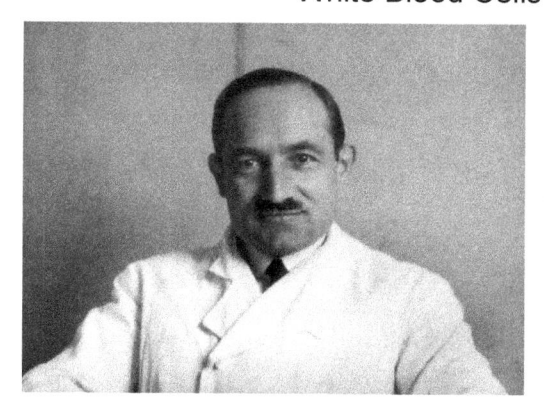

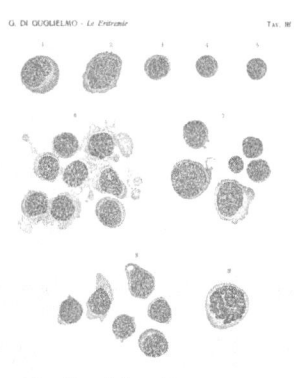

Erythroid cells as seen by Di Guglielmo

appointments. After he became independent, he continued to publish on neoplastic erythroid disorders including *myelosi eritremica cronica* (1942). One of the proponents of Di Guglielmo's syndrome was Dameshek (*p.188*), although Wintrobe remarked that Di Guglielmo himself would be surprised what Dameshek made of his disease! Dameshek saw a natural progression from erythremic myelosis through erythroleukemia to acute myeloblastic leukemia (1958). Even in 1969, Dameshek maintained his position and felt that RA and RARS were just part of the syndrome, which he now called a myeloproliferative disorder. The FAB classification scored the more chronic form as RA or RAEB, and the acute form as M6 (erythroleukemia). The WHO classification also scored the acute form as erythroleukemia. The *acute erythremic myelosis* of Di Guglielmo was difficult to classify, but is probably rare. By 2008, the WHO committee in their revision dropped the name refractory anemia in favor of refractory cytopenia with unilineage dysplasia (RCUD): RA, refractory neutropenia (RN) and refractory thrombocytopenia

(RT). In addition, a category between MDS and myeloproliferative neoplasms had already been added in 2002, and CMML had been transferred to that category. In the 2016 revision, the classification became more restrained again, by removing any mention of cytopenia (a *"sine qua non"*) and focusing on the lineage dysplasia (single: MDS-SLD or multiple lineages: MDS-MLD). These continuously changing classifications are undoubtedly good for academic credit, but are becoming too complicated for "simple" clinicians, unless they can be shown to have significant prognostic and/or therapeutic implications.

The International Prognostic Scoring System for MDS was introduced by Peter Greenberg (b.1937; Palo Alto CA) and colleagues in 1997. It was useful, although it underestimated the importance of life threatening neutropenia. The lowest score (0) had a median survival of >5 years, the highest score (2) of 0.4 years..

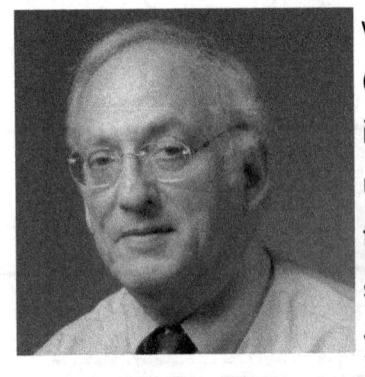

Peter Greenberg

The suggested therapy initially was "carefully doing nothing", but hypomethylating agents (azacitidine and decitabine) were introduced in the early 1980's; they promote myeloid differentiation. The drug azacitidine was approved in 2004 and decitabine in 2006. Growth factors were used with variable success. Patients with RA with low erythropoietin levels could benefit from erythropoietin (EPO), sometimes in

White Blood Cells

	Score				
	0	0.5	1	1.5	2
Marrow myeloblast percentage	<5	5-10	–	11-20	21-30
Karyotype	Good	Intermediate	Poor	–	–
Peripheral blood cytopenias	0 or 1	2 or 3	–	–	–
Risk groups	Total score	Median survival			
Low-risk	0 points	5.7			
Intermediate-1 risk	0.5-1 point	3.5			
Intermediate-2 risk	1.5-2 points	1.2			
High risk	2.5 or more points	0.4			

Karyotype: good—normal karyotype, -Y, del(5q), del(20q); intermediate—all karyotypes not good or poor risk; poor—abnormal chromosome 7, complex karyotype (three or more anomalies). Peripheral blood cytopenias: hemoglobin, <10 g/dl; absolute neutrophil count, <1500/mm^3; platelet count, <100,000/mm^3.

Table from Greenberg's 1997 paper

combination with filgrastim (1995). High-dose chemotherapy was rarely effective in this older population, as was lower dose chemotherapy (low-dose Ara-C).

Immunosuppression with ALG or cyclosporine was proposed for patients with hypoplastic MDS, *e.g.* by Bruno Speck's group in Basel SU in 1988, but was not studied in a randomized trial. Response to immunosuppression was found to be related to younger age, shorter duration and certain HLA types (John Barrett's group at NIH; 2003).

Thalidomide, the teratogenic antiangiogenic drug and immuno-modulator, and its analog lenalidomide (Revlimid®), appear to be particularly effective in the 5q¯syndrome (Alan List, Tucson AZ; 2005). Syngeneic or allogeneic stem-cell transplantation is the only treatment that can cure up to half the patients with higher risk MDS, and non-myeloablative allografts are attractive in the older population (*p.235*). Toxicity excludes most patients because of age or comorbidities.

Myeloproliferative Disorders (Mypro)

In 1951, William Dameshek (*p188*) suggested that a group of conditions were characterized by the self-perpetuating (*i.e.,* neoplastic) proliferation of one or more lines of bone-marrow elements: red cells, white cells, megakaryocytes, and reticulum cells-fibroblasts. He coined the name *myeloproliferative disorders* (*Mypro*). It occurred to various degrees in the bone

TABLE 1.—*The Myeloproliferative Disorders*
Myelostimulatory Factor's

Syndromes	Erythroblasts	Granulocytes	Megakaryocytes	Fibroblasts	Myeloid metaplasia of spleen and liver
Chronic Granulocytic Leukemia	±	+++	+ to +++	+	++
Polycythemia Vera	+++	++	++ to +++	+ to +++	+ to +++
Idiopathic or Agnogenic Myeloid Metaplasia of Spleen	±	±	+++	+ to +++	+++
Megakaryocytic Leukemia	±	±	+++	+	+ to +++
Erythroleukemia (including diGuglielmo syndrome)	+++	+	±	±	+ to +++

Degrees of Proliferation: + slight ++ moderate +++ marked

Table from Dameshek's 1951 Blood paper

marrow, spleen and liver. Sometimes one cell line predominated, whereas at other times a combination of several cell lines was involved. Relationships with various other bone marrow disorders exist or may develop as shown in the figure that Dameshek's co-author Friedrich W ("Frederick") Gunz published in 1958. Gunz was born in Munich GE in 1914, moved with his family to England in 1933, and did his medical training in London. He moved in 1950 to Christchurch NZ.

In 1956, he spent a sabbatical in Boston with Dameshek and he was invited to co-author the next edition of Dameshek's *Leukemia* (1960). In 1967, Gunz moved to Sydney AU. After his retirement in 1980, he was active in support groups and palliative services. He died in Sydney in 1990.

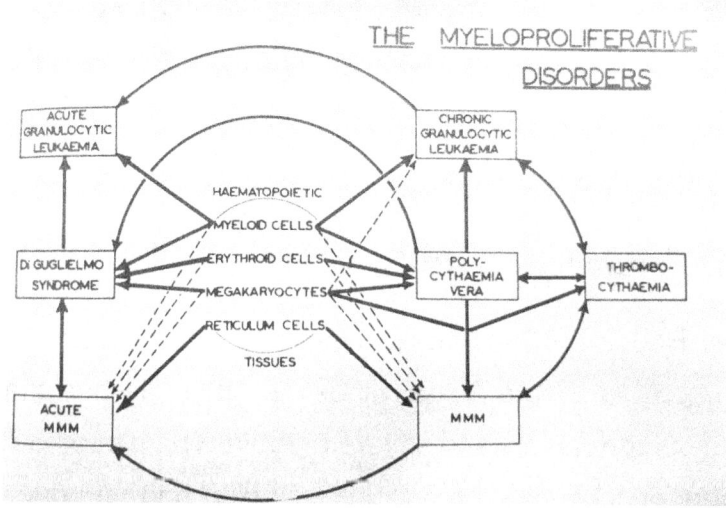

Figure from Gunz's 1958 paper

The myeloproliferative disorders listed by Dameshek included *Myelosclerosis with myeloid metaplasia (MMM), polycythemia vera, Di Guglielmo syndrome (p.176), Chronic myelogenous leukemia (CML; p.153) and thrombocythemia. AML (p.147)* and *acute myelosclerosis with myeloid metaplasia* were also included. Dameshek stressed that the various syndromes had so much overlap that it was difficult to draw clear-cut dividing lines. So many "transition forms" existed that a single term would be reasonable! The disease CML was already covered under the leukemias (*p.153*). In 1967, Philip Fialkow (1934-1996) in Seattle WA studied the X chromosome mosaicism, introduced by Ernest Beutler and Susumu Ohno in 1961 (*p.82*). Fialkow's group documented the clonal nature of CML (1967), polycythemia vera (1976), MMM (1978) and thrombocythemia (1981). They showed that a single G6PD isoenzyme type was present in different myeloid lineages, as well as in certain lymphoid cell types, establishing the common stem-cell origin of the clonal process (1980, 1985)

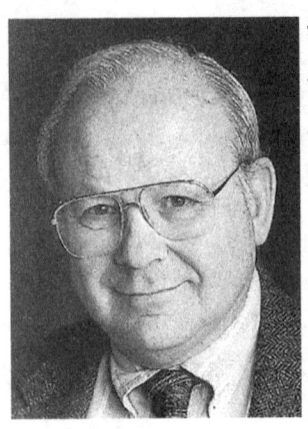

Philip Fialkow

Primary Myelofibrosis (PMF)

Gustav Heuck (1854-1940) in Germany reported on a young man who died after a 1-year illness in 1879. He had massive hepato-splenomegaly and severe anemia. The blood had large numbers of "colorless corpuscles" (Ehrlich had introduced his triacid stain just two years before!). The autopsy showed osteosclerosis, which was confirmed microscopically. The spleen had numerous nucleated red cells. In line with the then current concepts, Heuck considered this to be "splenic" leukemia, and an argument against Neumann's theory of myeloid leukemia. Neumann (*p.20*) countered by suggesting that the marrow had first been hyperplastic, before becoming sclerotic: the "burnt-out" marrow. In Germany, Georg Schmorl (1861-1932) and Max Askanazy (1865-1940) in 1904, and Herbert Assman (1882-1950) in 1907, published additional cases, and the name Heuck-Assman disease was introduced. Assman called it *"osteosclerotic anemia"*. Donhauser in Philadelphia PA reported on a patient with splenomegaly, but little anemia and leukocytosis in 1908. At autopsy, myelofibrosis and myeloid metaplasia were found. The author concluded that a toxin must have caused the osteosclerosis, and that the spleen reverted to its "fetal power to form blood". The discussion about whether the splenic hematopoiesis was part of the primary process, or a compensation for the myelofibrosis, was active for many years. Dameshek, in 1951, referred to a study from 1947 by Elwyn Heller (1911-1978) and colleagues in Pittsburgh PA, in which they claimed that myeloid metaplasia, occurring with or without myelofibrosis, was a peculiar form of leukemia. Dameshek used the name *idiopathic or "agnogenic" myeloid metaplasia*, which had been introduced in 1940 by Henry Jackson (1892-1968) and Frederic Parker in Boston MA. The name *chronic idiopathic myelofibrosis* was used in the WHO classification of hematopoietic and lymphoid tumors of 2002 Other authors used *MMM (myelofibrosis with myeloid metaplasia)*, but in 2006 an international group decided that the name *primary myelofibrosis (PMF)* should be used. PMF can be differentiated from CML by a normal neutrophil alkaline phosphatase (NAP) index, and obviously by the absence of the Ph' chromosome. Therapy was mainly supportive. Splenectomy carried the risk of the anemia becoming more severe. Allogeneic stem-cell transplantation would be a curative option, but most patients are elderly and at high risk of complications. In 2005, four independent groups reported that the majority of patients with non-CML myeloproliferative disorders carried a *JAK2* tyrosine-kinase mutation *(JAK2V617F)*. The laboratories were in Seattle WA, Cambridge UK, Basel SU, and Paris. *Janus kinase (JAK)* inhibitors, such as ruxilitinib, fedratinib and pacritinib, are showing effectiveness in reducing spleen size and constitutional symptoms. Histone deacetylase (HDAC) inhibitors, such as panibinostat, in combination with *JAK* inhibitor ruxolitinib, are being studied. Interferon-α, but in particular peginterferon-alfa 2a, was shown to be effective in several myeloproliferative disorders by the MD Anderson group in 2009.

Polycythemia Vera

Louis Vaquez (1860-1936) in Paris described a 40-year-old man with chronic "cyanosis", dyspnea, palpitations, pruritus and headaches in 1892. The red cell count was markedly elevated. Vaquez interpreted these as symptoms of congenital heart disease. The autopsy showed no heart problems, but marked hepatosplenomegaly. Vaquez concluded that hematopoietic hyperactivity had caused the increased red cell count. It was called "*la maladie de Vaquez*". Within a decade, several similar cases were reported

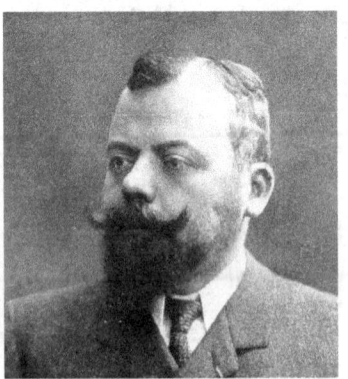

Louis Vaquez

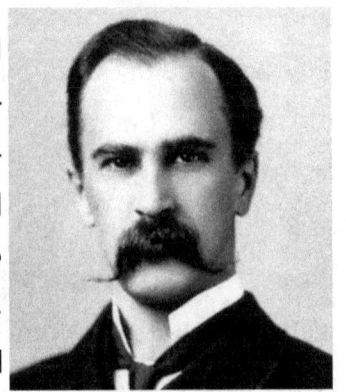

Willam Osler

from the USA (*e.g.*, Richard Cabot; 1868-1938) and England. In 1908, William Osler (1849-1919), perhaps one of the greatest and most male-chauvinist internists, added his own cases and reviewed the literature. Wilhelm Türk (1871-1916) in Vienna AT, recognized the generalized nature of the disease in 1904, by documenting leuko-erythroblastosis and increased production of granulocytes and platelets. Frederick Parkes-Weber (1863-1962), a dermatologist in London, confirmed this, and especially the granulocytic hyperplasia in 1908. Clearly the disease, now called Vaquez-Osler disease, was a panmyelopathy with "pancytosis" in the peripheral blood. Clinical symptoms included itching of the lower extremities, especially after bathing (*erythromelalgia*), caused by platelet-aggregation induced blood-vessel blockage (1994); low-dose aspirin helped here. Patients who did not receive therapy had a median survival of 1.5-3 years. Phlebotomy to bring the hematocrit under 45 (for men, 42 for women) was the primary treatment (1908), and markedly improved symptoms and survival. Then intravenous injection of radioactive isotopes (^{32}P) was introduced in 1940. Alkylating agents (nitrogen mustard (1950); busulfan (1958); chlorambucil (1965)) and hydroxyurea were used and supposed to improve overall survival. However, ^{32}P injections were suspected to be associated with an increased risk of AML since 1943. Louis Wasserman (1912-1999) in New York organized the first Polycythemia-Vera Study-Group randomized trial in 1967, comparing phlebotomy alone, with the combination of phlebotomy and chlorambucil or ^{32}P. Overall survival was better for the phlebotomy alone group, because of an increased risk of AML in the other two arms. The next study showed that hydroxyurea led to a lower risk of thrombosis and a lower risk of AML than chlorambucil or ^{32}P. When, in 2005, the molecular marker *JAK2V617V* was discovered, and found to be present in 95% of the patients with polycythemia vera (2006), the oral *JAK* inhibitor ruxolitinib (*Jakafi*®) was shown to be active by reducing spleen size and symptoms (approved in 2014).

Essential Thrombocythemia

Pathologists Emil Epstein (1875-1951) and Alfred Goedel in Vienna AT, described "hemorrhagic thrombocythemia" in 1934. The patient had extremely high platelet counts, mild increase in red blood cells, and recurrent mucocutaneous bleeding. In contrast with a case reported by Di Guglielmo, no prominent panmyelosis was found. Other descriptions of the disorder with extremely high platelet count, splenomegaly, bone-marrow megakaryocytic hyperplasia, and hemorrhage or thrombosis followed under a variety of names. In a review in 1954, the authors concluded that primary thrombocythemia (in contrast with thrombocytosis) was a myeloproliferative disorder, separate from polycythemia vera or megakaryocytic leukemia. Frederick Gunz in Christchurch NZ, suggested in 1960, that it was difficult to define the entity "primary" or "essential" thrombocythemia by pathology, but that the disorder clearly existed as clinical entity. The bone marrow would always show megakaryocytic hyperplasia, but occasionally was fibrotic. Clumped platelets were often found in bone-marrow aspirates. Splenomegaly was usually present with congestion and sometimes myeloid metaplasia. Leukocytosis was found in nearly all cases, and many cases had anemia at some stage of the disease. Treatment with ^{32}P was recommended in 1957 and would bring down the platelet count (and white cell count) and also the risk of bleeding. Busulfan was equally effective. Hydroxyurea proved effective, and in 1987 anagrelide (*Agrylin®*) was introduced. This phosphodiesterase inhibitor worked by inhibiting the maturation of platelets from megakaryocytes. A randomized study, in 2005 in England, suggested that hydroxyurea plus aspirin was superior to anagrelide plus aspirin. Since half the patients with essential thrombocythemia have the *JAK2V617F* molecular marker, therapy with a *JAK* inhibitor would become an option.

Other Myeloproliferative Disorders

Chronic Myelogenous Leukemia (CML) probably belongs with the Myeloproliferative disorders, but was already discussed with the leukemias *(p.151)*

Di Guglielmo's syndrome, if it exists as a separate entity, was discussed among the myelodysplastic syndromes *(p.176)*. The "syndrome" may well be a mixture of a myelodysplastic syndrome and acute erythroleukemia (FAB M6).

Chronic Myelomonocytic Leukemia (CMML) used to be among the myelodysplastic syndromes (1976), but is now (since 2002) listed in the category of MDS/Mypro. Environmental carcinogens, such as ionizing radiation and cytotoxic agents, may play a role in causing the disease. A high rate of *Ras* mutation is found in CMML with deregulation of this pathway. The most common cytogenetic abnormalities are +8, -7, del(7q), -Y and structural 12p abnormalities. Therapy consists of hypomethylating agents, hydroxyurea or allogeneic stem-cell transplantation for suitable candidates.

Acute Myelofibrosis is an acute panmyelosis with myelofibrosis. There is disagreement in the literature about the classification of the disorder. Some consider it to be equivalent to acute megakaryoblastic leukemia (FAB M7), while others see it as an acute variant of a myelodysplastic syndrome (acute panmyelosis with myelofibrosis; APMF).

William Dameshek, *born as Ze'ev in 1900 in Semliansk, near Voronezh in central Russia, moved with his family to the US during pogroms, when he was three years old. He graduated from Harvard College and Harvard Medical School in 1923 and then did a 2-year internship in Medicine at Boston City Hospital. There he had his first exposure to hematology,* *since Dr. Ralph C Larrabee had a small "Blood Laboratory". After completion of his internship, Dameshek continued at Boston City Hospital and the Blood Laboratory, and assisted with a Laboratory-Medicine class taught at Tufts University. When the new Beth-Israel Deaconess Medical Center opened in 1928, Dameshek became a (the?) hematologist there. He was active in establishing clinical hematology, and started his experimental work. In 1939, he moved to the Pratt Diagnostic Hospital to start the Blood Research Laboratory there. He studied acquired hemolytic anemia, particularly auto-immune hemolytic anemia and ITP. He pioneered the use of corticosteroids in ITP, and of anti-metabolites in auto-immune hemolytic anemia. He tried to achieve a synthesis of all auto-immune disorders. .*

Dameshek was a very dominant personality and often had a strained relationship with other early American hematologists. He was the founder, and first editor, of Blood *in 1946. It became the journal of the* American Society of Hematology (ASH) *upon the society's founding in 1958. To document his international interests, a summary of the articles was also given in Interlingua, a kind of simpler Romance language. The* International Society of Hematology (ISH) *had been founded in 1946, and in 1968 was subdivided into three divisions: Inter-American (IAD), European-African (EAD), and Asian-Pacific (APD). Dameshek was intimately involved with the early organization of ISH.*

In 1946, Dameshek participated in the first trial of nitrogen mustard in malignant lymphoma. In 1951, he described the concept of myeloproliferative disorders (polycythemia vera, essential thrombocytosis, primary myelofibrosis) as MPD. This concept is still being accepted today. In 1959, he was involved with the first autologous bone-marrow transplants for lymphoma using massive doses of nitrogen mustard. He proposed, in 1967, that chronic lymphocytic leukemia (CLL) is the result of a gradual accumulation of lymphocytes, just as both Gowers and Pinkus had proposed at the end of the 19th Century. The same year, he tried to find out what aplastic anemia, PNH, and "hypoplastic" leukemia have in common. He saw beneficial effects of oxymetholone in four children with aplastic anemia. He published the book Leukemia *in 1958. The next edition (1960) was co-authored by Frederick W Gunz of Christchurch NZ. Dameshek also published several other books. He thrived on controversy and loved the excitement of intellectual battle. He believed that William Hewson in England (1739-1774) was the father of hematology, because of his description of the lymphoid system. William Dameshek died in 1969, just shy of his 70th birthday.*

Lymphomas

Thomas Hodgkin was born in a town just north of London in 1798. He was the first child of his Quaker parents to survive infancy. In 1819, he started his medical training at Guy's Hospital, considered one of the finest in London, and the one most interested in scientific training. He transferred to the University of Edinburgh, the best medical school in Great Britain, and obtained his MD there in 1823. He then spent some time at Hôpital Necker in Paris with René Laennec, who had introduced the stethoscope; here he learned to combine physical examination with pathologic findings. In 1825, he returned to Guy's Hospital, where a Museum of Anatomic Pathology had to be started, since Guy's and St. Thomas' hospitals had decided to separate. Hodgkin became the inspector of the dead and curator of the new museum. About 3 years later, he was asked

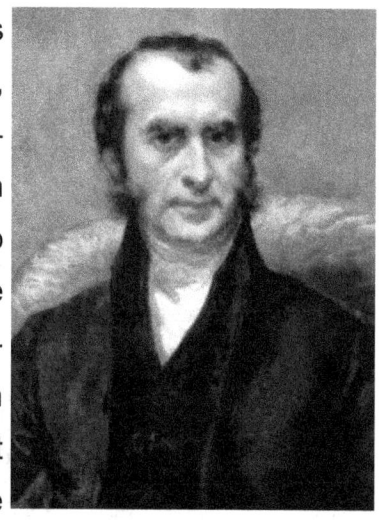

Thomas Hodgkin

ON SOME
MORBID APPEARANCES
OF
THE ABSORBENT GLANDS
AND
SPLEEN.

BY DR. HODGKIN.
PRESENTED
BY DR. R. LEE.

READ JANUARY 10TH AND 24TH, 1832.

THE morbid alterations of structure which I am about to describe are probably familiar to many

Hodgkin's presentation

to do autopsies on several patients who had extensive lymphadenopathy and splenomegaly. The patients had been treated by Richard Bright (*of nephrology fame*) and Thomas Addison (*of Addison's disease fame*). After he had collected 6 cases, he submitted his report "*On Some Morbid Appearances of the Absorbant Glands and Spleen*" to the Medical and Surgical Society in 1832, where it was received with indifference. He did not propose a name for the new disease, which he suspected to be a malignancy. He also did not publish his findings in a medical journal.

Around the same time, his position at Guy's had become difficult. As a Quaker, Hodgkin was quite active in the anti-slavery movement, and in opposition to mistreatment of Native Americans in the colonies. That put him into conflict with the treasurer of the hospital (Benjamin "King" Harrison), who was also a member of the Hudson Bay Company. Hodgkin's promotion was blocked, and he resigned from Guy's, leaving his collection of pathologic material behind in the Gordon museum of the hospital. After recovering from depression, he opened a small medical practice, but spent more time on his humanitarian efforts. With his wealthy friend Sir Moses Montefiore, he traveled the world to protest slavery and antisemitism. He died from cholera in Jaffa, Palestine in 1866.

His name would have been forgotten, if not for Samuel Wilks (1824-1911). In 1856, when he described amyloid for the first time ("*lardaceous disease*"), Wilks included four of Hodgkin's cases; he thought his observations were original. Before completing his paper, however, he found out that Bright, in a 1838 paper, had referred to Hodgkin's cases. He then searched for Hodgkin's original paper. He introduced the name Hodgkin's disease. In 1865, Wilks reported on fifteen cases under that name. Independently, Wunderlich in Germany, Trousseau in Paris, and Bonfils also in France, all reported similar cases, but under different names. Names that were used were *lymphogranuloma, adénie, granuloma malignum, lymphadenoma* and *lymphoblastoma*. Clearly, many of the reported cases were not, what we now call, Hodgkin's disease. Other types of lymph-node cancers were also called Hodgkin's disease in these early days.

In the mid 1840's, cases of leukemia were reported (*p.137*) and Rudolf Virchow already subdivided these in lienal (splenic) and lymphatic, and leukemic and aleukemic. The aleukemic variant presumably subsumed many cases of lymphoma and was also called "pseudo-leukemia". The terminology remained rather confusing. In the 1890's, Julius Dreschfeld (1845-1907), from Bavaria GE but mostly working in Manchester UK, and Hans Kundrat (1845-1893) in Vienna AT, independently reported cases of "aleukemic lymphatic leukemia", that remained for prolonged periods of time confined to the lymphatic system. Kundrat called it lymphosarcoma and put "lymphogranuloma malignum" in the differential diagnosis. Then in 1925, Nathan Brill (1860-1925) and his colleagues at Mount Sinai Hospital, New York reported two cases of "generalized giant lymph follicle hyperplasia of lymph nodes and spleen", an entity also described, two years later, also in New York, by Douglas Symmers (1879-1952).. Both believed the disorder to be non-malignant. For many years the disease was known as "Brill-Symmers disease", until Henry Rappaport (1913-2003) and colleagues in 1956 at the Armed Forces Institute of Pathology, Washington DC, pointed out that 5 types of follicular lymphoma existed.

Reticulum sarcoma was a difficult disease. In 1930, Frédéric Roulet (1902-1985) in Basel SU, described a group of reticulum-cell sarcomas of lymphoid tissue, which he gave the name "*Rethotelsarcom*". This was partly based on the concept of the Reticulo-Endothelial System (RES) propagated by Ludwig Aschoff in Freiburg GE, who between 1913 and 1923, had coined this name as a system of specialized cells that clear colloidal vital stains from the circulation.

In the meantime, Hodgkin's disease proved to be a group of diseases, even though Wilks had suggested that it was a single entity. In 1872, Theodor Langhans (1839-1915) in Marburg GE recognized "grössere Zellen mit 2-4 und mehr Kernen und etwas dunkelkörniger Zellsubstanz" (larger cells with 2-4 and more nuclei and slightly darker cellular substance) in some of the lymphomas, and Greenfield in England also referred to multinucleated cells containing 4-8-12 nuclei in 1878. Nevertheless, these cells have been named after Carl Sternberg (1872-1935) in Austria (1898) and Dorothy Reed (-Mendenhall) (1874-1964) at Johns Hopkins in 1902. She initially earned a Medicine internship there, but William Osler told her that it was "not a place for women"! She then chose a Pathology fellowship, and (after again

White Blood Cells

being discriminated because of her gender) finally Pediatrics. She ultimately focused on maternal and infant health in Madison WI and Washington DC. The Reed Sternberg cell became central to the diagnosis of Hodgkin's disease.

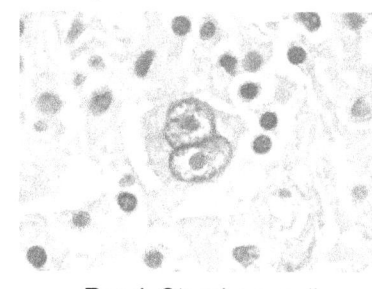

Reed–Sternberg cell

Herbert Fox was able to make slides of the original specimens of Thomas Hodgkin (1832) at the Gordon Museum of Guy's Hospital in 1926. He confirmed the diagnosis of Hodgkin's disease in at least two of the 6 cases! Hodgkin's disease had now been well established.

In 1937-1947, Henry Jackson and Frederic Parker at Harvard came up with the first histologic classification of Hodgkin's disease. They distinguished between "paragranuloma" with few Reed-Sternberg cells and slow progression, far more common "granuloma" with more Reed-Sternberg cells, and "sarcoma" with an abundance of anaplastic giant cells. Robert Lukes (1922-1994) in Los Angeles originally proposed six subtypes, but it was believed that clinicians would not be able to remember six types; therefore, it ultimately became four subtypes: lymphocyte predominance (the least aggressive), nodular sclerosis, mixed cellularity, and lymphocyte depletion.

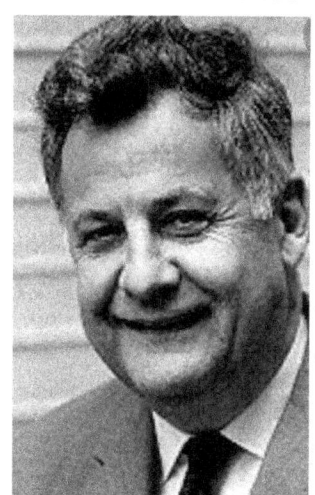

Robert Lukes

Rye classification	Histological features	Prognosis
Lymphocyte predominant	Lymphocytes and RSCs	Best
Nodular sclerosis	Nodules of lymphoreticular cells and lacunar RSCs	Good
Mixed cellularity	Mixture of lymphocytes, eosinophils, plasma cells, and RSCs	Fair
Lymphocyte depleted	Lymphocytes and RSCs	Poor

RSCs: Reed-Sternberg cells

The Rye classification of Hodgkin's disease as accepted in 1966

This subdivision was accepted by a nomenclature committee in 1966, at the conference organized by Henry Kaplan (*p.208*) at the Westchester Country Club in Rye NY. Sidney Farber (1903-1973) of Boston, the pediatric pathologist who established the *Jimmy Fund* for research in childhood cancers, chaired the meeting. The agreed-upon nomenclature has been generally used since then as the Rye classification. The Reed-Sternberg cells were shown to be hypermutated B-lymphocytes originating from the germinal center or post-germinal center ($CD30^+$, $CD15^+$, $CD20^-$, $CD45^-$). In many cases of Hodgkin's disease, the Reed-Sternberg cells also contain Epstein-Barr virus.

While Hodgkin's disease was now a separate disease, many other types of lymphoma remained. In 1942, Edward Gall (1906-1979) and Tracy Mallory (1896-1951) at Harvard made a clinicopathologic survey of 618 cases of lymphoma, diagnosed between 1917 and 1936. In addition to the 229 cases of Hodgkin's disease, they had 389 cases of other lymphomas. They divided them into 5 categories: 127 cases of reticulum-cell sarcoma, 85 cases of lymphoblastic lymphoma, 135 cases of lymphocytic lymphoma, and 42 cases of follicular lymphoma. Their reticulum-cell sarcoma had two subtypes: "stem-cell lymphoma" and "clasmatocytic lymphoma". The "stem-cell lymphoma" was named after James Ewing (1866-1943) who, in 1928, implied that reticulum-cell or large round-cell sarcoma was a tumor composed of cells less mature than the lymphocyte derived from the germinal centers of pulp cords. Similarly, Paul Klemperer (1888-1964), originally from Vienna AT but practicing at Mount Sinai in New York, claimed in 1932 that the reticulum cell was totipotent and similar with cells observed in the embryonic mesenchyme. The reticulum cells of stem-cell lymphoma had already had many names: *lymphoidocyte* of Artur Pappenheim (1912), *hemohistioblast* of Adolfo Ferrata (1918), and *hemocytoblast* of Hubert Turnbull (1936). The clasmatocytic lymphoma had cells resembling monocytes with irregular borders and suggested phagocytic qualities. Jackson and Parker in their 1947 book *"Hodgkin's Disease and Allied Disorders"* did not agree with the term "reticulum cell". They believed that "reticulum cells" should be interpreted either as supporting fibrous cells in lymphoid tissue, or as defining certain cellular elements of these tissues. Nevertheless, they continued to use the term "reticulum-cell sarcoma", in order not to add to the confusion. They also continued to use the terms lymphocytoma, lymphoblastoma, and giant-follicle lymphoma, but reintroduced the rare *"lymphosarcoma"*, as originally described by Kundrat In 1893.

The next major development in lymphoma classification was Henry Rappaport (1913-2003)'s terminology, originally from 1956, but published in 1966 in *"Tumors of the Hematopoietic System"*. Rappaport was born in Lemberg AT (now Lviv, Ukraine) and attended medical school in Vienna. In 1940, he came to the USA and headed the Reticulo-Endothelial Pathology and Hematology sections of the Armed Forces Institute of Pathology in Washington DC from 1949-1954. He then moved to the University of Chicago and ultimately to the City of Hope (Duarte CA). His classification was based strictly on morphological features. He used the terms nodular and diffuse, and regarded the large cells as "histiocytes".

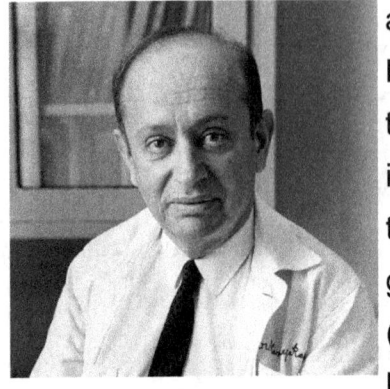

Henry Rappaport

Around the same time, however, studies showed that lymphocytes could transform into large proliferating cells in response to mitogens or antigens, which might have explained Rappaport's "histiocytes".

During this same time frame (1958), Denis Burkitt (1911-1993), an Irish missionary surgeon in Uganda, reported on children with swellings in the angle of the jaw. This malignancy, diagnosed as a lymphoma by Dennis Wright (1931-2020) of Makerere University in Kampala, was associated with endemic chronic malaria, and found to be caused by the Epstein-Barr virus. The non-endemic form of Burkitt's lymphoma was not caused by EBV.

White Blood Cells

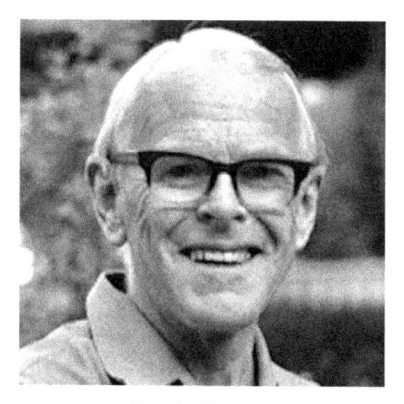

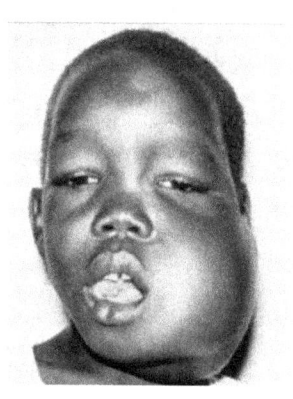

Denis Burkitt *Burkitt's lymphoma*

By 1970, the era of immunological diagnosis of lymphocytes had started. Victor Nussenzweig's group in New York demonstrated that lymphocytes under the control of the thymus, were able to form rosettes with sheep red blood cells. Ellen Vitetta's group in Dallas TX isolated surface immunoglobulin from mouse splenic lymphocytes. The subdivision into T-cells (T for *thymus*) and B-cells (B for *Bursa*, the avian equivalent of bone-marrow in mammals) allowed further subdivision of malignant lymphomas. Karl Lennert's (1921-2012) group in Kiel GE, developed the Kiel classification in 1975. With light and electron microscopy, the non-specific esterase stain, and immunoglobulin studies, they distinguished lymphomas based on their connection with the germinal center of the lymph node. Virtually all lymphomas proved to be of B-cell origin. Their classification was readily accepted in Europe and distinguished

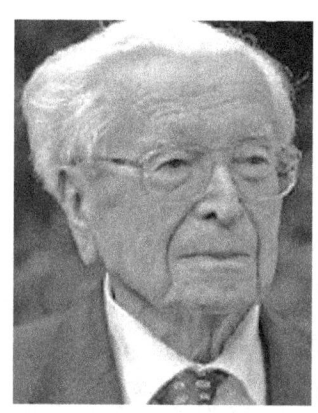

Karl Lennert

two grades of malignancy. In 1974, Robert Lukes in Los Angeles and Robert Collins (1928-2013) in Nashville TN, published their classification of non-Hodgkin lymphomas based on immunology, which also did away with "reticulosarcoma or histiocytic lymphoma", and also found virtually all lymphomas to be of B-cell origin. Their classification was mostly used in North America as the Working Formulation of 1982, which distinguished three grades of malignancy. Discussions about terminology and classification were fierce. I recall that at a meeting of the American Society of Hematology, a clinician proposed a separate meeting about the nomenclature, preferably in the Caribbean! That same year, Dennis Weisenburger (b.1948) and colleagues in Omaha NE described mantle-cell lymphoma (MCL), histologically low grade, but clinically quite aggressive. Ultimately in 1991, an international study group came up with the REAL (**R**evised **E**uropean-**A**merican Classification of **L**ymphoid **N**eoplasms) classification.

George Klein (1925-2016), a Hungarian working at the Karolinska Institute in Stockholm SW, identified t(8;14)(q24;q32) as the recurrent chromosomal translocation in Burkitt's lymphoma in 1976, and Philip Leder (1934-2020) at Harvard cloned the *MYC* gene and identified *MYC* and *IGH@* as reciprocal partners in t(8;14)(q24;q32) in 1982. In 1979, Janet Rowley's group in Chicago found t(14;18)(q32;q21) as the recurrent translocation in follicular lymphoma. Carlo Croce (b.1944) and his colleagues in Philadelphia PA identified *BCL2* and *IGH@* as its reciprocal partners.

White Blood Cells

The initial results of radiation therapy for patients with Hodgkin's disease made clear that only patients with very localized disease could be cured. The first report of radiation therapy in lymphoma came from William Pusey (1865-1940) in 1902, just six years after Wilhelm Röntgen (1845-1923) had discovered X-rays. Pusey, in Chicago IL, mainly used his radiation for skin diseases, but also treated a young man with cervical lymphadenopathy (probably non-Hodgkin lymphoma). Within 23 days of radiation, the circumference of the neck had decreased by 4½ inches and the tumor had decreased to the size of an olive. No recurrence occurred in the next 3 months. The effect was also good in two cases of Hodgkin's disease. The next year, Nicholas Senn (1844-1908), a surgeon also in Chicago, reported great success in two cases of lymphoma, without giving credit to the radiologists who were responsible for the therapy; he also did not mention Dr. Pusey's work! The real efforts with radiation therapy started in the 1950's. In the early years, calculation of the dose was still difficult and often relied on the Human Erythema Dose (HED); the radiation was limited to the involved field. In the 1930's, René Gilbert (1898-1962) in Geneva SU started to irradiate not only the involved lymph nodes, but also the adjacent lymph nodes to a lower dose. Similar approaches were taken at Princess Margaret Hospital in Toronto CN, and Vera Peters (1911-1993) was able to enhance the treatment and she obtained actual cures in Hodgkin's disease. That Hodgkin's disease was potentially a curable disease was first broached by Eric Easson and

Blood is LIfe

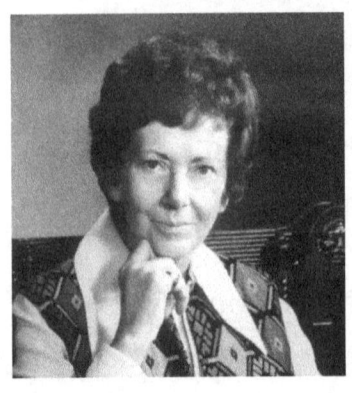

Vera Peters

Marion Russell of The Christie Hospital in Manchester UK in an article in the British Medical Journal in 1960: *The Cure of Hodgkin's disease*. They based this on their assumption that Hodgkin's disease started in a single site, and spread along lymphatic channels in an orderly fashion. Henry Kaplan at Stanford University was a great supporter of this concept, and he asserted that one could construct a "road map" for successive sites of involvement. However, distinct gaps between areas of lymph nodes involved were found in many patients. Sir David Smithers (1908-1995) of the Royal Marsden Hospital in London, had a completely opposite opinion. He believed that Hodgkin's disease was truly multifocal, but that the Reed-Sternberg cell had certain preferential sites where it could grow favorably in the early stages of the disease. He assumed that regional radiation therapy would also destroy these preferential sites. I remember having been taught only about the Kaplan concept. If one assumes an orderly spread, staging becomes of major importance. At the Rye conference of 1966, a first attempt was made to introduce a staging system of 4 stages and systemic symptoms. After international objections, followed by negotiations, in 1971 a conference was held in Ann Arbor MI. There, the Ann-Arbor staging system was accepted. Attempts by Vera Peters to propose the use of the TNM system, as used for other tumors, were torpedoed by Réné

White Blood Cells

Ann Arbor staging	
Stage I:	Single lymph node region (I) or single extranodal organ or site (IE).
Stage II:	Two or more lymph node regions on the same side of the diaphragm alone (II) or with involvement of limited, contiguous extralymphatic organ or tissue (II$_E$).
Stage III:	Lymph node regions on both sides of the diaphragm (III), including one organ or area near the lymph nodes or the spleen (III$_E$).
Stage IV:	Dissemination to one or more extralymphatic organs or tissues, with or without involvement of nearby lymph nodes.
Modifying features:	
A:	Asymptomatic.
B:	Unexplained fever (> 38C); night sweats; loss of more than 10% body weight in 6 months.
E:	Involvement of a single, contiguous or proximal extranodal site.
X:	Bulky disease (mass >10 cm; >0.33).

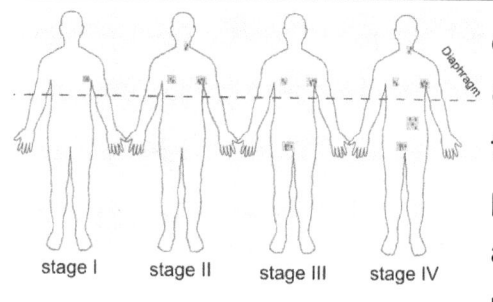

stage I   stage II   stage III   stage IV

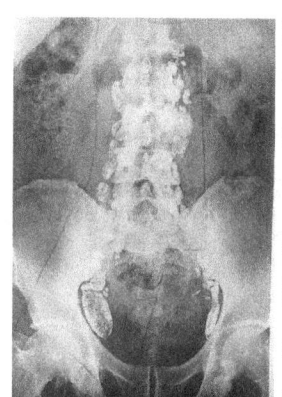

Positive lymphangiogram

Tubiana (1920-2013) of Villejuif FR. Undoubtedly, Kaplan wanted his staging system to become generally accepted. To rule out abdominal and retroperitoneal involvement, extensive staging procedures were needed. The first pedal lymphangiography was done by Hernani Monteiro (1891-1963) of the University of Porto PT in 1931. The procedure received more attention, when John Kinmonth (1916-1982) described the technique in 1952, especially when better oily contrast media became available around 1960. Manuscripts about lymphangiography peaked between 1965 and 1975. When even this procedure did not reveal retroperitoneal involvement by Hodgkin's disease, the suspicion of splenic involvement led many centers to perform a staging laparotomy. The Cotswolds modification of the Ann Arbor staging was introduced in 1988 to address extranodal and/or bulky disease, and more recently in 2014, the Lugano classification that relies on PET-CT or CT scans. With the improved radiological techniques, lymphangiogram and staging laparotomy became techniques of the past.

Réné Gilbert (1925,1939) and Vera Peters (1950, 1966) had introduced curative radiation therapy for localized Hodgkin's disease, but Henry Kaplan (*p.210*) of Stanford deserves credit for further developing it. The introduction of new radiotherapy equipment, allowing megavoltage radiation, was also important. These energy source included ^{60}Co (3 MeV) and linear accelerators (4-8MeV), and they came on line in the mid 1950's. After the Stanford group had shown that stages I and II could be cured with radiation therapy using their 6MeV linear accelerator, they used this therapy also for stage III disease, starting in 1962.

Already in 1946, Leon Jacobson, and Goodman and Gilman, had shown that nitrogen mustard (NH_2; Mustargen) elicited dramatic clinical responses in patients with Hodgkin's disease. Around the same time, it was shown that corticosteroids can lead to lymphoid atrophy in mice and regression of transplanted lymphosarcoma. New chemotherapy drugs were introduced in the 1960's: cyclophosphamide, Thio-

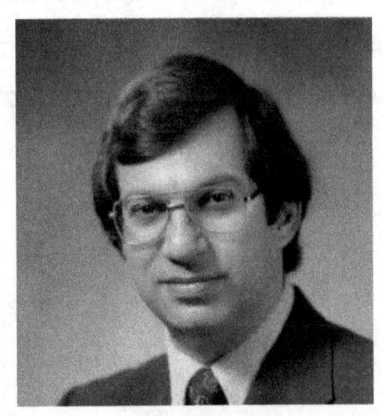

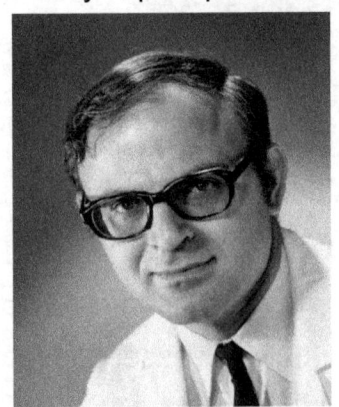

Vince DeVita *George Canellos*

TEPA, Vinca alkaloids, procarbazine, and nitrosoureas. They all had activity in lymphomas, but it took combining some of them to obtain long-lasting responses. Vincent DeVita (b.1935), George Canellos (b.1934) and their group at the National Cancer Institute (Bethesda, MD) took the courageous step of combining four active drugs with different dose-limiting toxicities. The study with nitrogen mustard, vincristine, methotrexate, and prednisone started in 1963. Even when a good response was obtained, therapy was continued for 6 months. The regimen was replaced by MOPP, in which procarbazine was substituted for methotrexate. The complete remission rate jumped from 20% to 80% with many cures. Clearly, Hodgkin's disease could now be cured by either radiotherapy (early stages) or chemotherapy (advanced stages). Kaplan and Saul Rosenberg (b.1928) at Stanford started to successfully combine radiation and chemotherapy. On the other hand, studies also suggested that chemotherapy alone could be curative for early-stage Hodgkin's disease. Particularly in settings where no good radiation therapy was available, this became an attractive option *(e.g.* Uganda). Since MOPP therapy increased the risk of therapy induced acute leukemia/myelodysplasia, Gianni Bonadonna (1934-2015) in Milan IT introduced the ABVD (**A**driamycin, **B**leomycin **V**inblastine, **D**acarbazine) regimen around 1974.

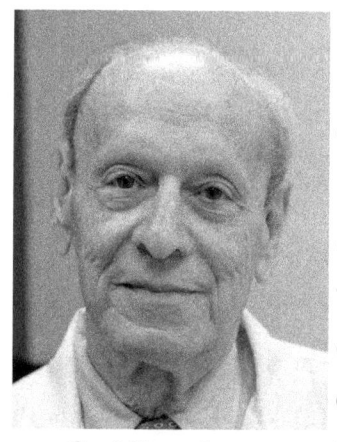

Saul Rosenberg

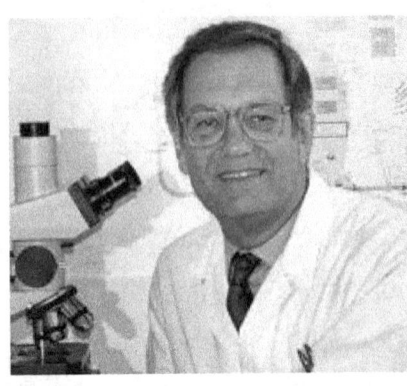

Gianni Bonnadonna

ABVD proved superior to MOPP in randomized studies. ABVD became first-line chemotherapy for advanced Hodgkin's disease, although alternating ABVD and MOPP was also still recommended. Overall, in the early 21st Century, Hodgkin's disease had become a curable disease for the vast majority of patients. For patients with relapsed disease, high-dose chemotherapy with autologous stem-cell transplantation (*p.240*) still was a viable option. Immune therapy also became an option here. Brentuximab, an antibody-drug combination targeting CD30 was approved for relapsed and later also for newly diagnosed patients. PD-1 inhibitors (*e.g.*, nivolumab, pembrolizumab) were also approved in combination with other therapeutic modalities.

The non-Hodgkin lymphomas spread in a less orderly fashion. Although the Ann-Arbor staging system could be used, it became more logical to distinguish between localized lymphoma (often a single lesion) and more widespread disease. Lymphangiogram and staging laparotomy were not of great benefit for the staging, but the bone-marrow biopsy was of great importance. When CT-, MRI-, and PET-scans became available, they were of importance to document abdominal and/or CNS disease and the response to therapy. In the 1970's, gallium-citrate (^{67}Ga) scans were of benefit, particularly to document the response to therapy.

Radiation therapy was of minor importance for non-Hodgkin lymphomas, except perhaps for a documented single lesion, CNS disease, or to help with the treatment of bulky disease.

Chemotherapy was the primary form of therapy and the choice was dependent upon the histological grade (low grade vs intermediate or high grade) and the immunophenotype of the tumor.

The low-grade lymphomas were often followed as long as possible without therapeutic intervention ("watchful waiting"), treated with single-agent oral chemotherapy (*e.g.*, chlorambucil), or more aggressive intravenous chemotherapy (*e.g.*, **C**yclophosphamide, **V**incristine, **P**rednisone; *CVP*). The disease would mostly respond well to treatment, but would relapse invariably. Even randomized studies failed to demonstrate a survival advantage of the more intensive therapy. That started to change when Ronald Levy (b.1941)'s group at Stanford University developed tumor-specific idiotype vaccines for patients with B-cell non-Hodgkin lymphoma in 1997. This was followed rapidly by the humanized anti-CD20 monoclonal antibody rituximab (Rituxan®), developed by Nabil Hanna and Mitchell Reff at IDEC Pharmaceuticals, or the ^{131}I-labeled mouse monoclonal anti-CD20 (tositumomab) studied in 2000 by Mark Kaminski (b. 1952)'s group in Ann Arbor MI. Rituximab proved to be a true game changer for low grade lymphoma, even though its use also suppressed normal B-cell function for a prolonged period of time.

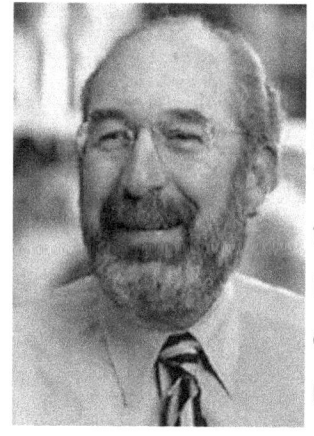

Ron Levy

Another promising drug was fludarabine, originally produced by John Montgomery and Kathleen Hewson in 1968; the drug showed very potent lympholytic action in chronic lymphocytic leukemia and low-grade lymphoma, but also against healthy B lymphocytes.

For intermediate or high-grade malignant lymphoma, combination chemotherapy became the primary form of therapy. Denis Burkitt in Kampala UG had been successful in Burkitt's lymphoma with pulsed single-dose cyclophosphamide in 1965. The first cures in aggressive lymphoma were reported around 1975 by the NCI with C-MOPP, in which nitrogen mustard was replaced by cyclophosphamide. With combination chemotherapy (*e.g.*, *CHOP*: **C**yclophosphamide, adriamycin (**H**ydroxydaunorubicin or doxorubicin), vincristine (**O**ncovin®) and **P**rednisone), continuous complete remissions of up to 60% were obtained in the 1980's. Even more aggressive regimens were proposed (*e.g.*, *MACOP-B, m-BACOD, ProMACE/Cyta-BOM*), but were not found to be more effective than CHOP. In 1993, a predictive model for aggressive non-Hodgkin lymphoma was introduced, based on age, stage, performance status, and bulk of disease: *International Prognostic Index* (IPI), to permit comparison of various therapeutic interventions. Rituximab was often added to the CHOP therapy: *R-CHOP.*

In relapsed lymphoma, high-dose chemotherapy with autologous or allogeneic stem-cell transplantation was successful in salvaging a considerable proportion of the patients (*p.240*).

White Blood Cells

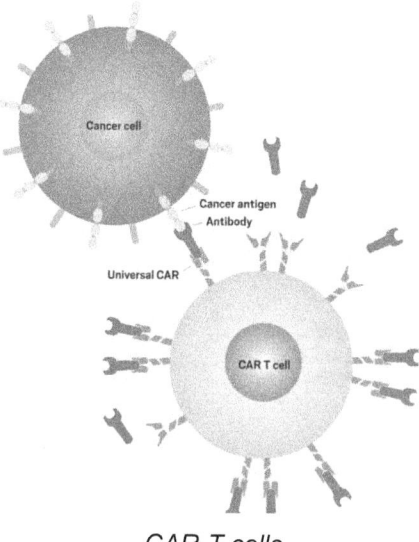

The most recent approach has been to produce autologous CAR-T cells (**C**himeric **A**ntigen **R**eceptor - T). The basic concept of CAR was to link an extracellular ligand recognition domain, typically a single-chain variable fragment (scFv), to an intracellular signaling module, to induce T-cell activation upon antigen binding. Subsequent generations added molecules to mimic co-stimulation. The approach of co-stimulation augmented cytokine production and proliferation of T-cells *in vitro*. In B-cell lymphoma, potent *in-vivo* anti-tumor activity was demonstrated. These studies were started, around 2002, by the laboratories of Philip Greenberg (b.1945) at the Fred Hutchinson Cancer Research Center in Seattle WA, and of Renier Brentjens and Michel Sadelain at Memorial Sloan Kettering Cancer Center in New York. The first clinical study in 2010, at the latter institution, showed that patients with refractory CLL or B-cell ALL tolerated the infusions well. Steven Rosenberg (b.1940)'s group at the NCI saw a dramatic response in a patient with bulky B-cell lymphoma, although normal B-cells disappeared for about 10 months. The same group reported in 2015, that 8 of 15 patients with B-cell malignancies achieved complete remissions. Many other groups and centers (*e.g.*, Philadelphia PA) contributed to the further development of CAR-T cells. The interest in CAR-T therapy for hematological and non-hematological neoplasms rapidly expanded, and commercial companies became heavily involved.

The success with the treatment of Hodgkin's disease and non-Hodgkin lymphomas was instrumental in the acceptance of Medical Oncology as a recognized subspecialty of Internal Medicine by the American Board of Internal Medicine. Most continental Europeans obviously continue to consider the lymphomas to belong to the field of Hematology!

Henry Seymour Kaplan was born in Chicago in 1918. He graduated from Rush Medical College and then trained in radiology in Minneapolis MN. In 1945, he received his first academic appointment at Yale University (New Haven CT). In 1948, Kaplan was recruited to Stanford University as chairman of Radiology. Stanford was then still located in San Francisco, but Kaplan helped orchestrate the move to a new campus in Palo Alto CA. He had to fight hard to recruit outstanding researchers. The only radiation machine available was a ^{60}Co source. Kaplan developed the first linear

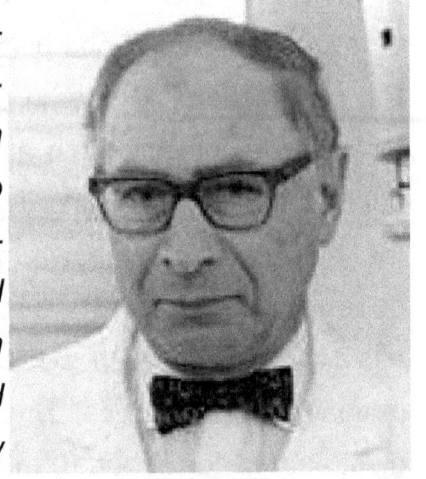

accelerator together with electrical engineer Edward Ginzton in 1954 (6MeV). In the laboratory, he continued to work on the radiation-induced (TBI) leukemia and lymphoma; he discovered that local radiation of the mouse thymus, where the leukemia started, was curative. This was about the same time, that Ludwik Gross (1904-1999) in New York isolated the murine leukemia virus named after him (1951). Kaplan discovered that radiation induced the leukemia in mice, by triggering a latent RNA virus into activity. This established a link between an external cancer-causing agent and a virus. Clinically he focused on Hodgkin's disease. When he started, only 5% of patients with Hodgkin's disease survived. He gathered around him a team of a surgeon, a pathologist, a radiologist and an oncologist (Saul Rosenberg in 1961). Randomized clinical trials were started in 1962. High-dose radiation therapy (4-5,000 cGy) was given, as needed, through two ports: mantle field and inverted Y. Kaplan helped develop the Ann Arbor staging system. When Vince DeVita and George Canellos showed, in 1967, that multi-agent chemotherapy (MOPP) achieved high response rates, Stanford started combined-modality treatment. In 1975 Kaplan became Director of the new Cancer Biology Research Laboratory at Stanford, where he tried to isolate a human lymphoma virus. So far that attempt has been unsuccessful. Kaplan died from lung cancer in 1984.

Paraproteinemias

The existence of antibodies was known since the late 19th century. The production of *diphtheria antitoxin* (=antibodies) by Behring and Ehrlich, in the 1890's, were an excellent therapeutic example. Ehrlich also already proposed his "magic bullet" by binding toxic drugs to antibodies to treat infectious diseases (and cancer?).

The modern era of antibody research started in 1948, when Örjan Ouchterlony (1914-2004) at the Karolinska Institute in Stockholm SW created the Ouchterlony double immune-diffusion test. This test, based on precipitation of the antigen-antibody complex in agarose gel, was used in the detection, identification and quantification of antibodies and antigens. Before him, Arne Tiselius (1902-1971), who studied with Theodor Svedberg (1884-1971) at Uppsala University SW, had made his doctoral thesis on electrophoresis of proteins in 1930. In 1937, he separated serum globulins into three fractions, which he called α-, β-, and γ-globulin. Two years later, he demonstrated antibody activity in the gamma-globulin fraction. He received the Nobel Prize for Chemistry in 1948.

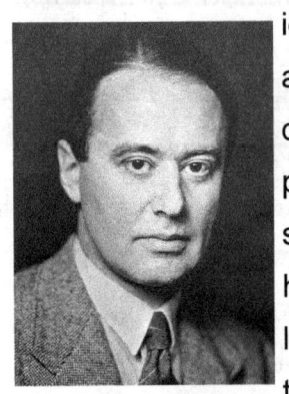

Arne Tiselius

His electrophoresis apparatus was cumbersome, and was replaced by filter paper and then by agarose gel. Immunofixation was introduced in 1964.

Jan Waldenström (1906-1996), also in Sweden (first

at Uppsala, then at the University of Lund), analyzed cases of high gammaglobulin and distinguished between mono- and polyclonal hypergammaglobulinemia. In 1944, he reported on the disease that is named after him. Waldenström's macroglobulinemia is a subtype of malignant lymphoma "with a large amount of a single unknown blood protein with an extremely high molecular weight, a "macroglobulin"". Polyclonal hypergammaglobulinemia was mostly associated with infections/inflammation, but the monoclonal variant was associated with hematologic malignancy (multiple myeloma or Waldenström's disease), with light-chain amyloid, or with no disease at all. The latter condition was called "benign monoclonal protein" or, after 1978, MGUS (*Monoclonal Gammopathy of Unknown Significance*), as described by Robert Kyle (b.1928) of the Mayo Clinic in Rochester MN. MGUS incidence increases with age. I recall that Willy Hijmans (1921-2018), a gerontology immunologist in Leiden NL, and one of my mentors, told me that in their studies at least 10% of healthy adults over 90 years of age had a monoclonal gammopathy.

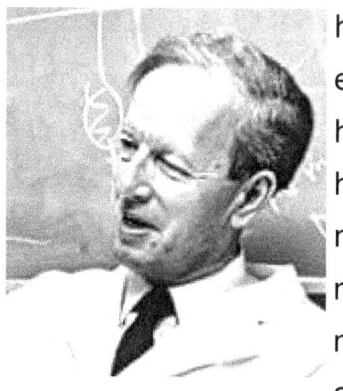

Jan Waldenström

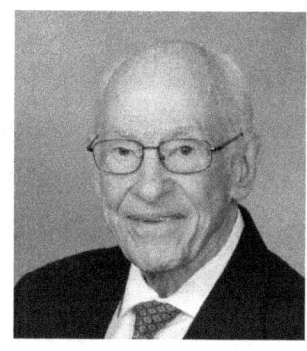

Robert Kyle

In 1959, Gerald Edelman (1929-2014) and colleagues at Rockefeller University, New York, discovered that antibody molecules were made up of multiple polypeptide chains, rather than of a single chain. This held true for all major human immunoglobulin classes. Using a reducing agent to break the disulfide bonds, they were able to separate the polypeptide chains and obtain heavy (H) chains and light (L) chains. The heavy chains are A (found in serum as well in saliva and other secretions), M (high-molecular weight and present during early stage after antigenic challenge), and G (present during later stages after antigenic challenge, and representing about 70% of normal human immunoglobulins). The light chains are κ (kappa) or λ (lambda), named after Leonhard **K**orngold and his technician Rose **L**ipari of Sloan Kettering Institute in New York, who identified them in Bence Jones protein with the Ouchterlony technique in 1956. Bence Jones protein (*not Bence-Jones protein!*) was first reported in 1845 by Henry Bence Jones (1813-1873), a chemical pathologist at St. George's Hospital London. Samuel Solly (1805-1871), a surgeon at St. Thomas' Hospital London, admitted a 39 year-old woman in 1844. She had a 4 year history of bone pains, at times excruciating, bone fractures, and developing deformity of ribs and spine. She died 5 days after admission. Autopsy revealed multiple bone fractures, and a compressed chest cavity to one-quarter of its normal size. Sections of the bones revealed a "red grumous matter" and marked thinning of the bones. The majority of nucleated cells in the red matter had

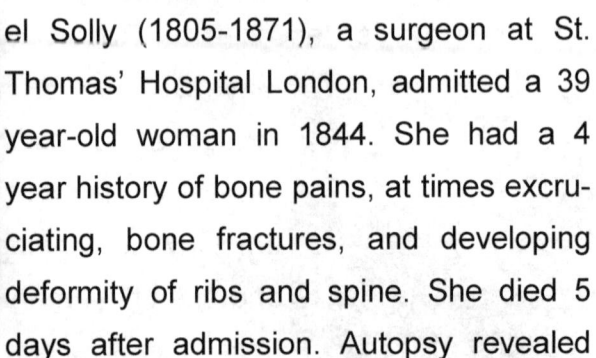

Henry Bence Jones

a clear oval outline and one bright central nucleolus. A similar patient, a 46-year-old man, was seen in consultation by William McIntyre, a Harley Street consultant, later that year. In the preceding two years, the patient had acute episodes of chest pain, but he recovered several times. He became debilitated and developed sciatic pain. His urine was of high density; with nitric acid the urine became clear, but a precipitate developed after an hour. When heated, the precipitate underwent complete solution, but again consolidated upon cooling. He died on January 1, 1846. The autopsy showed brittle bones filled with a soft "gelatiniform substance of blood-red colour and unctuous feel". A urine specimen had also been sent to Dr Bence Jones. He confirmed that the urine contained a precipitate that formed after the addition of nitric acid, dissolved upon heating, but formed again upon cooling. He calculated that the patient excreted more than 60 grams of protein per day and he concluded that the protein was "hydrated deutoxide of albumin". The disease was called "*mollities ossium*" (softness of the bones). Von Rusitzky of Kiev RU introduced the name "multiple myeloma" when he observed 8 separate tumors of the bones at autopsy. In 1875, Heinrich von Waldeyer Hartz (1836-1921), mainly known from his work in neuroanatomy at the Charité in Berlin, introduced the term "plasma cell" to describe the round cells as seen by Solly, but he probably described tissue mast cells. Santiago Ramon y Cajal (1862-1934), the great Spanish neuroscientist, described the plasma cells more clearly in 1890 (*cyanophilic cells of Cajal*). Five years later, Tamás Marschalkó (1862-1915) in Budapest HU, gave an excellent description of plasma cells, with eccentric nucleus, perinuclear halo *("Hof")* and spherical cytoplasm. James Wright (1869-1928; *of Wright's stain fame*) in Boston, identified the myeloma cells as plasma cells in 1900. He also detected these cells in normal bone marrow and emphasized that myeloma was a neoplasm originating in only one type of bone-marrow cell, *i.e.*, the plasma cell. Whereas some authors (*e.g.*, Ludwig Aschoff;1928 and James Ewing;1940) considered plasmacytoma to be a bone tumor, others (*e.g.*, Artur Pappenheim;1907; Von Witzleben;1925) regarded it a hematologic malignancy. Charles Geschickter (1901-1987) and Murray Copeland (1903-1982) surveyed the 425 recorded cases of multiple myeloma in 1928, and emphasized pathologic fractures, Bence Jones proteinuria, anemia, and chronic renal disease. They did not recognize the abnormality of blood proteins yet. The hyperproteinemia of myeloma was first described the same year by Perlzweig at Johns Hopkins in Baltimore. In 1947, Astrid Fagraeus (1913-1997) at Karolinska Institute in Stock-

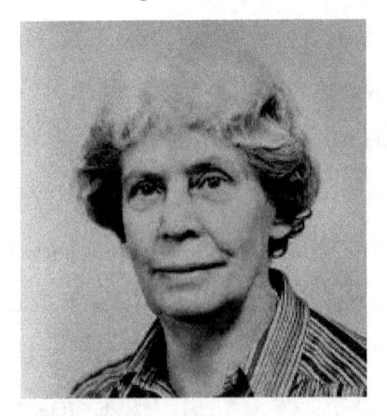

Astrid Fagraeus

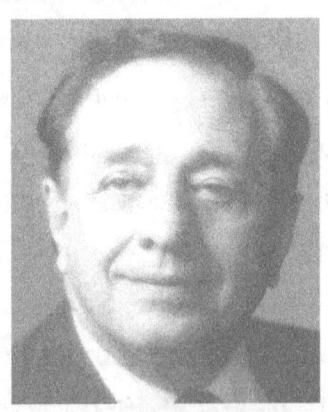

Bob Good

holm SW, and in 1948, Robert Good (1922-2003) in Minneapolis MN, independently demonstrated that plasma cells were the major source of immunoglobulins. With the features of plasma-cell tumors in the bone-marrow cavity, monoclonal gammopathy (serum and/or Bence Jones proteinuria), and renal problems coming together, multiple myeloma was now clearly established as a distinct entity. It was also called Morbus Kahler (Kahler's disease) after Otto Kahler (1849-1893), who in 1885, while Professor at the University of Prague AT (now Czech Republic), saw a 46-year-old physician with severe chest pain. Bone pains increased over the next couple of years, albuminuria was found, followed by anemia. The kyphosis that he developed, made him look dwarf like. When he died in 1887, deformity and softening of the bones and masses of plasma cells were found at autopsy. Whereas (multiple) myeloma has become the name most frequently used, in several countries the name Kahler's disease is still predominant.

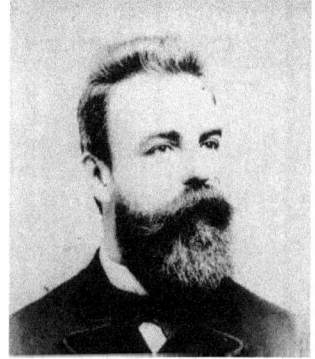

Otto Kahler

Multiple myeloma is a relatively frequent disease, accounting for about 10% of hematological malignancies. It is rare below the age of 30 years and increases with age. The age distribution is quite similar with chronic lymphocytic leukemia. Isadore Snapper (1889-1973), one of the great bedside teachers, published a monograph *Multiple Myeloma* with Turner and Moscovitz in 1953. Snapper had moved in

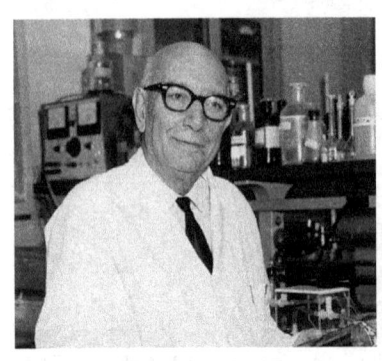

Isadore Snapper

1938 from Amsterdam to New York to escape likely Nazi invasion, but then spent several years in Beijing for the Rockefeller Foundation. After Pearl Harbor, he was interned by the Japanese. He was exchanged for Japanese diplomats; he returned to the USA in 1942, and then taught and practiced mainly in New York.

Based on levels of hemoglobin and calcium, bone lesions, amount of monoclonal protein in serum and/or urine, and renal function, Brian Durie (b.1943) and Sydney Salmon (1933-1999) in Tucson AZ, developed a staging system in 1975. This was followed, in 2005, by the International Staging System (ISS) that relied only on serum levels of $\beta2$-microglobulin and albumin; this staging system predicted survival rather well.

In 1947, N Alwell treated two patients with myeloma with urethane (ethyl carbamate). One of them had a nearly complete recovery. Subsequent studies of this drug in myeloma were less positive and a randomized study, published in 1966, showed it to be no better than placebo. Before that time, Snapper had treated a series of patients with intravenous stilbamidine, an anti kala-azar drug. About half the patients had temporary partial or complete relief of their bone pains, but interest in the drug disappeared when an oral alkylator was introduced.

Melphalan (Alkeran®) is a L-phenylalanine-linked nitrogen mustard, developed in 1954 in England and, almost simultaneously as L-sarcolysin, in Russia. Blokhin and his colleagues in Moscow published that the drug was effective in 3 of 6 patients with myeloma in 1958. Four years later, Daniel Bergsagel (1925-2007) and colleagues at MD Anderson Hospital in Houston TX, saw good results in one third of the patients treated with melphalan. With a one week loading dose, Barth Hoogstraten (b.1924) for the Acute Leukemia Group B, found objective improvement in 78% of patients, with responders surviving much longer than non responders (1967). During the same period, prednisone was shown to be effective in reducing serum globulin, but not in improving survival. The combination of melphalan and prednisone proved superior in a study published in 1969. The combination of carmustine (BCNU), cyclophosphamide, melphalan, vincristine and prednisone (M-2 protocol) at Memorial Sloan Kettering in New York proved very effective in the 1970's. A meta-analysis in 1998 showed that combination chemotherapy active in myeloma led to higher response rates than melphalan + prednisone, but not to longer survival. In 1983, Tim McElwain (1937-1990) and Ray Powles (b.1938) at the Royal Marsden in London, demonstrated that high-dose intravenous melphalan could induce complete biochemical

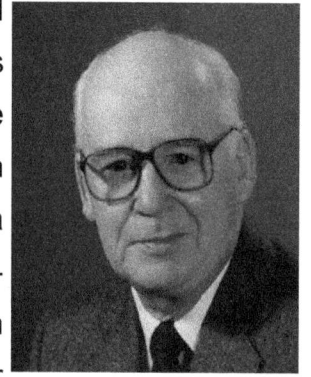

Daniel Bergsagel

remission at the expense of high therapy-related mortality. This became the basis for stem-cell transplantation for multiple myeloma (*p.241*) .

For patients who were not candidates for stem-cell transplantation, or who relapsed, new drugs were introduced. Thalidomide, the Softenon® of fetal-malformation infamy, was introduced in 1957 as a sedative, but taken off the market in late 1961. The drug showed activity against leprosy, graft-versus-host disease, and was being used in the USA more of less illegally, until the FDA approved it in 1998 for erythema nodosum leprosum (leprosy). Since thalidomide has strong anti-angiogenic effects, Bart Barlogie (b.1944) in Little Rock, AK was talked into using it for relapsed myeloma by the spouse of a patient in 1997. The treatment had success and the effect was confirmed in a series of patients. The thalidomide analog lenalidomide (Revlimid®) was studied at the Dana Farber Cancer Center in Boston and was found to have activity in refractory/relapsed patients. In combination with dexamethasone, the drug was approved in 2006. Bortezomib (Velcade®), a proteasome inhibitor, was shown to have activity in myeloma by Barlogie's group in 2003. Proteasome inhibitors lead to cellular apoptosis via the ubiquitin-proteasome pathway responsible for the orderly

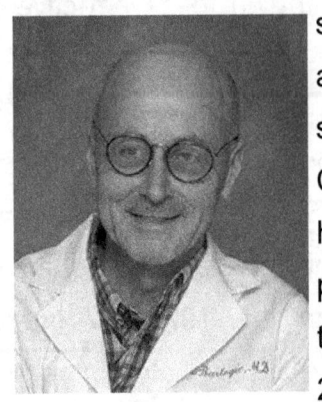

Bart Barlogie

degradation of eukaryotic cellular proteins. Both bortezomib based regimens, and lenalidomide-dexamethasone are now first-line treatment for patients on the road to stem-cell transplantation

For patients who are not candidates for transplant, melphalan + prednisone continued to be standard of care, but bortezomib-based regimens became more popular. As with other B-lymphocyte malignancies, monoclonal antibodies (*e.g.*, daratumumab or isatuximab, both against CD38), selective pathway inhibitors, and CAR-T cells are now also under study. Daratumumab has been particularly important in both relapsed and newly diagnosed myeloma when used in combination with various (up to 4) different therapeutic modalities.

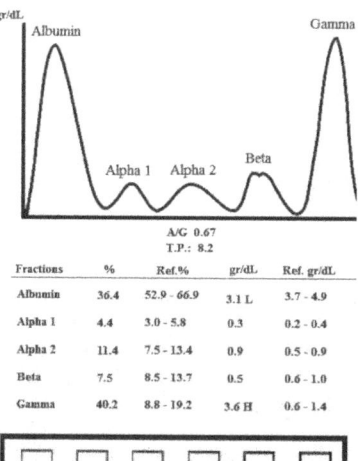

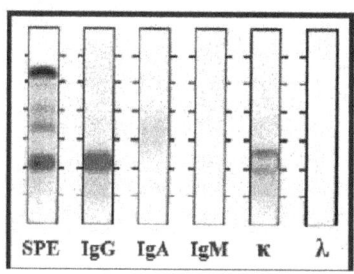

Fractions	%	Ref.%	gr/dL	Ref. gr/dL
Albumin	36.4	52.9 - 66.9	3.1 L	3.7 - 4.9
Alpha 1	4.4	3.0 - 5.8	0.3	0.2 - 0.4
Alpha 2	11.4	7.5 - 13.4	0.9	0.5 - 0.9
Beta	7.5	8.5 - 13.7	0.5	0.6 - 1.0
Gamma	40.2	8.8 - 19.2	3.6 H	0.6 - 1.4

A/G 0.67
T.P.: 8.2

Serum protein electrophoresis and immunofixation of monoclonal IgGk protein

Blood is Life

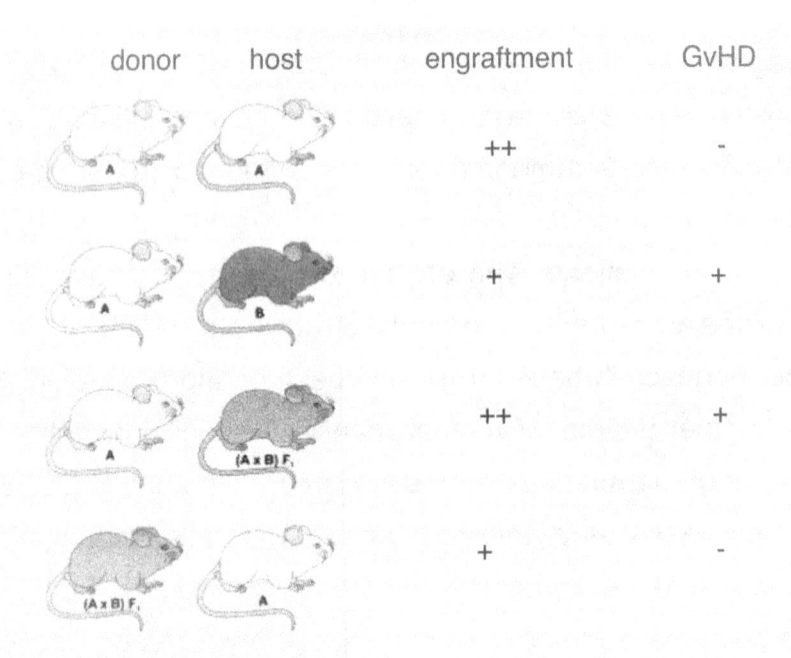

donor	host	engraftment	GvHD
A	A	++	−
A	B	+	+
A	(A x B) F1	++	+
(A x B) F1	A	+	−

Parent into F1 bone-marrow transplant, illustrating graft-vs-host disease

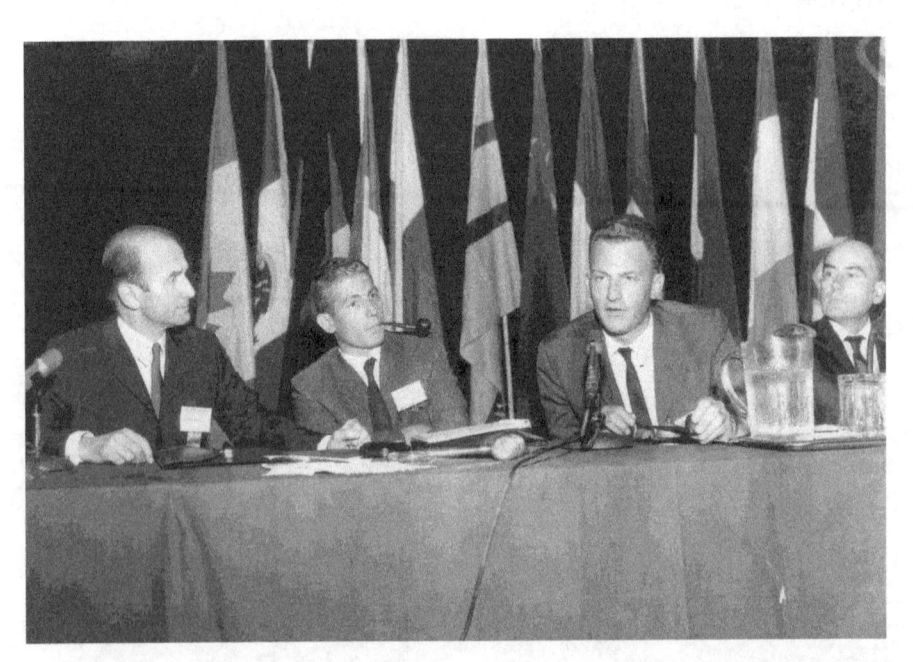

Georges Mathé, Dick van Bekkum, George Santos and Don Thomas.
International Society of Experimental Hematology, Davis CA 1971

STEM CELL TRANSPLANTATION

In 1937, Albert Schretzenmayr (1906-1995) in Cologne GE gave intramuscular injections of 1-2 ml of donor bone marrow to patients with anemia to "provide a missing factor". He claimed that the patients improved rapidly. The same year, Edwin Osgood in Portland OR treated a girl with aplastic anemia with liver extract, pentose nucleotide, blood transfusions and intravenous infusion of 18 ml of sternal marrow from her ABO-compatible brother. The patient died 5 days later. Maurice Morrison and Andrew Samwick in Brooklyn NY, treated a 42 year-old man with pancytopenia and hypocellular bone marrow, with intra-sternal infusion of small (3 and 5 ml) volumes of sternal bone marrow from his ABO-compatible brother and an unrelated donor in 1940. The patient started to improve within one week, and the authors believed that they had replaced a "missing factor". They envisaged in leukemia, where "the deficiency perhaps does not allow the myeloblast to mature", one might be tempted to "exsanguinate the bone marrow of the sternum, immediately followed by the introduction of healthy bone marrow"!

Bone-marrow transplantation received its scientific basis after World War II based on animal experiments. In 1922, the Danish radiologist Jan Fabricius-Møller had already documented that the decrease of platelets in the peripheral blood of guinea pigs after total body irradiation (TBI), did not occur when the legs were shielded. After the war, with its conclusion by nuclear bombs on Hiroshima and Nagasaki, the interest in the effects of radiation on living tissues markedly increased. Leon Jacobson in Chicago IL, rediscovered the effect of shielding part of the body during TBI in 1949. His group shielded the spleen of mice during TBI and saw that the mice survived, documenting that in the mouse the spleen is a hematopoietic organ. They confirmed that by being able to rescue irradiated mice with spleen-cell injection. Egon Lorenz (1892-1954) and colleagues at the NCI (Bethesda, MD) reported, also in 1952, that mice and guinea pigs could be rescued after TBI, by the intravenous injection of donor bone marrow from the same inbred strain (= syngeneic or isologous). The discussion started whether this was caused by cells or by a humoral factor. Finally in 1956, cytogeneticist Charles Ford and colleagues in Harwell UK, demonstrated that the rescue was by donor cells. They also introduced the term "radiation chimaera" for an animal carrying a foreign hematopoietic system after TBI. Studies with donor cells from different strains of mice (= allogeneic or homologous), or from different species (= xenogeneic or heterologous), followed with irradiated mice, rats, guinea pigs, dogs and monkeys. Many of these studies were reviewed in the 1967 book *Radiation Chimaeras* by Dick Van Bekkum (*p.15*) and pathologist Marco de Vries (1937-2009) in Rijswijk NL. While many investigators were satisfied that

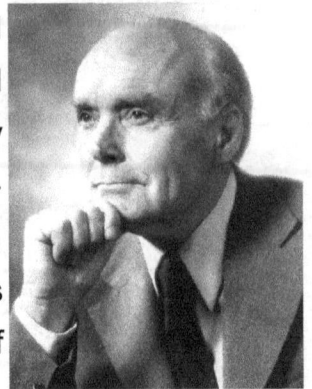

Charles Ford

Stem Cell Transplantation

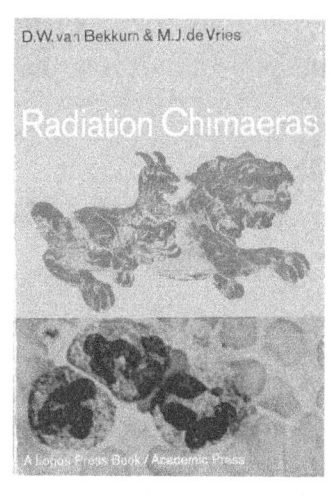

Dust cover of Radiation Chimaeras

they could establish radiation chimeras even in the xenogeneic setting, a large proportion of the recipients of allogeneic and xenogeneic stem-cell grafts died within several weeks after transplant. Radiobiologists David Barnes (1923-1998) and John Loutit (1910-1992) in Harwell UK were the first to document this. They suggested an immunological reaction, which was later called "secondary disease". John Trentin (1918-2005) in Houston TX, studied the issue in 1956 with parent into F1 transplants (*p.222*). It took several years, before it was determined that secondary disease was a graft-versus-host reaction, not a host-versus graft reaction. By the late 1960's, the problem had been solved, and donor lymphocytes were held responsible for the graft-versus-host disease (GvHD). Rupert Billingham (1921-2002), a student of Peter Medawar in London, but working in Philadelphia PA in 1967, summarized the requirements for GvHD: 1) the graft must contain immunologically active cells; 2) the host must possess important transplantation antigens that are lacking in the donor; 3) the host must be incapable of rejecting the donor cells, at least during the immediate period after transplant.

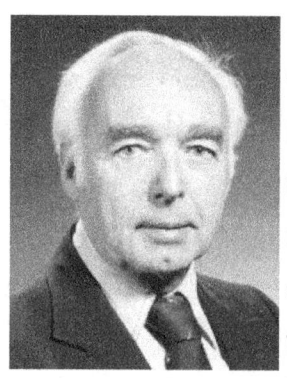

Rupert Billingham

While these animal studies elucidated the immunological aspects of stem-cell transplantation, early clinical studies had started. The group of Joseph Ferrebee (1908-2001) in Cooperstown NY, demonstrated that large volumes of bone marrow could be transfused intravenously without causing bone-marrow emboli in 1957. The next year, two children with refractory ALL received grafts from their identical-twin donors after TBI. Both had hematologic recovery, but relapsed after 7 and 12 weeks. Don Thomas (*p.243*) was the first author of these papers. In 1958, the most heavily irradiated physicists of the Vinca Nuclear-Reactor accident in (now) Serbia received allografts from ABO-compatible unrelated donors in Paris by Georges Mathé (*p.123*). No evidence of durable engraftment was found, but four of the patients had autologous recovery. Both in Paris and in Cooperstown, additional patients were treated with TBI and allografts without the benefit of HLA-typing. Mathé used bone marrow from several family members, up to six, to allow the patient to determine which donor was best! One of his patients, a 26-year-old physician with refractory ALL, received TBI and marrow grafts from his parents and 4 siblings. He attained complete remission that continued for 18 months. Marrow cells from one of his brothers had fully engrafted. The patient survived severe GvHD, but ultimately died from a viral infection while in complete remission. This first successful allograft occurred in 1963.

Patients with aplastic anemia received allografts without a preparative regimen. None engrafted.

Stem Cell Transplantation

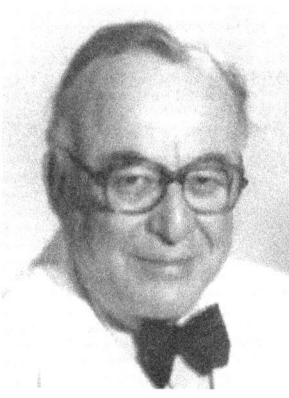

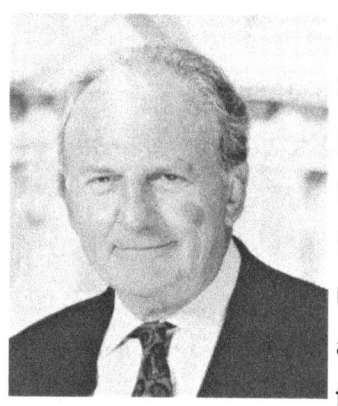

In 1970, Mortimer Bortin (1922-1994) in Milwaukee WI reviewed all human bone-marrow transplants until 1969. Except for Mathé's patient and 3 children receiving allografts for immunodeficiency, all 203 patients had died. When HLA-typing became available, HLA-matched siblings could be identified. Allografts with these donors were far more successful. Don Thomas had moved to Seattle WA in 1963, and was building a large bone-marrow transplantation (BMT) program there. With a combination of TBI and cyclophosphamide, they had about 15% long-term survival in patients with relapsed leukemia who received either syngeneic or HLA-identical sibling allografts (1977). In 1976, they started doing transplants for acute myelogenous leukemia in first remission. Now the long-term survival rate became 60% (1979). Many centers followed their approach, either with TBI and cyclophosphamide, or with busulfan and cyclophosphamide as preparative regimen, as used by the group of George Santos (1928-2001) at Johns Hopkins in Baltimore MD. To prevent GvHD, the Seattle team mainly used methotrexate, the Baltimore group used low-dose cyclophosphamide. In 1978, cyclosporine was introduced as immunosuppressant. This calcineurin inhibitor decreased the incidence and severity of GvHD, especially in combination with short-course methotrexate. An alternative method of preventing GvHD was tested in London and in Minneapolis MN in 1982: T-cell depletion of the bone-marrow graft. The mouse work for this approach had already been done in the 1960's. The introduction of monoclonal antibodies made this approach more practical for clinical work. Following the first positive reports, many centers jumped on the bandwagon, to avoid the side effects of methotrexate and cyclosporine. Unfortunately, it became clear before 1990, that total T-cell depletion was effective for the prevention of GvHD, but resulted in higher risks of graft rejection and recurrence of the leukemia. The latter was particularly true for chronic myelogenous leukemia. Subset specific T-cell depletion was tried (1991), as was *in-vivo* instead of *in-vitro* T-cell depletion (alemtuzumab). Since 2008, the use of high-dose cyclophosphamide shortly after transplant has been shown to be effective in the prevention of acute and chronic GvHD, and is increasingly used.

Studies in Seattle had already shown in 1979, that patients who developed GvHD, had a lower risk of relapse than patients without GvHD. This confirmed Mathé's 1965 concept of "adoptive immunotherapy". It also led to the use of donor lymphocyte infusion (*DLI*) by Hans Joachim Kolb and colleagues in Munich GE in 1987. These donor lymphocyte infusions were successful in restoring complete remission in many relapsed patients, but at the expense of the risk of occurrence or recurrence of GvHD.

Stem Cell Transplantation

The first reported allografts were done in the era before HLA typing and were nearly all unsuccessful. When HLA-typing permitted the selection of HLA-identical sibling donors (*p.39*), the results became much better. That raised the hope that HLA-identical unrelated donors would also be worthwhile pursuing. Bruno Speck (1934-1998), while working in Leiden in 1972, performed the first transplant from an HLA-matched unrelated donor from Denmark for a Dutch patient with aplastic anemia. The preparative regimen was insufficient and the donor bone marrow did not engraft. In 1980, the Seattle team performed a successful unrelated transplant in a patient with ALL. Earlier, some transplants from unrelated donors into children with severe combined immunodeficiency (SCID) had been successful (1975-1977).

The team at the University of Iowa developed a pool of volunteer unrelated donors (1985), and had some patients with leukemia or aplastic anemia who became long-term survivors after matched unrelated transplants. In England, between 1977 and 1987, among four transplant centers, 51 patients received unrelated allografts from donors of the Anthony Nolan Register, that had been started in London in 1974. In the USA, smaller registries were started in Seattle WA, Milwaukee WI and Minneapolis MN. In 1985, the US government decided to fund the National Marrow Donor Program; it started in Minneapolis in 1986. In Europe, registries were also organized, *e.g.*, in France (*Greffe de Moelle*; 1986), the Netherlands (*Europdonor*, 1988) and Germany (*DKMS*; 1991). Overall, the results of HLA-identical unrelated bone-marrow transplants were good, but not quite as good as transplants from HLA-identical siblings: GvHD and rejection were more frequent. The ever increasing complexity of the HLA system made it increasingly difficult to find an HLA fully-identical unrelated donor.

An alternative for an HLA-matched unrelated donor would be a haploidentical related donor. If such transplants were possible, nearly every patient could find a donor rapidly. Haplo-identical bone-marrow transplants in children with severe immunodeficiency became possible if the MLC (mixed lymphocyte culture) was non-reactive (1983). For older patients, the results in Seattle with partially-matched related donors in the late 1970's gave some hope, although rejection was more frequent; GvHD was more frequent too, and occurred earlier after transplant. The group in Milwaukee WI addressed these issues by increasing the preparative regimen and performing T-cell depletion of the donor bone marrow. Some of their patients survived (1985). This approach was attractive for countries with limited family size (China!), a homogeneous population (Japan, Israel, China), or with limited money to be spent on unrelated-donor searches (all non-industrialized countries). Marcello Martini's group in Perugia IT, started a study in patients with acute leukemia using haplo-identical related donors in 1996. Their

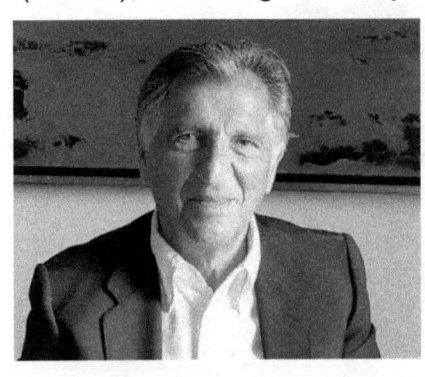

Marcello Martini

preparative regimen consisted of TBI, thioTEPA, fludarabine and anti-thymocyte globulin. The graft consisted of massive doses of stem cells from T-cell depleted G-CSF - stimulated peripheral-blood cells with/without bone marrow. All patients engrafted and GvHD did not develop, but nearly half the patients died in transplant. Transplants from the mother proved better than from the father. In 2002, Yu Wang and her colleagues at Beijing University CH, started a program of haploidentical bone-marrow and peripheral-blood transplants for patients with leukemia. They collected bone marrow and peripheral blood stem cells after stimulation with filgrastim (G-CSF), and they used a preparative regimen of cytarabine, busulfan, cyclophosphamide, methyl-CCNU, and anti-thymocyte globulin. Virtually all patients engrafted, and less than half the patients developed significant GvHD. Leukemia-free survival was 50-65%, depending on the risk group. Even in first complete remission AML, the results were quite comparable with those of HLA-identical sibling transplants! In several other countries similar results were obtained with various preparative regimens and various GvHD prophylaxis protocols.

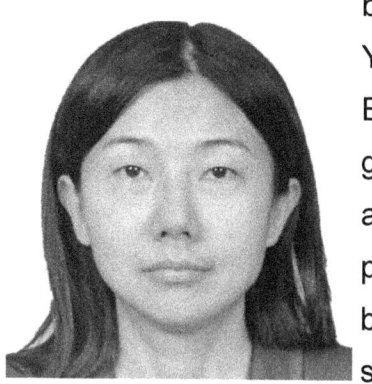

Yu Wang

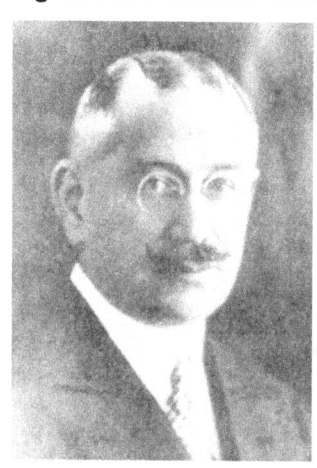

Alexander Maximov

As mentioned above, peripheral-blood stem cells were being used in several of these studies. Alexander Maximov (1874-1928) in St. Petersburg RU, had postulated in 1909, that among the lymphocytes in the peripheral blood, a population of common stem cells circulated that had, or could regain, pluripotency ("gemeinsame Stamzellen"). Joan Goodman and George Hodgson in Oak Ridge TN found evidence of stem cells in the peripheral blood of mice in 1962. Paul Chervenick and Dale Boggs in Pittsburgh PA, demonstrated in 1971 that in humans the stem cells in the peripheral blood were rare, but they were more frequent in myelofibrosis and CML. The latter was used by John Goldman (1938-2013) in London for collection and use for autologous stem-cell transplantation (SCT) in CML (1981). Massive collections of unstimulated peripheral blood stem cells were occasionally used (Omaha NE,1988), but the situation drastically changed when it was shown that stem cells in the peripheral blood markedly increased after aggressive chemotherapy. This was studied by Chris Juttner in Adelaide AU, and Ted Fliedner (1929-2015) in Ulm GE, in 1985. In 1989, sargramostim (GM CSF) was found to increase circulating stem cells, and the same year filgrastim (G-CSF) proved even more active for stem-cell collection. When chemotherapy and sargramostim were combined, Alessandro Gianni (b.1943) and colleagues in Milan IT, obtained a 1,000-fold increase in CFU-GM (1989). For stem cell collection in donors not requiring chemotherapy, filgrastim appeared

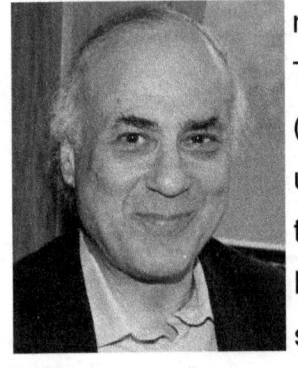

John Goldman

more active than sargramostim and could be administered subcutaneously (1993). The large dose of stem cells, defined as CFU-GM, or as $CD34^+$ cells, - after Curt Civin (b.1948) at John Hopkins had documented that cell-surface glycoprotein on lympho-hematopoietic progenitor cells in 1984 -, that could be collected from growth-factor stimulated peripheral blood, resulted in faster engraftment than seen after unstimulated bone marrow, both in the autologous and allogeneic setting: engraftment was about one week faster. This resulted in a lower risk of infection, and even allowed many patients to undergo their transplant completely as outpatients. By 1993, the vast majority of autologous transplants were done with peripheral blood stem cells (PBSC) only. PBSC were probably also less likely to harbor neoplastic cells and made the use of "purged" bone marrow redundant. Malcolm Brenner (b.1951) from Cambridge UK, while working in Memphis TN, showed in 1992, that retrovirally transduced leukemia cells could indeed contribute to relapse after autologous SCT. The bone-marrow purging during the 1980's had mainly been performed with pharmacological techniques (4-hydroperoxyy-cyclophosphamide (4-HC) or mafosfamide) or with immunological methods (monoclonal antibodies with complement or ricin). For allogeneic transplants the issue was more complex, since PBSC contained far more T-cells, increasing the risk of GvHD.

In 1974, Søren Knudtzon in Copenhagen DE showed that circulating cells in human cord blood were able to grow CFU-GM *in vitro*. This was picked up by investigators at Memorial Sloan Kettering in New York and in Indianapolis IN, in the 1980's. Hal Broxmeyer (b.1944) had just moved from the former to the latter city. In 1988, he provided the umbilical-cord blood cells (UCB) from an HLA-identical newborn sister of a 5-year-old boy with Fanconi's anemia, to Éliane Gluckman (b.1940) in Paris. The mild preparative regimen and allogeneic transplant led to hematologic recovery after 3 weeks, and the patient was alive and well without GvHD 9 months later. This led to an enormous interest in UCB, since these immunologically naïve cells were expected to cause less GvHD and perhaps would require less strict HLA-identity between donor and patient. UCB banks were set up in many countries, both for allogeneic transplants and for commercial autologous storage.

By the early 1990's, the situation for autologous and syngeneic SCT was clear: PBSC were the way to go. In the allogeneic setting, HLA-identical siblings were still first choice as donors. For patients who did not have a healthy HLA identical sibling donor, several options had to be considered: single or double UCB, sufficiently HLA-matched unrelated donor, or haplo-identical related donor? Allowable interval until transplant, age of the patient and donor, and need of antitumor effect of the allograft remained important issues.

As mentioned before, in 1965 Georges Mathé in Paris had introduced the concept of "adoptive immunotherapy": the transfer of allogeneic lymphocytes and/or stem cells with the primary goal of immunotherapy. His concept originated from his studies with L_{1210} mouse leukemia. He saw that after TBI, the infusion of allogeneic mouse bone marrow could cure the leukemia, but syngeneic (same strain) bone-marrow cells could not. Mathé prematurely left the bone-marrow transplantation field to focus on more general leukemia immunotherapy with irradiated leukemic blast cells and BCG.

Interestingly, the use of donor leukocytes to induce an immunological reaction was not new. Transfusion of granulocytes *(p.306)* was used for many years to fight bacterial infections in patients with severe neutropenia. With the granulocytes, donor lymphocytes were also transfused. When such granulocyte transfusions had not been irradiated, the donor lymphocytes could cause GvHD, and even some complete remissions, as shown by Mathé's group in 1965.

Would complete engraftment of donor cells be necessary to see this anti-tumor effect? Samuel Strober (b.1940)'s group at Stanford University showed in the mouse model in 1978, that total lymphoid irradiation (TLI) allowed allogeneic bone-marrow transplantation without GvHD and mostly with mixed chimerism (part donor, part recipient). This model, and their results in an outbred dog model (1979), were suggested for organ allotransplantation in man. Ten years later, Megan Sykes and David Sachs (b.1942) at NCI, demonstrated that mixed chimeras could be converted into full chimeras with donor-lymphocyte infusions (*DLI*). The hope was that the anti tumor effect could be separated from the GvHD effect by first achieving mixed chimerism with a non-myeloablative preparative regimen. The drug that held the most promise for that endeavor proved to be fludarabine, developed in 1968. This strongly lympholytic drug was associated with transfusion induced GvHD after its FDA approval for the treatment of chronic lymphocytic leukemia in 1991.

As is usual the case, several investigators claimed primacy for the developments of non-myeloablative stem cell transplants (NST). Shimon Slavin (b.1941) in Jerusalem IS referred to his mouse work with Sam Strober (b.1940) at Stanford. The group at MD Anderson in Houston referred to Emil Freireich's studies of transfusion-induced GvHD after fludarabine. Rainer Storb (b.1935) and the Seattle group also claimed priority. In my interview with him in Paris in 2001, Georges Mathė considered non-myeloablative stem-cell transplants his greatest contribution to the field. Alternative names for NST have been *"transplant lite"* (Houston), *"mini transplant"* (Seattle) and *"reduced-intensity conditioning (RIC) transplant"*. Particularly for patients who are older or otherwise intolerant of an aggressive preparative regimen, NST is an extremely attractive option. Instead of fludarabine, low(er) doses of TBI, busulfan, cyclophosphamide, and anti-thymocyte globulin (ATG) have also been used.

Large numbers of hematologic diseases, and even some solid tumors have been treated with SCT. Severe aplastic anemia was among the first. Moreno Robbins and Noyes at the University of Washington in Seattle performed the first SCT from an identical twin donor in 1960. The donor bone marrow engrafted without a preparative regimen. When larger numbers of syngeneic SCT for aplastic anemia had been performed, it became apparent that only a minority were successful without preparative regimen. After a preparative regimen, nearly all were successful. Allografts were unsuccessful until HLA-identical siblings could be identified. In 1973, the Seattle group reported the first series of patients who had received allografts for aplastic anemia. About half of them became long-term survivors. Early transplant, and absence of sensitization by multiple transfusions, resulted in better outcomes. For younger patients (<25 years?) with aplastic anemia and an HLA-identical sibling, allografting became the standard therapy.

Acute leukemia became an important indication for SCT. In 1958, Don Thomas and his colleagues at Cooperstown NY performed the first syngeneic SCT for a child with refractory ALL. When ALL patients received their syngeneic SCT earlier in the course of their disease, a minority had long-term survival (20%; Seattle 1986). A single allograft with a related donor not selected by HLA typing survived (Mathé; Paris 1963), but all others failed. When HLA-identical siblings could be used as donors, the Seattle group in 1979 reported about 50% survival in patients with ALL transplanted in complete remission and 20% for patients in relapse. Several registries (IBMTR: *International Bone Marrow Transplant Registry;* EBMT: *European Bone Marrow Transplantation Group)* reported similar results among large numbers of patients. Autologous SCT for ALL was unsuccessful before bone-marrow purging became available. John Kersey (1938

John Kersey

-2013)'s group in Minneapolis MN reported in 1987 that outcomes after HLA-identical sibling transplants and autologous transplant with antibody-purged bone marrow were quite similar.

For AML, the Seattle group started to use SCT with HLA-matched-sibling donors in 1970. When patients with advanced AML underwent allografting, only about 15% became long-term survivors. In 1976, this group started performing allografts for patients with AML in complete remission. Now the long-term survival became 60%. Again, registries confirmed the difference between SCT in relapse and remission. A point of discussion became whether the Seattle preparative regimen of TBI and cyclophosphamide should be followed, or the John Hopkins regimen of busulfan and cyclophosphamide.

For patients without an HLA-identical donor, the group of Karel Dicke (b.1939) at MD Anderson in Houston TX, introduced autologous SCT in 1979. Bone marrow had been harvested during remission and stored after cryopreservation. This approach became more attractive when purging of the bone-marrow graft with 4-hydroperoxycyclophosphamide (4-HC; Johns Hopkins, 1985) or mafosfamide (Claude Gorin; Paris, b.1946; 1986) became available. Interestingly, autologous SCT with purged bone marrow became far more popular in Europe than in North America. When PBSC were introduced, purged bone marrow lost most of its appeal.

In chronic myelogenous leukemia (CML), autologous SCT during blast crisis with cells obtained during chronic phase was introduced by Dean Buckner and the Seattle team in 1974. They harvested bone marrow during chronic phase. When the cryopreserved bone marrow was used after TBI, only a small percentage attained a second chronic phase, and all patients died within a couple of months. John Goldman and his group in London collected and cryopreserved PBSC during chronic phase. When used after transformation of the disease, SCT resulted in a second chronic phase in most of the patients, but survival was still only several months. With double transplants and post-SCT therapy, or with *in-vitro* treatment of the collected graft, the results were somewhat better. With syngeneic SCT, studied by Alex Fefer (1938-2010) and colleagues in Seattle, engraftment and remission were good; about a quarter of the patients had recurrence of their disease when transplanted in chronic phase. In the late 1970's, the Seattle group started doing allografts from HLA-identical sibling donors in patients with advanced CML, with only an occasional long-term survivor. Around 1980, they started doing these transplants in chronic phase with around 50% long-term survival. Many groups followed their example, with similar results. T-cell depletion of the allografts resulted in less GvHD, but more recurrence of the leukemia, as reported by several groups in the late 1980's. Allografts from matched unrelated donors gave results that were only slightly worse than from HLA identical siblings. Then in the late 1990's, tyrosine-kinase inhibitors (imatinib was the first) were introduced and started to replace allogeneic SCT as first-line therapy for CML (2001).

    The first SCTs for lymphoma were done by

Dameshek's group in Boston in 1959. They collected autologous bone marrow, treated the patients with high-dose nitrogen mustard, and reinfused the bone marrow the next day. Bone-marrow function recovered in 3 of the 5 patients, but remissions were only brief. More serious was the approach by the group at NCI (Bethesda MD) in children with relapsed Burkitt's lymphoma in 1978. They received high dose chemotherapy and cryopreserved bone marrow. About a quarter of the patients remained in remission. Alberto Marmont's group in Genova IT, reported in 1984 on 10 patients with relapsed or primary-resistant lymphoma who received high-dose chemotherapy and autologous non cryopreserved bone marrow. Nine patients had bone-marrow recovery and 5 continued in complete remission. Many studies followed, both in Hodgkin's disease and in intermediate or high-grade non-Hodgkin's lymphoma. In chemotherapy sensitive non-Hodgkin's lymphoma, the PARMA study in Europe showed that high-dose chemotherapy with autologous bone-marrow rescue was superior to conventional salvage chemotherapy (1995). This had also been found in relapsed Hodgkin's disease (1989). The introduction of PBSC around 1990, decreased the therapy related mortality of the procedures. Karl Blume (1937-2013) and colleagues in Duarte CA reported excellent results with autologous SCT for high-risk patients in first remission (1992). Syngeneic SCT for malignant lymphoma was not clearly better than autolo-

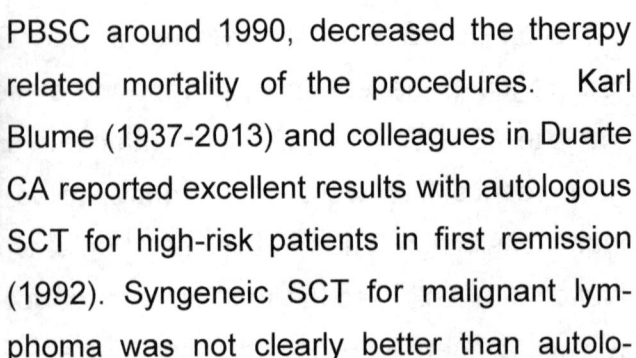

Karl Blume

gous SCT. Allogeneic SCT was fraught with the usual complications of GvHD *etc.*. In cases where the bone marrow was involved (*e.g.*, low grade lymphoma), allografts were clearly an option, particularly when NST came along.

Multiple Myeloma proved sensitive to high-dose melphalan, as shown in 1983 by McElwain and Powles at the Royal Marsden in London. They, and particularly Bart Barlogie in Houston, used it in combination with autologous SCT (1988). When PBSC became available, such autologous SCT became even easier with less toxicity in the mostly older patient population. In subsequent years, Barlogie's group, now in Little Rock AK, found that better supportive care (PBSC, GM-CSF) and double (=tandem) transplants led to better results (1994), and that melphalan by itself was better than melphalan plus TBI. Similar results were reported from France by Jean-Luc Harousseau (b.1948) of Nantes on behalf of a collaborative group (1995, 2002). In a randomized study, this group showed that autologous SCT improved the response rate, event-free survival, and overall survival (1996). Barlogie's group developed their "total therapy" concept for newly

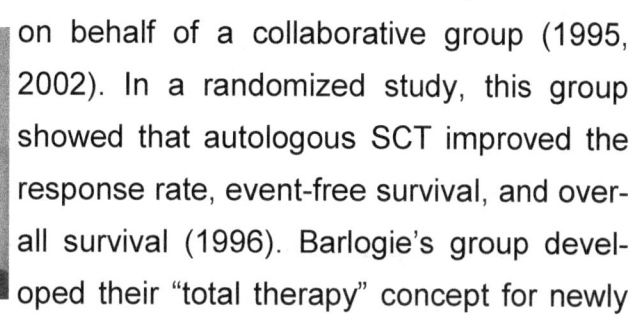

Jean-Luc Harousseau diagnosed myeloma, consisting of remission induction with vincristine, adriamycin and dexamethasone (VAD), followed by high-dose cyclophosphamide and GM-CSF for PBSC collection. This again was followed by high-dose melphalan and the first transplant. Patients in remission underwent a second transplant. Median event-free survival was 43 months, and overall survival was 68 months (1999). Selection of $CD34^+$ cells or bone-marrow purging were possible, but did not appear to improve the results (2001). Post transplant maintenance therapy with bortezomib (2012) or lenalidomide (2017) were found to extent event free and overall survival. Allogeneic transplant was not attractive in most instances, because of the age of the patients. Nevertheless, for some patients it proved curative. Our group just celebrated the 35-year disease-free survival of a patient after an allograft from her HLA-identical sister! Non-myeloablative transplants made allografts more feasible for the higher-age group.

Stem-cell transplantation for solid tumors falls outside the scope of this book. Yet, in the late 1980's and 1990's, autologous SCT for breast cancer was the most frequent indication for SCT, particularly in the USA. By 1998, this indication had disappeared again, for a variety of reasons, some medical and some socio-economical. Autologous SCT for the few patients with testicular cancer who were not cured, or not likely to be cured, with first-line therapy, appeared more productive.

Stem-cell transplantation became an important tool in the armamentarium of hematology. With rapid changes in molecular and immunological therapies in the last decade, the long-term future of current SCT is uncertain. In 2006, 50,417 first stem-cell transplants were performed world-wide: 57% autologous and 43% allogeneic (12,000 from family donors and the rest from unrelated donors). The main indications were lymphoproliferative disorders (55%) and leukemia (34%). About half occurred in Europe and 36% in the Americas. In 2014, the WMDA (*World Marrow Donor Association*) reported 20,600 unrelated transplants (4,149 bone-marrow donations, 12,506 peripheral-blood stem-cell donations, and 3,949 cord-blood units). SCT had become a growth industry after the 1970's.

Edward Donnall ("Don") Thomas *was born in 1920 in rural Texas, where his physician father still made house calls with horse and buggy. He first did a MS in chemistry, and then went to Harvard medical school. This was followed by an internship and Hematology fellowship with Clement Finch (1915-2010) on iron metabolism. After military service, a fellowship at MIT in Boston, and Internal Medicine, he joined the faculty of Brigham and Women's Hospital in Boston. Two year later, he joined Joseph W Ferrebee (1909-2001) in Cooperstown NY, where his interest in bone-marrow transplantation started. The group showed that considerable volumes of bone marrow could be infused intravenously, and they also did syngeneic bone-marrow transplants in children with ALL, and allogeneic transplants in dogs. In 1963, he was recruited to the University of Washington in Seattle as Head of Oncology. He continued his work with allografts in dogs and*

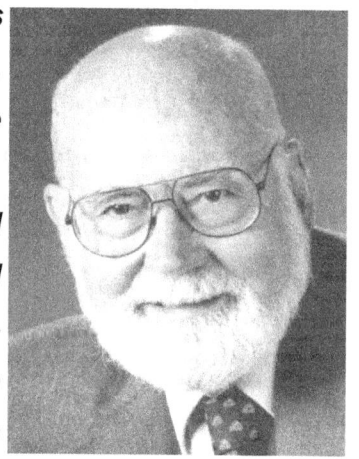

syngeneic grafts in children. Several important members were added to the team (e.g., Robert Epstein, Dean Buckner, Reginald Clift, Paul Neiman, Alex Fefer and Rainer Storb). When HLA-typing became possible, allografts from HLA-identical siblings were started in 1969. In 1975, the new Fred Hutchinson Cancer Research Center was opened. It became the largest bone-marrow transplant program in the world and remained that for at least 20 years. Allografts in patients with refractory leukemia resulted in about 15% long term survival. In 1976, they took the courageous step to perform allografts much earlier during the course of AML (first complete remission). The long-term survival rate now went up to about 60%. Chronic Myelogenous Leukemia also proved curable with allografts. The Seattle team made important contributions to the staging, prevention and therapy of graft-versus-host disease. Their program size allowed randomized studies. Their main preparative regimen was and remained total-body irradiation based. In 1989, Don Thomas went into partial retirement. During his entire career he was supported by his wife Dottie, both in the laboratory and in program administration. He shared in the Nobel Prize in Physiology/Medicine in 1990. He died in 2012 at the age of 92.

PLATELETS

Whereas Van Leeuwenhoek saw red cells and Hewson saw white cells, nobody saw platelets (*thrombocytes*) in the blood until the mid 19th century. That was largely caused by the limitations of the microscope, until achromatic lenses became available around 1825-1830. Alfred Donné in Paris reported in 1845 in his "*Cours de microscopie complémentaire des études médicales*" (his microscopy course for physicians) "there exist in the blood three types of particles". Red and white blood cells were clearly defined, but the third one was more elusive. William Addison in Malvern UK (*p.129*) thought that among the "pus" colorless particles he saw in 1842, some were "so minute that I am not aware that similar molecules have ever before been noticed in human blood". It took another 30 years before William Osler saw bacteria-like particles in the blood of normal humans and animals. He had no idea about their function, but did provide illustrations of the cells "$\frac{1}{8}$-$\frac{1}{2}$ the size of a red corpuscle". The particles did not stick together in a blood smear, but accumulated together in a drop of blood. Georges Hayem (*p.48*) in Paris studied platelets far more extensively in 1878. He believed his "*hématoblastes*", shown as biconvex discs that had a great tendency to change their form and to aggregate and interact with fibrin strands, were probably destined to become erythrocytes! He kept that opinion for almost half a century (1923), unwilling to accept facts from other investigators. This also happened with his dualistic opinion about the origin of stem cells (*p.8*). Hayem was the first to count platelets in the peripheral blood accurately. Giulio Bizzozero in Pavia IT published in 1882 a monograph on platelets ("Blutplättchen" or later only "Plättchen") in German. He stressed that these new cells were an independent line, with a specialized function, *i.e.*, hemostasis. He reported how the platelets accumulated to form the hemostatic plug when blood vessels were severed or damaged. He indicated that hemostasis and coagulation were not synonymous. He supposed that the platelets would produce a substance to initiate the formation of a clot! Pathologists Karl Eberth (1835-1926) and Curt Schimmelbusch (1860-1895) in Halle GE confirmed the aggregation of platelets after damage to the vessel wall in 1885, and demonstrated the "viscous metamorphosis" of platelets when they aggregated. James Wright in Boston MA (*p.216*) documented the origin of platelets ("*plates*" as he called them) from megakaryocytes in 1916. He did not find a correlation between the number of megakaryocytes in the bone marrow and the number of platelets in the blood.

Hayem had shown that (horse) blood, when prevented from clotting by cooling, sedimented into three different layers: the top was cell poor, the middle was platelet rich, and the bottom had mainly red cells. Upon warming all clotted, but only the middle layer gave clot retraction. When

Giulio Bizzozero

platelets were removed by filtration, the retraction was greatly reduced. Le Sourd and Pagniez in France showed that only "living" platelets were capable of clot retraction in 1906. The efficiency of clot retraction was proportional to the platelet concentration. Biochemist Ernst Lüscher (1916-2002) in Bern SU showed that glycolysis was necessary for clot retraction in 1956, and in 1959 that a contractile protein was involved.

Around the same time, the adhesion of platelets to the damaged vessel wall was studied. Bounameaux and Hugues, working in the laboratory of Jacques Roskam in Liège BE (*p.43*), demonstrated that platelets adhered to certain non-biological surfaces and suggested that the thrombogenic surface of a damaged vessel was collagen. Hugues also found hat the adhesion reaction was not the same as the aggregation event. The aggregation of platelets went back to Bizzozero's work of the 1880's. The laboratory of Paul Owren (1905-1990) in Oslo NO was active in that field. Arvid Hellem published in 1960 on the effect of a column with glass beads on platelet rich plasma. He believed that the reduction in platelet number after the column was due to platelet adhesion to the beads and that the loss in platelets became more extensive as more red cells were left in the plasma. The retention was also accomplished with red-cell hemolysate.

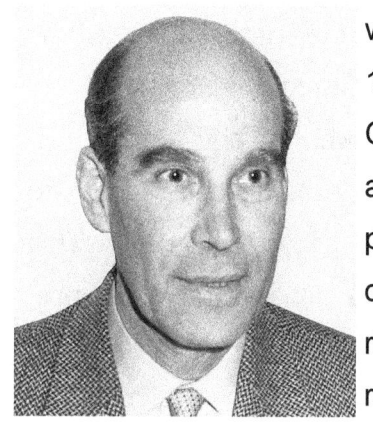

Paul Owren

This "aggregating" agent was called "factor R" for "red cells", even though Ollgaard in Copenhagen DE found that similar material was present in platelets in 1964. Gaarder in Owren's group showed that the "factor R" was adenosine diphosphate (ADP) in 1964. In the early 1960's, the aggregometer had been developed (*p.45*) and could now be used to study platelet aggregation *in-vitro*.

Hayem had already observed that his "*hématoblastes*" interacted with fibrin strands. Yet, blood appeared to clot with equal facility, whether or not platelets were abundant. Biochemist Erwin Chargaff (1905-2002) in New York prepared a lipid extract from (horse) platelets that accelerated clotting in cell-free (chicken) plasma in 1936. The activity was in the phospholipid fraction. In 1947, the group of Kenneth Brinkhous (*p.283*) in Chapel Hill NC, demonstrated that low-temperature high-speed centrifugation produced plasma with a progressively longer clotting time, proportional to the reduction in platelets. Simon van Creveld (1894-1971) in Amsterdam NL separated a fraction with an anti-heparin effect from platelet extracts, which he called "platelet factor" in 1951. This turned out to be "platelet factor 3", present in all cells; when made available by platelets, it acted as a central event for blood coagulation. This protein factor, encoded by the *F3* gene on chromosome 1 (1995), can be recognized by monoclonal antibodies

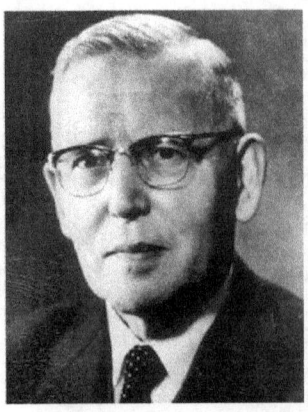

Simon van Creveld

(CD142). It initiates thrombin formation from the proenzyme prothrombin. Platelet agonists, such as thrombin, collagen, and epinephrine were shown to release ADP from platelet dense granules; collagen-induced platelet aggregation was shown to be mediated by either ADP or thromboxane A_2 (TxA_2). Alan Nurden and Jacques Caen (b.1927) in Paris found glycoprotein IIb/IIIa, now known as integrin $\alpha_{IIb}\beta_3$, on platelets in 1974. Binding of these receptors leads to a cascade of events resulting in an increase in intracellular calcium. Platelet activation by ADP leads to changes in the platelet gpIIb/IIIa receptors that induce binding to fibrinogen (1999). Many platelets then stick together resulting in a clot. The coagulation cascade follows to stabilize the clot, as thrombin converts the soluble fibrinogen into insoluble fibrin strands. In 1994, the humoral substance responsible for causing the platelet count to rise was purified and cloned as thrombopoietin (TPO). This again led to the development of pharmaceutical TPO mimetics.

HEREDITARY PLATELET DISORDERS

Glanzmann's Thrombasthenia

Eduard Glanzmann (1887-1959), a Swiss pediatrician who was doing postgraduate work at the Charité in Berlin, noted in 1918 that some of his patients had many symptoms of thrombocytopenic purpura (mucocutaneous bleeding), but normal platelet counts . Their bleeding times were longer than normal and their blood did not show normal clot retraction. He concluded that the patients had defective platelets. In the following decades, clinical observations of the few patients who were diagnosed, revealed that the disease was probably inherited in an autosomal recessive manner, but could also occur as an autoimmune disease (Barry Coller, b.1944; 1986). The clinical manifestations varied from mild to fatal.

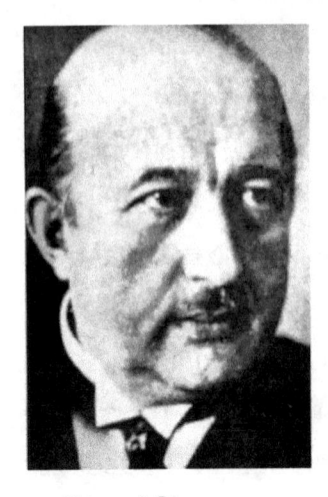

Eduard Glanzmann

Heterozygotes were asymptomatic. Clusters of patients with thrombasthenia were found in France, India, among Iraqi Jews, and among Arabs in Israel and Jordan (Coller, 1986). Various gene mutations (now >100!) have been detected. A major advance was when Alan Nurden and Jacques Caen demonstrated in 1974 that the platelets in this disease contain defective or low levels of gpIIb/IIIa, the receptor for fibrinogen. As a result, no fibrinogen bridging of platelets to other platelets occurred and the bleeding

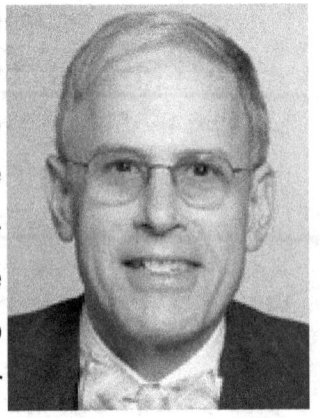

Barry Coller

time was significantly prolonged. Even before that receptor discovery, the introduction of the aggregometer had allowed the study of thrombasthenia platelets. It was shown that the aggregation induced by ADP, collagen, and epinephrine was markedly decreased. The therapy of thrombasthenia consisted of topical therapy (gelfoam, good dental hygiene, *etc.*), platelet transfusions in case of heavy bleeding, ε-aminocaproic acid, or recombinant factor VIIa. In some patients desmopressin was effective, even though their bleeding times were not normalized; this drug can also counteract anti-platelet agents (2016).

Von Willebrand's disease

Erik Adolf von Willebrand (1870-1949) was a Swedish speaking Finn at the University of Helsinki. He was consulted in 1924 on a young girl with a bleeding disorder. He reported in 1926, that the disease was different from hemophilia since it occurred in both sexes. The disease, soon named after him, appeared in successive generations on the Finnish Åland islands. The disease was autosomal dominant. The patients had a long bleeding time. George Minot (*p.90*) reported a similar case two years later. Von Willebrand thought that the long bleeding time reflected a defect in the platelets, but Robert Macfarlane (1907-1987) in England and Armand Quick (*p.45*) in the USA thought, in the early 1940's, that the disorder was due to a vascular abnormality. In 1953, several groups reported similar patients who also had a deficient titer of antihemophilic factor. Margaret Howard and Barry Firkin in Melbourne AU showed in 1971 that the antibiotic ristocetin causes clumping

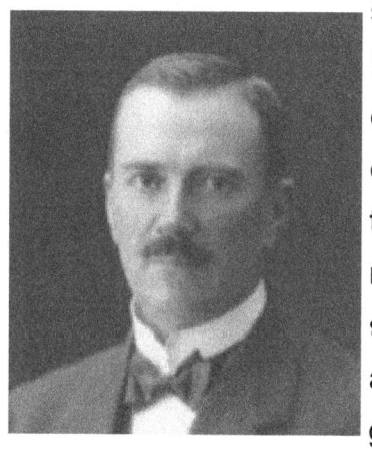

Erik von Willebrand

of normal platelets, but not of platelets from Von Willebrand's patients . Platelet aggregation after ADP, collagen, and epinephrine was normal, but decreased after ristocetin. Inga Marie Nilsson (1923-1999) and colleagues in Malmö SW detected in 1960, that transfusion of normal plasma was followed, several hours later, by an increase in the titer of antihemophilic factor to levels much higher than expected. Harvey Weiss (b.1929) and Leon Hoyer in New York isolated the Von Willebrand Factor (VWF) in 1973, and it was later identified as a 2,050-amino acid monomer with several different domains. For example, one domain binds to factor VIII, another to the platelet GP1b-receptor, heparin, and possibly collagen. Multimers are the functional units and can be extremely large (>20,000 kDa). The VWF was located on the short arm of chromosome 12. In 2008, a new diagnostic category of "low VWF" was introduced, with levels higher than Von Willebrand's disease, but sometimes still with bleeding episodes. In addition to the plasma-type Von Willebrand's disease, a platelet type has also been recognized. In this autosomal-dominant genetic defect, VWF is qualitatively normal, but the GP1b receptor of the platelet membrane is altered which increases the binding of VWF. Large platelet aggregates are removed from the circulation resulting in thrombocytopenia. Desmopressin (intranasal or intravenous) was found to stimulate the release

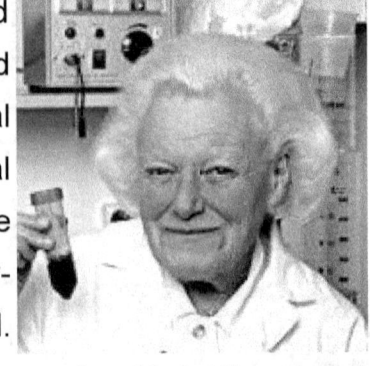

Inga Marie Nilsson

of VWF from endothelial cells. Human-derived factor VIII concentrates, which also contain VWF, can be used for bleeding or surgery. A recombinant VWF was approved by the FDA in 2015 and in Europe (EMA) in 2018.

Giant platelet disorders

Bernard-Soulier syndrome. In 1948, Jean Bernard (*p.169*) and Jean-Pierre Soulier (1915-2003) in Paris described a young man with a prolonged bleeding time, a low platelet count and very large platelets (*macrothrombocytopenia*). They called it "*dystrophie thrombocytaire-hémorragipare congénitale*". Rare additional cases were reported, and the clinical manifestations usually were epistaxis and gingival bleeding occurring in early childhood. Later also menorrhagia or even gastrointestinal bleeding. It was shown to be an autosomal recessive genetic disorder with a prevalence of <1 per 1,000,000 people. Platelet aggregation is normal after ADP, collagen, and epinephrine as agonists, but decreased after ristocetin. The disease was shown to be caused by one of several (47?) mutations in three genes (17p12, 22q11.2, 3q29 and 3q21) responsible for the multi-subunit nature of the affected GP1b-V-IX receptor. Therapy consisted of topical measures, and platelet transfusions for surgery or severe bleeding.

May-Hegglin anomaly was named after the German physician Richard May (1863-1936), who saw the anomaly in 1909, and Swiss physician Robert Hegglin (1907-1969) who saw the same anomaly in 1945. The platelets were abnormally large, and the leukocytes had small rods (Döhle-like bodies) in their cytoplasm. Döhle bodies, named after Karl Döhle (1855-1928), who saw them in 1892, are often present in conjunction with toxic granulation (infection, burns, leukemoid reaction). The anomaly is probably associated with the *MYH9* gene on chromosome 22q12.3 that is responsible for the production of the myosin-9 protein. Treatment consisted of tranexamic acid or desmopressin.

ACQUIRED PLATELET DISORDERS

Idiopathic thrombocytopenic purpura (ITP)

The first description of acquired purpura probably came from Amato Lusitano (1511-1568), a Marrano physician born in Castelo Branco PT as João Rodrigues. Fear of the Inquisition made him travel and work all over Europe, until he ultimately landed in Salonica (now Thessaloniki GR), where the Ottoman Empire was a safe haven for Jews. The disease was named after Paul Gottlieb Werlhof (1699-1767), who

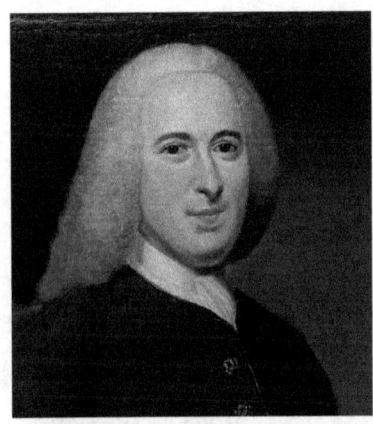

Paul Werlhof

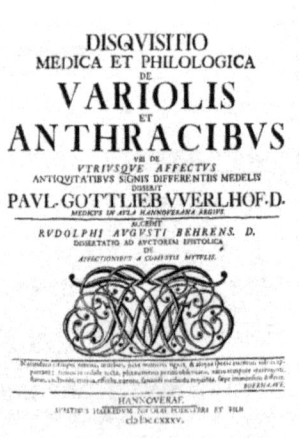

Werlhof's publicatiom

practiced in Hanover GE. He described the disease in two young girls in a paper of 1735, even though platelets were still unknown. His *"morbus maculosus haemorrhagicus"* was not linked to platelets until one year after Bizzozero had published his monograph in 1882: Brohm in Germany made the link between low platelets and purpura in 1883. Similar observations were made by Denys in Louvain BE in 1887. The disease, reported both in children and adults, was now well documented as ITP, but few improvements in pathophysiology and therapy were made. It was shown that the bone marrow had normal or increased megakaryopoiesis, and that the disease could occur rather suddenly. Whereas many cases were mild, fatal cases could occur when the platelet count was very low (<5,000/mm^3?). With platelet counts >20,000/mm^3, serious bleeding was unusual. Ernest Frank in Germany suggested in 1915, that decreased production of platelets was responsible for ITP, perhaps caused by a toxin. On the other hand, the first successful therapy was the splenectomy reported by Paul Kaznelson (1898-1959) from Poland in a medical journal in Vienna AT in 1916. He was still a medical student in Prague CZ; he observed the improvement of a young woman with chronic purpura treated with splenectomy. He interpreted that the spleen had been the graveyard of the platelets. Maxwell Wintrobe and his colleagues in Salt Lake City UT reported on the beneficial effect of injections with ACTH on platelet counts and symptoms in a patient with ITP in 1950 . The next year, William Harrington (1924-1992) in St Louis MO observed a child with transient purpura, born to a mother with ITP. He suspected that the passage of a humoral factor from mother to child was responsible for platelet destruction. He infused himself with the plasma of a patient with ITP in 1950. Within three hours, his platelets dropped to dangerously low levels and remained there for 4 days. This *Harrington-Hollingsworth experiment* demonstrated that a circulating factor was responsible for the low platelets.

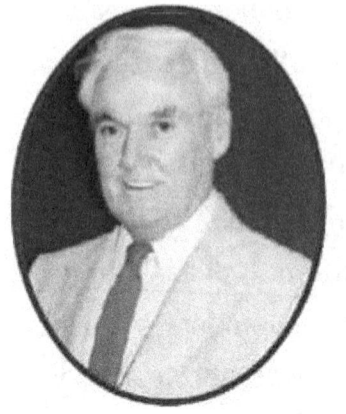

Bill Harrington

Robert Evans and colleagues in San Francisco CA, who described the combination of ITP and Coombs-positive hemolytic anemia in 1951, concluded that both had an immune genesis, paving the way to immunosuppressants as effective treatment. That changed the name ITP from "*idiopathic thrombocytopenic purpura*" to "*immune thrombocytopenic purpura*". Additional studies showed that the circulating factor was a collection of immunoglobulins. These antibodies could be directed against thrombopoietin (2001) or against platelet-specific receptors (2005). Most of the antibodies were of IgG class and directed against GpIIb/IIIa or GpIb-IX. The coating of platelets rendered them susceptible to opsonization and phagocytosis by splenic macrophages and/or liver Kuppfer cells. Platelet-kinetics studies in the 1980's suggested that decreased production in the bone marrow may be a factor in some cases of ITP.

Following the early studies with ACTH injections in

1950, corticosteroids became first-line treatment of ITP. A randomized study in children was done by Jörg Sartorius in Switzerland in 1972. Because of his untimely death, the study was not published until 1983. Most patients responded to steroids, but tapering the dose could result in a relapse of the symptoms. For some years, treatment with Rho(D) globulin was recommended for Rh-positive patients with functional spleens. This led to destruction of red cells and leaving the Fcγ receptor of macrophages saturated (Salama, 1984). This effect could also be accomplished with intravenous immunoglobulin, without the risk of hemolysis (1981). For emergency use (*e.g.*, surgery) i.v. immunoglobulin works fast. Various immunosuppressants have been used. Splenectomy is effective, but recommended mainly for patients who have relapsed frequently. The use of rituximab to avoid splenectomy had its own drawbacks (2008). Thrombopoietic agonists (romiplostim, elthrombopag) would stimulate the production of platelets, not decrease their destruction (2006).

Thrombotic Thrombocytopenic Purpura (TTP)

In 1924, Eli Moschcowitz (1879-1964) in New York (Beth Israel Hospital) reported on a 16-year-old girl, who presented with anemia, small and large bruises, microscopic hematuria, fever and, at autopsy, disseminated intravascular thrombi. Cases of what became called "Moschcowitz disease" were

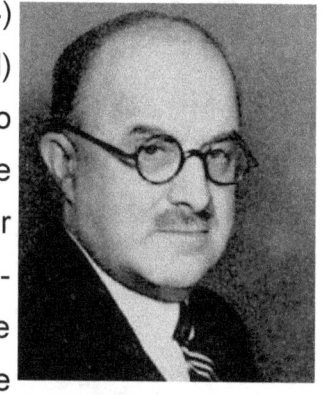

Eli Moschcowitz

reported over the years, and in 1966 John Ultmann (1925-2000)'s group in Chicago wrote a 20-page review of about 270 cases of, what they now called, *thrombotic thrombocytopenic purpura (TTP)* in the journal *Medicine.* The syndrome consisted of thrombocytopenia, micro-angiopathic hemolytic anemia, fever and mostly neurological and renal impairment. The mortality was 90%! A close connection with hemolytic uremic syndrome (HUS) existed. The incidence was about 5 per million per year. The causes were multiple. A genetic variant became known as the *Upshaw-Shulman syndrome*, reported by Lawrence Shulman in 1960 and Jefferson Upshaw in 1978. The auto-immune variant was more difficult to pinpoint. It had already been assumed for years that a missing factor in the blood was the cause of the syndrome, and several case reports showed that blood transfusion had been beneficial; the first ones were reported by Moschcowitz in 1925. Then in 1978, Jefferson Upshaw showed that in a child with "his syndrome", whom he had followed for 11 years, the 32 episodes she had experienced, responded well to plasma infusions. The episodes had been precipitated by infections, surgery, childbirth *etc.* Plasma infusions proved also useful in other patients with TTP. In 1982, Moake and colleagues of Baylor in Houston TX reported a link of Von Willebrand's disease and TTP. They found unusually large or "ultralarge" VWF multimers in

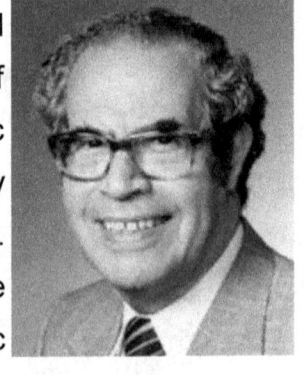

John Ultmann

chronic relapsing TTP, and they proposed that the patients lacked a VWF depolymerase, possibly a protease, that normally would cleave ultra-large VWF, to prevent it from causing intravascular platelet aggregation and thrombosis. Plasma infusions would replace the depolymerase or remove an inciting cofactor. In 1996, a candidate VWF-cleaving protease was identified in human plasma by Han-Mou Tsai in New York, and independently by Miha Furlan and coworkers in Bern SU. The VWF-cleaving protease was shown to be missing from the blood of congenital TTP, and inhibited by

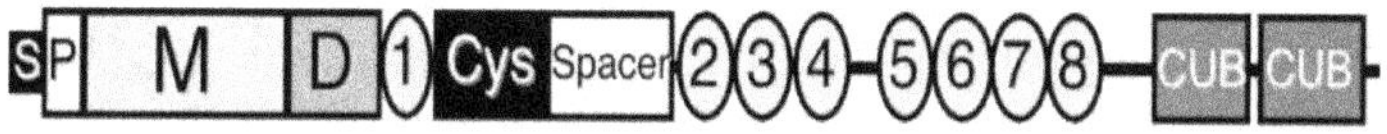

Figure 1. Structure of ADAMTS13. The primary translation product consists of 1427 amino acid residues. Motifs include a signal peptide (S), propeptide (P), metalloprotease (M), disintegrin (D), Cys-rich, spacer, CUB, and thrombospondin (TSP1) domains (1-8).

IgG autoantibodies in patients with acquired TTP. The protease was purified, cloned (2001) and named ADAMTS13 (1999). The name came from "*a d*isintegrin-like *a*nd *m*etalloprotease with *t*hrombo*s*pondin repeats". Mutations in the ADAMTS13 gene were shown to cause congenital TTP. The inhibition of ADAMTS13 was considered the underlying mechanism of TTP, and leads to an increase in circulating VWF multimers. Increased platelet adhesion to areas of endothelial injury, particularly where arterioles and capillaries

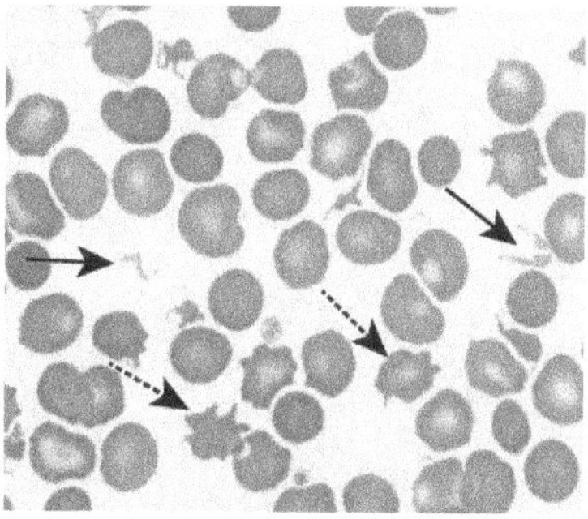

Schistocytes

meet, leads to small platelets clots. Red cells passing the microscopic clots are subjected to shear stress, which damages their membranes and leads to schistocyte formation. The clots lead to end-organ damage (brain, kidney *etc.*). Although plasma infusions were of value, in the early 1990's plasmapheresis was shown to be superior. Immunosuppression with corticosteroids was recommended to decrease the number of days that plasmapheresis was needed.

Rituximab, by killing the B lymphocytes that produce the autoantibody, was found to help in cases failing to respond to steroids and plasmapheresis. In 2019, caplacizumab-yhdp (Cablivi®) was approved. This humanized monoclonal antibody reduces the platelets binding to VWF, preventing blood clots. Monitoring the disease involved following the schistocytes and the LDH (lactate dehydrogenase) levels in the peripheral blood. With appropriate and prompt therapy the survival rate should now be >80%. James George (b.1937)'s group in Oklahoma City has been prominent in establishing guidelines for the therapy of both TTP and ITP.

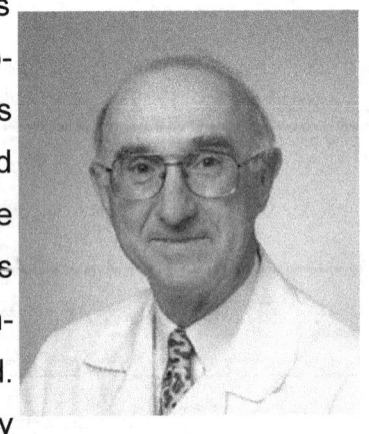

Jim George

COAGULATION

Plato (ca.425-348 BCE), in his dialogue Τιμαιος (Timaeus), thought that blood contained fibers that caused it to congeal when it left the warmth of the body. His pupil Aristotle (384-322 BCE) believed that those fibers were composed of earth and were solid; blood from which the fibers were removed, would not solidify. Little happened until the 17th century, when Marcello Malpighi (*p.24*) in Italy washed clotted blood to remove the red cells, and was left with the fibrous strands. Under the microscope they looked like a "network of nerve-like threads". William Hewson (*p.25*) localized the source of the fibers to the "coagulable lymph", which we now call plasma. He also found that cooling blood slowed the clotting process, contrary to Plato's opinion. Hewson believed that exposure to air made the blood clot. John Hunter (1728-1793) in London, however, showed that blood also clotted in a vacuum. In his posthumous *A treatise on the blood, inflammation and gun-shot wounds* of 1817, he reported that blood clotted most readily "round the edge of the dish which it contained". He believed that coagulation was due to a "vital principle" in blood. This concept was supported by Charles Thackrah (*p.30*) in 1819 and by many others. Thackrah also confirmed Hewson's view that blood

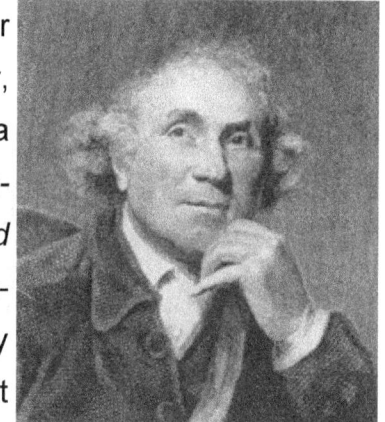

John Hunter

clotted very slowly in rest, by studying coagulation in a segment of vein between two ligatures. Rudolf Virchow (p.168) demonstrated that blood clotted rapidly when a drop of mercury was introduced, demonstrating that the roughness of surfaces was not necessary for clotting to start.

Johannes Müller (1801-1858) in Berlin described fibrin, the substance of a thrombus, in 1837. The early authors thought that insoluble fibrin existed in the circulating blood and that coagulation was a gelation of the preexisting fibrin. Benjamin Babington (1794-1866) in Cambridge UK, had suggested in 1830, that fibrin formed from a precursor that was later called *fibrinogen* by Virchow (1856), and was chemically isolated by Prosper Denis de Commercy in Toul FR (1799-1863). Where the fibrinogen originated was not clear (red cells? leukocytes? albumin?) until the earty 20th century, when Olaf Hammersten (1841-1932) in Uppsala SW isolated it from plasma in 1911. It had already been known then for about a decade that the liver was the source of fibrinogen. In 1892, Alexander Schmidt (1831-1894) in Dorpat (now Tartu ES) identified an enzyme in fresh plasma that forms fibrin out of fibrinogen; he called it "fibrin ferment" and later *thrombin*. He realized that the thrombin also needed to come from a precursor. Two years later, Cornelius Pekelharing (1848-1922) in Utrecht NL named that precursor *prothrombin*. The source of prothrombin was not completely

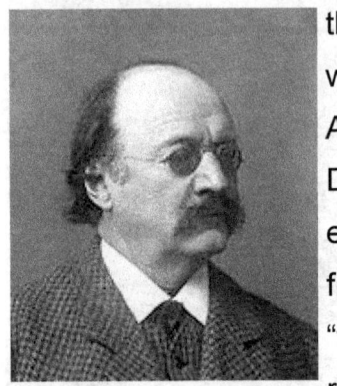

Alexander Schmidt

solved, until Harry Smith (1895-1972)'s group in Iowa City IA determined in 1936 that the liver produced prothrombin. Immunologist Jules Bordet (1870-1961) in Brussels BE started the purification of the enzymes in 1921, and biochemist Walter Seegers (1910-1996) finished it in Detroit MI in 1962. Thrombin proved to be a proteolytic enzyme that severs several small fragments off fibrinogen. What remains was the fibrin monomer. The monomers join by aggregation to form the insoluble fibers of the clot. Although calcium ions were not necessary for this coagulation, they definitely accelerated fibrin formation.

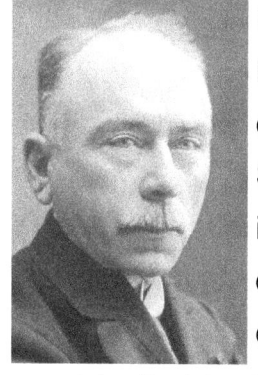

Jules Bordet

Zoologist Henri de Blainville (1777-1850) in Paris reported at a meeting in 1832, that the intravenous injection of a suspension of brain tissue was immediately fatal, by clotting off the animal's blood vessels. This was confirmed by Andrew Buchanan (1798-1882) in Glasgow UK in 1845, and it was extensively studied for the rest of the 19th century. Alexander Schmidt assumed that tissue was a "zymoplastic", *i.e.*, an enzyme-forming substance, to convert prothrombin into thrombin. Paul Morawitz (1879-1936) in Tübingen GE confirmed in 1905 that the tissue extracts did not clot fibrinogen directly, but rather by changing prothrombin to thrombin. He called Schmidt's

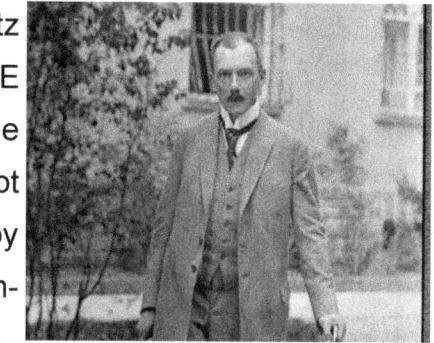

Paul Morawitz

zymoplastic substance *thrombokinase*. Other names were *tissue factor* (1935) and *thromboplastin* (1938). The thromboplastin was dependent upon calcium salts, and found to consist of phospholipoproteins (1944). Paul Morawitz proposed the coagulation pathway that is now called the *extrinsic pathway*. Despite many other theories, Morawitz' classic concept survived. Major developments occurred around 1940, when the technology had improved. The group of Harry Smith in Iowa devised a two-stage assay for measuring prothrombin in plasma. Prothrombin was converted to thrombin by the *in-vitro* addition of tissue thromboplastin and calcium, and then the generated thrombin was quantified. Armand Quick in New York introduced a one-stage assay named after him, the PT (*p.45*). This test became of great importance for the study of liver disease and for the dosing of oral anticoagulant agents. The results of the two-stage and one-stage tests were sometimes discordant, such as in early infancy and when blood was stored at 4°C. This suggested that the conversion of prothrombin to thrombin was dependent upon additional plasma agents. This led to the discovery of these additional clotting factors.

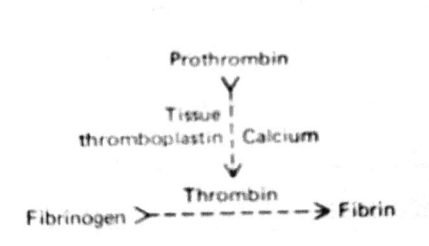

Quick showed in 1943 that an agent in plasma corrected the prolonged PT of oxalated plasma stored in the refrigerator: the *labile factor*. Paul Owren, during World War

II in Norway, observed a woman with a life-long bleeding tendency. Her PT was long, but was corrected by prothrombin-depleted plasma. He called the substance *factor V.* (fibrinogen, prothrombin, thromboplastin, and calcium being the first four). An alternative name was *proaccelerin.* In 1947, Owren showed that another factor was necessary for tissue thromboplastin to change prothrombin to thrombin. This became *factor VII* (*Factor VI* remained unassigned). Then in the mid 1950's, groups in Chapel Hill NC and London, based on two patients with prolonged PT, found a needed factor that was not factor VII. This factor could also be supplied by the venom of Russell's viper. The factor was named after the patients: the Stuart(-Prower) factor (factor X). Factors VII and X were rapidly purified. Both are synthesized in the liver, and their genes are located on chromosome 13. Factor VII became available in a recombinant form (eptacog alfa; Novoseven®) in 1999, and factor X has been available as a concentrate since 2015. Factors VII and X both need vitamin K for their synthesis. Vitamin K had been discovered around 1930, when chickens that were fed an ether-extracted diet started bleeding: "Koagulations-Vitamin". The defect in vitamin-K deficient chicks was soon attributed to a prothrombin deficiency. Later studies also associated vitamin K with factor VII, Stuart factor, Christmas factor (Factor IX) and proteins C and S. The vitamin was formally synthesized in 1939.

In 1922, Canadian veterinarian Frank Schofield (1889-1970) discovered that a hemorrhagic disease in cattle was caused by a clotting defect, associated with the feeding of spoiled sweet clover. During the Great Depression, farmer Ed Carson in Wisconsin was forced to feed his cattle spoiled sweet clover. When a cow died, he transported the dead cow, a milk can containing incoagulable blood, and a lot of spoiled sweet clover to the University of Wisconsin in Madison. The biochemist Karl Paul Link (1901-1978) identified the toxic component of the clover as bishydroxycoumarin (Dicumarol). This led to warfarin (**W**isconsin **A**lumni **Re**search **F**oundation), better known as coumadin (1954). In the absence of vitamin K, post-translational carboxylation of the prothrombin precursor does not occur, leading to an abnormal and non-functional prothrombin variant: PIVKA-II (**P**rotein **I**nduced by **V**itamin **K** **A**bsence/**A**gonist-II).

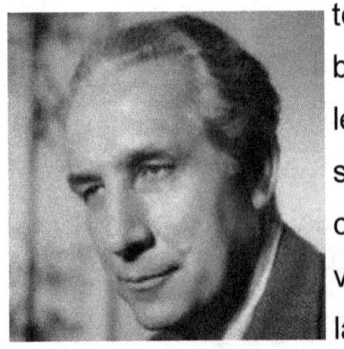

Karl Paul Link

In 1842, Jones in England wondered why the circulating blood did not coagulate? Joseph Lister (1827-1912) in Glasgow UK, not a great surgeon but pivotal for his antisepsis work, found that blood remained partially fluid for several hours in a vulcanized Indian-rubber tube in 1863. He concluded that blood clotted after contact with certain, but not all, surfaces. The lining cells of blood vessels were perhaps non-coagulant? Hayem and Bizzozero both had claimed that platelets were necessary for clotting, but cell-depleted plasma also clotted. Morawitz held thromboplastic substances responsible for this, and in the late 1930's, several investigators (*e.g.*, Jules Bordet) developed the view that plasma itself contained all the factors needed for coagulation and could provide a "thromboplastin" to initiate the process.

Lockard Conley (1915-2010) at Johns Hopkins demonstrated in 1949, that normal plasma (inside silicone coated tubes) remained liquid indefinitely, but clotted quickly when exposed to glass. Haskell Milstone in New Haven CT suggested in the late 1940's, that the conversion of prothrombin to thrombin was brought about by a "thrombokinase complex" derived during clotting from a "prothrombokinase complex". This precursor complex was supposedly composed of tissue, platelet factors, and plasma agents such as phospholipids, antihemophilic factor (factor VIII), proaccelerin (factor V), and proconvertin (factor VII).

The events through which glass initiates coagulation in plasma, is now considered the *intrinsic pathway* of thrombin formation, described as a cascade (Oscar Ratnoff) or waterfall (Robert Macfarlane 1907-1987; Oxford UK). The study of this cascade was made possible by the *thromboplastin-generation test* of Rosemary Biggs (1912-2001) and Stuart Douglas(1921-1998) in Oxford UK in 1953, and simultaneously by Kenneth Brinkhous' group in Chapel Hill NC as the *partial thromboplastin time (PTT)* (p.45).

The plasma factor that was activated by contact with glass was named in 1955 after John Hageman,

Rosemary Biggs

a railroad-brake man, who was found to have too slowly

clotting blood before surgery. His diagnosis was made by Oscar Ratnoff (1916-2008) in Cleveland OH. The autosomal recessive Hageman-factor deficiency could be corrected by the factor (now called factor XII) that remained after all known clotting factors had been removed from plasma. The factor was purified in 1962. Three years later, it was shown that the Hageman factor had to be activated by "warping" to a clot-promoting form. Tannins and the bark of plants (in ancient Egypt and Greece!) could activate the Hageman factor. The activated Hageman factor would mediate the activation of *plasma thromboplastin antecedent (PTA, factor XI)*, as documented by the Oxford UK group in 1956, and by Leo Vroman (1915-2014), a biologist and poet in Utrecht NL, in 1958. PTA deficiency is an autosomal recessive disorder, more frequently found in Ashkenazi Jews and in Japanese. It turned out to be a serine protease of 596 amino acids encoded by a gene on chromosome 13. Activated Hageman factor also caused the release of small fragments of protein, *kinins*, from its precursors in plasma, the *kininogens*. Joel Margolis in Oxford UK proposed in 1956, that the activated Hageman factor changed a plasma enzyme *kallikrein* to an active form. The latter would bring about the release of kinins from kininogens. Other investigators supported this concept.

In 1965, William Hathaway (b. 1929) and colleagues

in Lexington KY, studied members of the Fletcher family. Four children had abnormal blood clotting, but no clinical evidence of bleeding. Their Fletcher trait, and several similar traits reported by other centers under different names, was based on an as yet unknown factor, that turned out to be prekallikrein as detected in 1975.

The issue of hemophilia was already mentioned in the Introduction (*p.4*), and will be discussed again later (*p.274*). For now, it is mainly important that Georges Hayem had already suggested that hemophilia was due to a defect in blood clotting. Almroth Wright (1861-1947) in London observed in 1893 that the clotting time in hemophilia was abnormally long. The same year, Von Manteuffel in Germany found that tissue extracts (the *zymoplastic substance* of his teacher Alexander Schmidt) shortened the clotting time of hemophilic blood. Thomas Addis (1881-1949) in Edinburgh UK suggested in 1911 that the conversion of prothrombin to thrombin was impaired in hemophilia. The discussion whether the defect in hemophilia was localized in plasma or in platelets, occupied the first 30 years of the 20th century, until in 1937 Arthur Patek and colleagues at Harvard University demonstrated that the addition of normal plasma corrected the defect in hemophilic plasma. They produced a crude fraction of normal plasma that corrected hemophilic plasma. It took until 1979, before Edward Tuddenham (b.1944) in London purified factor VIII. It turned

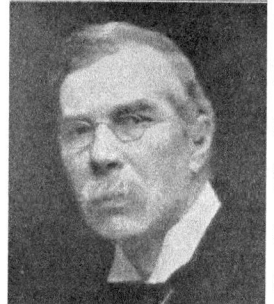

Almroth Wright

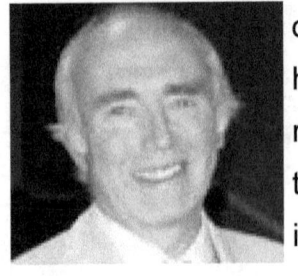

out to consist of six domains, and to be homologous to factor V. The A domains resemble those of ceruloplasmin. Activation of factor VIII is done by cleavage into two protein chains. Factor VIII is a glycoprotein pro-cofactor, synthesized by endothelium and the sinusoidal cells of the liver. It circulates in a stable non-covalent complex with VWF. The *F8* gene is located on the X chromosome. Upon activation by thrombin, it dissociates from VWF and interacts with factor IXa to activate factor X.

Edward Tuddenham

Alfredo Pavlovsky (1907-1984) and his colleagues in Buenos Aires AG observed in 1944 that the blood of two hemophiliacs seemed to be mutually corrective in the test tube. In one case, transfusion of plasma from one corrected the clotting time of the other. Then in 1952, two papers described patients with a hemophilia-like syndrome, but with a deficiency different from anti-hemophilia factor. Later that same year, Rosemary Biggs and colleagues reported it as Christmas factor, after a patient Stephen Christmas, and published this as close to Christmas as possible (*p.122*). Christmas factor became factor IX. The numbering of the clotting factors in Roman numerals was decided by consensus in 1962 and represented the sequence of reporting. Factor IX is synthesized in the liver and requires vitamin K. The gene was cloned in 1982 by biochemist Earl

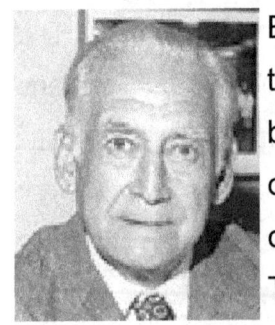

Alfredo Pavlovsky

Davie (1927-2020) in Seattle WA and found to be on the X chromosome. The final steps of the intrinsic pathway cascade involve thrombin greatly enhancing the functional activity of factor VIII and factor V. Thrombin also brings about the clumping of platelets, thus furnishing the bulk of the phospholipids required for the intrinsic pathway, via Van Creveld's *platelet factor 3*.

With so many factors involved with clotting, why does blood still circulate? Alexander Schmidt suggested that the fluidity of blood was maintained by the presence of inhibitors of clotting, which he believed were derived from tissues. Several investigators around 1930 (*e.g.*, William Howell (1860-1945) at Johns Hopkins) hypothesized that clotting was a consequence of the removal of the inhibition. This theory was not validated, and later studies showed that the effects of thrombin, the enzyme ultimately responsible for the formation of the clot, are limited. That had already been suggested in 1905 by Morawitz, when he observed that fibrin itself removed thrombin from the surrounding plasma. He also suggested that the plasma had antithrombin properties. After some confusion, Walter Seegers in Detroit MI documented that the inhibitor of thrombin in plasma was a specific protein, which he called antithrombin III. The nature of

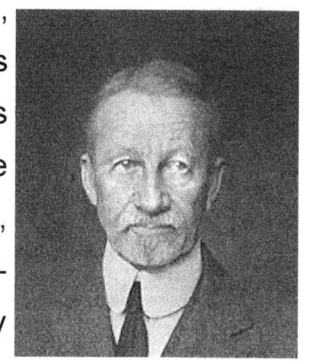

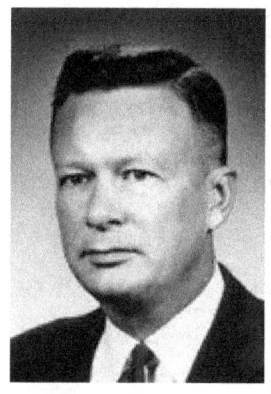

William Howell

Walter Seegers

antithrombin III had waited for the discovery of heparin by Jay McLean (1890-1957) at Johns Hopkins in 1916. He studied a crude fraction of hepatic tissue that showed a "marked power to inhibit coagulation". His mentor Howell called it *heparin*. It turned out to be a complex sugar, elucidated by Erik Jorpes (1894-1973) in Stockholm SW in 1936. He localized it in the mast cells of tissues. Heparin does not inhibit thrombin in the absence of antithrombin III. Several groups showed that antithrombin III is an even more potent inhibitor of the formation of thrombin than of thrombin itself. Heparin was used clinically for the first time in 1937. Antithrombin III is a glycoprotein of 432 amino acids produced by the liver. Its gene is located on chromosome 1. A recombinant antithrombin was produced in 1987 and approved in 1989. Additional inhibitors (*e.g.*, C1 inactivator) were isolated and were capable of neutralizing activated clotting factors.

Once a clot has been formed, it needs to be dissolved. Gabriel Andral in Paris believed that during the dissolution, the plasma would contain less clotting material (fibrinogen was not described until 12 years later by Virchow!) than usual in 1844. John Hunter had already reported in 1811, that some postmortem blood was fluid, particularly in people who had died suddenly (*e.g.*, anger or lightning). Morawitz attributed this to the plasma's intrinsic proteolytic activity. Albert Dastre (1844-1917) in Paris introduced the term *fibrinolysis* in 1893, when he observed that fibrin was digested by serum. Sven Gustav Hedin in London located this proteolytic activity in the ox to a crude fraction of serum in 1903. *Plasmin*, a serine protease different from trypsin, is released by the liver as plasminogen. In addition to fibrinolysis, the enzyme is also important in the complement system and in inflammation. It cleaves fibrin, fibronectin, and VWF. Plasminogen was purified in the early 1940's (Millstone in New Haven CT). The production of plasminogen is regulated by the *PLG* gene on chromosome 6. Plasminogen is activated by a serine protease of 527 amino-acids produced by endothelial cells, the *tissue plasminogen activator* (t-PA). In the late 1970's, purification was completed. The fibrin specificity of t-PA was stressed and the basis was laid for the use of t-PA as fibrinolytic agent. The gene for t-PA is located on chromosome 8. The clinical studies started in the early 1980's, in acute myocardial infarction and renal-vein thrombosis. T-PA was cloned in 1982 and it became commercially available as Activase® or Actlyse®. The drug was approved for ischemic-stroke treatment in 1996.

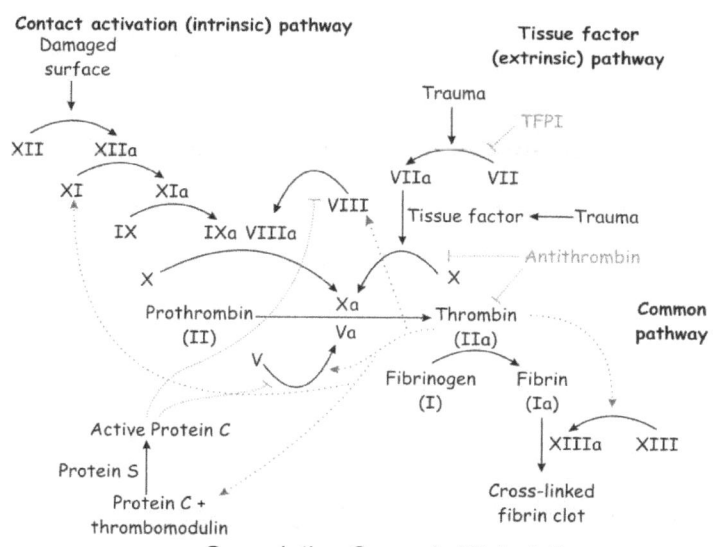

Coagulation Cascade/Waterfall

Bleeding disorders

Hemophilia

As mentioned in the Introduction *(p.4)*, the Babylonian Talmud, written in the 6th century, indicated that by the end of the 2nd century, the risks of circumcision in babies with a bleeding disorder were already known. In the 10th century, the Moorish surgeon Abu-'l' Qasim Khalaf Ibn 'Abbis al-Zarawi (also known as Albucasis) in Cordoba SP described a village where many males bled severely after a trivial injury. During the Middle Ages, scattered reports of males with severe life-long bleeding were reported. In 1791, a newspaper reported on a man who had hemophilic sons by one woman, but healthy sons by another. The first "modern" report came from John Otto in Philadelphia PA *(p.5)* in 1803. He used the common English term "bleeders". This report stirred increased interest in the problem. Christian Friedrich Nasse (1778-1851) in Bonn GE formalized the observations of John Otto and John Hay (Boston MA; 1813) about the heredity of hemophilia in Nasse's law: *hemophilia occurs only in males, but is transmitted through females.* John Hay had shown that the daughter of a hemophiliac could transmit the disorders to her sons. Friedrich Hopff and his professor Johann Lukas Schönlein (1793-1864) in Zürich SU, named the disease *haemorrhaphilia* in 1828, later shortened to *haemophilia*. Although some earlier studies had reported hemophilia also in occasional women, a review in 1911 of about 1,000 cases and 224 pedigrees, could not find a single authentic case of hemophilia in a female. The sex-linked inheritance of a hemophilia-like disease in Queen Victoria's descendants (*the Royal Disease*) became the fascination of physicians and non-physicians alike; it had a dramatic effect on political changes in Russia.

The inheritance pattern was explained when the gene theory of heredity was established (*p.35*), and inheritance through the X-chromosome was determined: *hemizygous state* (*p.82*). As described before (*p.269*), the clotting defects in hemophilia were detected and factor VIII (hemophilia A), factor IX (hemophilia B, Christmas factor) and Von Willebrand factor (*p.251*) were identified. Hemophilias A and B were clinically indistinguishable and occurred in mild, moderate, or severe forms (plasma factor levels 6-30%, 2-5%, and ≤1%, respectively). The prevalence of hemophilia A is about 1 in 10,000 and of hemophilia B 1 in 50,000 with no significant racial differences.

Purification of factor VIII (AHF) to biochemical homogeneity remained elusive through the 1970's. In 1964, two important developments occurred. Ken Brinkhous' group in Chapel Hill NC was able to separate antihemophilic factor (AHF) from plasma by precipitation with neutral amino acids. Judith Graham Pool (1919-1975) of Stanford (Palo Alto CA), serendipitously discovered that a large proportion of AHF was present in "cryoprecipitate", the fraction that

Judith Pool

remained insoluble after fresh-frozen plasma was allowed to thaw at 4°C. Both preparations could be lyophilized. This dramatically changed the quality of life of patients with hemophilia A. They could now self-administer the cryoprecipitate, and even use the material prophylactically. The 1970's were a gratifying example of a chronic disease that now could be treated/prevented. Two problems arose, though. The first was that about 20% of the patients became refractory to therapy, because of the appearance of inhibitors of *(= alloantibodies against)* AHF. Non-AHF treatments became available (see below) and attempts to build tolerance through repeated exposure to the antigen were successful. Brackmann in Bonn GE and Van Leeuwen and colleagues in Utrecht NL, both in 1986, were capable of making the patient inhibitor-free over a time span of 1-3 years.

The second problem was even more dangerous. Commercial interests led to pooled cryoprecipitate from thousands of donors; these enormous pools could more easily contain viruses not (yet?) detected by testing. In the early 1980's, 60-70% of US patients with severe hemophilia A became infected with HIV. We experienced the 1984-1990 Ryan White story from very up-close in Indiana. Both Baxter International and Bayer pharmaceutical companies sparked controversy by the forced withdrawal of the unheated product from the US markets, but still selling it to other countries. Countries where the cryoprecipitate was produced by local blood banks had much lower infection rates. Attempts were made to select very low-risk donors and PCR-based virus detection were introduced and became mandatory in Europe in 1999. Virucidal methods were introduced: "dry heating", pasteurization, nanofiltration and detergents.

For patients with mild hemophilia A, desmopressin, a synthetic derivative of anti-diuretic hormone (ADH), could increase the level of factor VIII in hemophilia A and in Von Willebrand disease, as shown by Pier Mannucci in Milan IT in 1977. In 1984, factor VIII was cloned by several groups and recombinant factors VIII (*e.g.*, Recombinate® by Bayer) went into clinical trial in 1987. The recombinant factor VIII was FDA approved in 1992. Inhibitors were about as frequent after recombinant factor VIII as after plasma-derived factor VIII (10-15%).

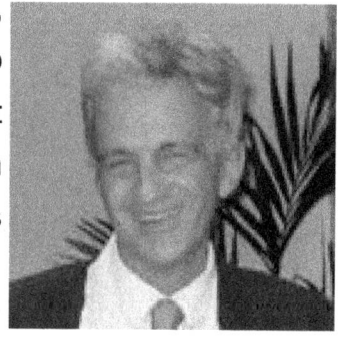

Pier Mannucci

Recombinant factor IX was produced in 1997, and is now available from several sources. Before that, plasma derived concentrates were used.

For patients with inhibitors, factor VIII or IX could be circumvented by activated factors VII, IX and X contained in factor IX complex concentrates as shown in 1980 by Jeanne Lusher (1935-2016) in Ann Arbor MI. In 1993, a recombinant activated factor VII was introduced by Novo Nordisk in Denmark as Novoseven RT®; it was approved in 1996.

Diffuse Intravascular Coagulation (DIC)

The first physician to describe DIC (diffuse/disseminated intravascular coagulation/consumption) was Franciscus Sylvius (born Franz de le Boë), a German who lived from 1614 until 1672, and who was Professor of Medicine in Leiden NL. He was the teacher of Jan Swammerdam (*p.25*) and Regnier de Graaf (*of reproductive biology fame*). Sylvius was best known from his studies of the pulmonary circulation, but he also tried to

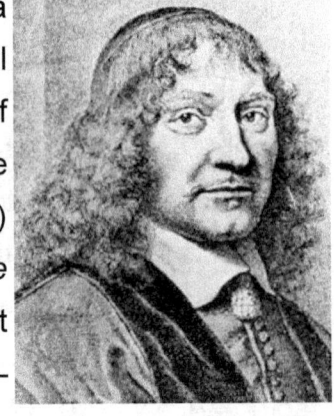

Franciscus Sylvius

explain the fluidity of blood in malignant fevers and in the plague by the presence of excess alkaline substances. Henri de Blainville's observation in 1832, that the intravenous injection of brain tissue immediately killed the animal by massive clotting (*p.263*), was confirmed. When the infusion was slow, few big clots were found, but the blood was incoagulable. Mills in Cincinnati OH observed that the blood of these animals was depleted of fibrinogen in 1921. Probably, the brain tissue had provided thromboplastin, which induced clotting via the extrinsic pathway. Few thrombi were found, perhaps because fibrin, before or after polymerization, was removed from the bloodstream. The clearest example in humans may be amniotic-fluid embolism during childbirth. This was already reported by John Hunter in 1817: a woman who died suddenly during childbirth had incoagulable blood. Various snake venoms could do the same, particularly the

Malayan pit viper. The bleeding tendency after a snake bite leads to hypofibrinogemia. In hematology, a good example is acute promyelocytic leukemia: the procoagulants in the azurophilic granules can initiate DIC (*p.151*), a frequently fatal complication. In clinical practice, the most frequent causes of DIC are sepsis, surgery, major trauma, burns, malignancy or pregnancy. The laboratory tests show low platelets and fibrinogen, high PT (*p.45*) and high D-dimer (*p.47*). Treatment should be directed towards the underlying condition. Despite support with platelets, fresh frozen plasma and heparin, the mortality is still 20-50%. Drotrecogin alfa (Xigris®), activated protein C (APC), was approved for the treatment of (DIC in) sepsis/septic shock in 2001. The expensive drug was heavily marketed, but failed to decrease mortality in a large randomized trial. The drug was then withdrawn from all markets.

Thrombosis

Thrombosis is a common medical problem, not limited to the field of hematology. It affects about 0.1% of the population annually and has done so probably for a long time. More than 2,500 years ago, Huang Ti in China wrote: "....when the blood coagulates within the foot, it causes pain and chills". Diocles of Carystus (ca. 375-ca. 295 BCE) observed that obstruction of the lumen of blood vessels may occur during inflammation. Galen supposedly used the word *thrombosis*. During the "modern" times of Medicine (starting in the 17th century CE), autopsies showed clotted blood in the heart and blood vessels, but the physicians could not distinguish yet between *thrombosis, embolism,* and *post-mortem coagulation*. Franciscus Sylvius (*p.278*) was the first to induce thrombosis in the experimental setting. In his *Praxeos Medicae Idea Nova* (New Idea in Medical Practice) of 1671, he reported that injection of acid substances into the veins of a living animal resulted in immediate coagulation of blood. Richard Wiseman, who was the sergeant surgeon of King Charles II of England, described the coagulation in varicose veins in 1686. He attributed it to "... either the coagulation of the serum...., or to obstruction of the vein by narrowing". John Hunter (*p.261*) described gangrene distal to a clot in the iliac artery in 1817. In 1856, Rudolf Virchow described three categories of factors contributing to venous thrombosis and pulmonary embolism: alterations in the blood flow, changes in the constitution of blood and changes in the vessel wall: *Virchow's triad*. It is still a useful concept for *thrombophilia*. Bizzozero (*p.246*) and Hayem (*p.48*) focused on the role of platelets, as did Karl Eberth (*p.246*). William Welch (1850-1934) at Johns Hopkins, focused on the role of leukocytes (mainly neutrophils) in

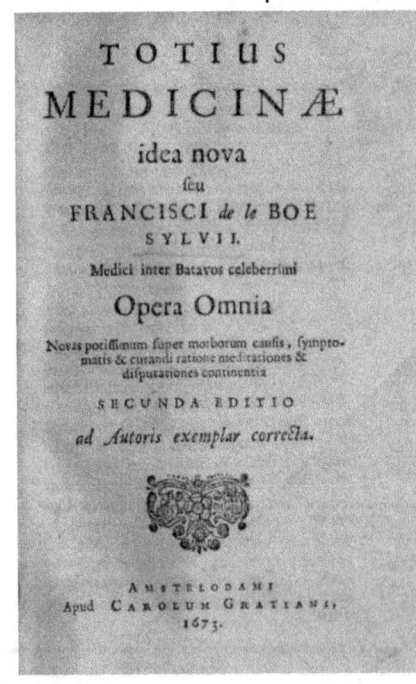

Sylvius' book

the formation of clots; this *"white clot"* adheres to the vessel wall and starts the formation of the *"red clot or tail"*, which usually grows in the direction of the current of blood. This forms the *"lines of Zahn"* (p.44).

Hewson had concluded that stagnation of blood was a poor stimulus to clotting (p.261). Eberth, however, documented that stasis of blood and damage to the vessel wall were potent initiators of clotting. In rapidly flowing blood, the elements flow in the central portion of the lumen, whereas in slowly moving blood the platelets wander toward the vessel wall. With damaged endothelium the platelets aggregate and adhere to the damage site, forming the *white clot*.

It took more time to determine the effect of changes in the constitution of the blood, the third part of Virchow's triad. Antithrombin deficiency was the first identified genetic factor for venous thrombosis. Whereas Morawitz had proposed the concept of antithrombin (AT) already in 1905, it took until 1963 before an assay for AT in plasma was presented. Two years later, Roger Egeberg (1902-1997) in Los Angeles CA, reported AT deficiency in a family having many members suffering from venous thrombosis. No case of homozygous AT deficiency has been described, suggesting that complete AT deficiency is incompatible with life. Heterozygous type I AT deficiency is present in about 1 in 2,000 people and is associated with a 10-fold increased risk of thrombosis (1-2% of thrombosis events). Many different mutations have been described, resulting either in functional defects or low plasma levels.

Functional protein C deficiency is a far more frequent cause of *thrombophilia*. Many proteins in blood coagulation are vitamin-K dependent (*p.265*) and vitamin-K antagonists have been used to treat thrombosis since the 1950's (*p.266*). In 1974, several groups described the post-translationally modified γ-carboxyglutamic acid present in vitamin-K dependent proteins, and also a vitamin-K dependent anticoagulant pathway, now called protein C. Protein C was isolated in 1976 by Johan Stenflo (b.1940) in Lund SW, and was shown the next year by Walter Kisiel to have anticoagulant activity. It turned out to be identical to the autoprothrombin IIa reported by Walter Seegers's group (*p.271*) in the 1960's. In 1981, John Griffin and colleagues in San Diego CA reported heterozygous protein-C deficiency in a family with recurring thrombosis. Two years later, homozygous protein C deficiency was found to be associated with severe neonatal purpura fulminans. Although more common than antithrombin deficiency, it was still present in <5% of the patients with thrombosis.

In 1987, however, Joseph Miletich and colleagues in St. Louis MO found protein-C deficiency in 1:250 blood donors. Thrombosis was rare in these donors or in their family members. Studies of thrombosis cohorts showed that <10% had deficiencies of AT, protein C or protein S, but 40% had a positive family history. In 1993, Björn Dahlbäck (b.1949) and his group in Lund SW came up with the concept of

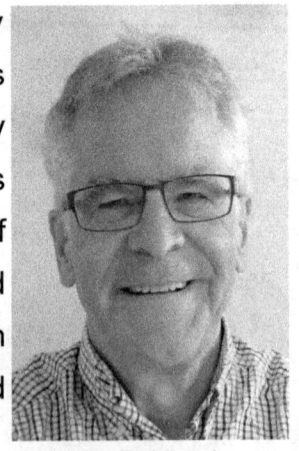

Björn Dahlbäck

activated protein-C (APC) resistance. This resistance turned out to be inherited; it was found in 20-60% of thrombosis patients and in 5-10% of healthy individuals. The APC resistance protein was purified and in 1994 identified as factor V. The genetic mutation of factor V, on chromosome 1, was first reported by Rogier Bertina and colleagues in Leiden NL in 1994, and is now known as factor V Leiden. The prevalence of factor V Leiden, which is based on a mutation probably about 21,000 years ago, varies from 0-15%. It is absent or rare in East Asia, black Africa, and among Native Americans. In Europe, it is frequent in Sweden, Germany, Cyprus and also in many Middle Eastern countries. Heterozygosity yields a lifelong hypercoagulable state with a 5-10 fold increased risk of venous thrombosis, particularly in combination with other risk factors (pregnancy, surgery, oral contraception *etc.*). Homozygous individuals have a 50-fold higher risk of venous thrombosis. The risk of arterial thrombosis is not increased.

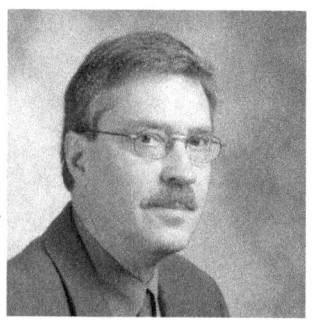

Rogier Bertina

Kenneth Merle Brinkhous *was born in Iowa in 1908. He graduated from the University of Iowa Medical School in 1932 and then trained in pathology. His mentor, Harry P Smith, led a training program that combined clinical pathology with research, primarily in blood coagulation. Brinkhous worked on hemophilia and was among the firsts to discover antihemophilic factor (factor VIII). During World War II, he* *commanded an army laboratory in Australia as the reference laboratory for the US Forces in the Pacific. He returned to Iowa, but in 1946 he was recruited to be the Chairman of the Pathology Laboratory at the University of North Carolina in Chapel Hill. He expanded the department of 2 people without research, to a large department with extensive research, again mainly in the field of coagulation. The new university hospital opened in 1952. His team developed the partial thromboplastin test (p.47) to test the intrinsic pathway of coagulation. They worked on treating hemophilia A with plasma containing factor VIII and on purifying factor VIII as a therapeutic agent. They also studied Von Willebrand's disease, and the effect of snake venom on blood clotting. His laboratory had colonies of dogs and pigs with genetically determined bleeding disorders. He continued to lead gene-therapy studies in these animals until almost the end of his life. He retired from the chairmanship of Pathology in 1973, but continued his research. He was continuously funded by the National Institutes of Health from 1947-1997, a record. He died in 2000 at the age of 93.*

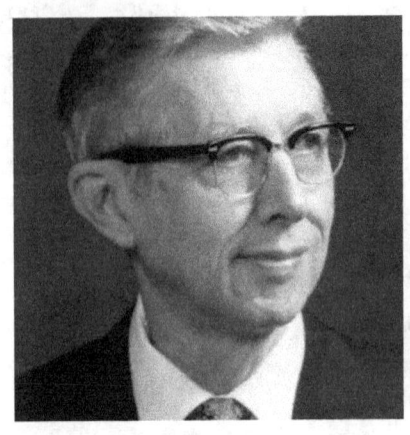

TRANSFUSION

Even though gladiators drank the blood of their slain adversaries to acquire their strength (*p.3*), that can hardly be considered a blood transfusion! Paul Ehrlich treated a patient with pancytopenia with subcutaneous injections of blood in 1888 (*p.106*). Here we will not consider that to be a blood transfusion either. In the 17th century, several authors claimed that transfusion from one individual (human or animal) to a patient was possible (*e.g.* Francesco Folli (1624-1685) in Florence IT) and they even described all funnels, tubes, animal bladders and cannulas needed. There is no evidence, however, that most of them really tried their methods. The few who actually did try, were unsuccessful (*e.g.*, Francis Potter of Kilmington UK in 1652).

The British architect Christopher Wren (1632-1723), who built St. Paul's cathedral in London but was also an anatomist, performed intravenous injections of fluids and drugs into dogs. One of his admirers, physician Richard Lower (1631-1691) in London, continued the experiments by injecting drugs intravenously into animals. This led him to consider injecting animal blood into other animals. In early 1665, he transferred blood from the cervical artery of one dog into the jugular vein of another dog that had been almost fully exsanguinated first. The recipient recovered rapidly and fully. He was successful partly because dogs do not have natural iso-agglutinins. Two years later, Jean-Baptiste Denys (1643-1704) in Paris transfused a 5-year-old boy with

Blood is Life

prolonged fever and lethargy, who had survived 20 phlebotomies (!), with 9 ounces of sheep's blood. He "cured' the boy of his disease. Next, he transfused a healthy paid volunteer with 20 ounces of blood. The recipient survived, but felt "great heat" along the vein in his arm, and later voided "black urine". A third recipient, already moribund, died after an attempted transfusion. Not to be outdone by a Frenchman, Richard Lower performed his first human transfusion in front of the Royal Society in late 1667. The patient, a 22-year-old clergyman, was bled for 7 ounces from his antecubital vein. Then he was connected via silver tubes and quills to a sheep's carotid artery. About 20 ounces of blood were transfused in 2 minutes. Six days later, the patient told the Society how much better he felt! About 3 weeks later, the transfusion was repeated into the same patient. This led to some fever, attributed to "drinking too much wine after the procedure". The international debate about priority started. The publication of Denys' letter to the Royal Society was delayed because of an "extraordinary accident": the editor was in jail at the time on suspicion of treason! Sporadic

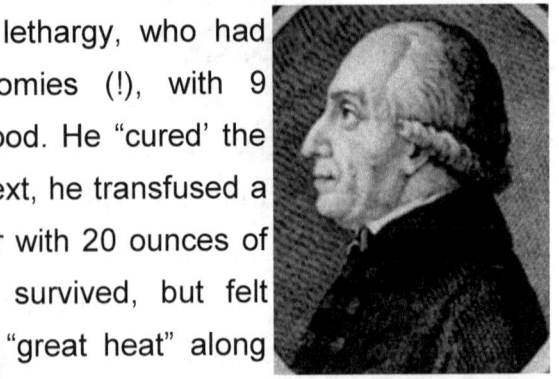

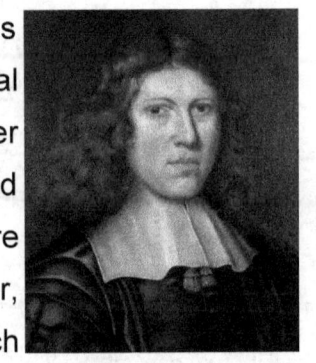

Jean-Baptiste Denys

Sheep to human transfusion

Richard Lower

Transfusion

reports about transfusions continued for indications such as insanity, mania, and long-lasting diseases. They all used animal blood donors. Since the oxygen carrying capacity of blood was not known yet, the danger of blood loss was not known either.

A more realistic report of the first clinical transfusion came from obstetrician James Blundell (1790-1878) in London. He was frustrated about massive puerperal hemorrhage. In 1817, he first experimented on exsanguinated dogs by transfusion of blood from other dogs, and he found that a small(er) transfusion was often sufficient to save the recipient. He found that species lines could not be crossed, and that venous blood was as efficacious as arterial blood. He developed special instruments for human transfusion: a warm-water-jacketed funnel, cannulas, syringes and even three-way stopcocks! He treated ten patients, two of them already moribund. Five of the remaining eight improved. He published his results in *The Lancet* in 1828. His example was soon followed by a few other obstetricians. At age 48, Blundell left Guy's Hospital after a dispute and he lived for 40

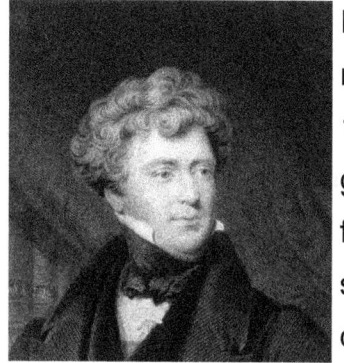

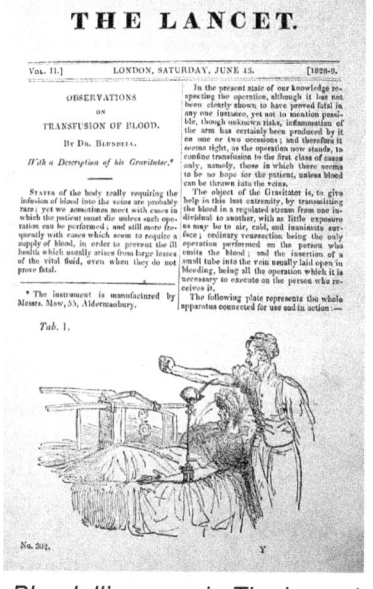

James Blundell

Blundell's paper in The Lancet

more years as a country squire.

Transfusions of milk, in the hope of producing white blood cells (as in lymph), were tried in the last quarter of the 19th century, but were uniformly unsuccessful and often fatal. Infusion of isotonic saline was found to be safer and was used increasingly in seriously ill patients. Infection control became only possible after 1867, when Joseph Lister had introduced antisepsis.

To prevent the donor blood from clotting, immediate transfer from donor to patient was necessary. Surgeon George Crile (1864-1943) in Cleveland OH started in 1898 using artery-to-vein anastomoses for direct transfusion, using a small metal tube. He performed 61 transfusions in 55 patients, as he reported in 1909. He did not do blood-group typing or cross matching, but mixed donor and recipient blood and observed them for 24 hours. The transfusion reaction rate was 35%, about what to be expected without ABO typing. A single successful transfusion was done by Alexis Carrel (1873-1944).

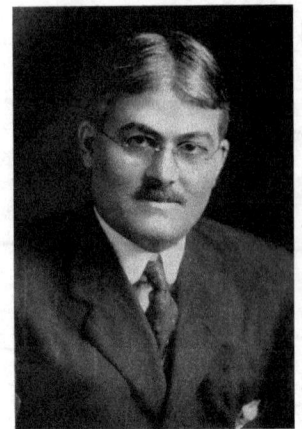

George Crile

Carrel, a French surgeon and later an eugenics-policy supporter back in France, was working in New York on tissue culture and organ transplantation experiments. He was famous for vascular sutures and received the 1912 Nobel prize in Physiology/Medicine for this. In 1908, a 5-day-old daughter of a famous surgeon in New York was bleeding from hemorrhagic disease of the newborn.

Transfusion

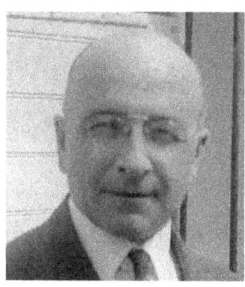

Alexis Carrel

Carrel was persuaded to try to rescue the infant. He connected her popliteal vein to her father's radial artery on the kitchen table! The bleeding stopped and the child recovered. New York obviously claimed this as the first successful transfusion! The direct donor-to-patient transfusions were cumbersome. Keeping the blood from clotting would be a major step. William Hewson (*p.25*) found that sodium sulphate prevented clotting and kept the blood bright red. In 1868, John Braxton-Hicks (1823-1897), another English obstetrician, tried to prevent clotting by adding "phosphate of soda" to the blood as it was drawn. He tried it in three bleeding women. The blood kept flowing, but all three women died in shock. Leonard Landois (*p.38*) used *hirudin*, extracted from leeches in 1892, and his approach was followed by Henry Satterlee and Ransom Hooker in New York in 1916. Making pure preparations of hirudin proved too difficult, though.

Alternatively, blood could be allowed to clot and the remaining serum transfused. This technique was also capable of resuscitating bled animals, as shown already in France in 1821. Whipped or twirled blood would be strained and injected. These defibrinated-blood transfusions remained popular until the early 20th century. The difficult techniques often led to fevers caused by pyrogens, or perhaps by damaged red cells.

Blood is Life

Animal-to-human transfusions started to disappear when Emil Ponfick (1844-1913) in Rostock GE showed in 1875 that xenogeneic (=heterologous) transfusions led to destruction of red cells, hemoglobinuria and kidney damage. The same year, Leonard Landois demonstrated that human serum lysed sheep red blood cells *in-vitro* and *in-vivo*. He also recognized the danger of hyperkalemia and emboli. He reviewed almost 500 cases of transfusion, including 129 from animals. With his analysis, animal-to-human transfusions disappeared, although a publication in France in 1928 still advocated them.

To avoid direct donor-artery to patient-vein transfusions, paraffin-coated Y-shaped cannulas were introduced by Curtis and David in Chicago IL in 1911. Lester Unger (1889-1974) in New York simplified the procedure by introducing a syringe and a four-way stopcock in 1915. An alternative was the paraffin coated glass cylinder with a fine cannula to be inserted into the patient's vein, introduced by Kimpton and Brown in Boston MA in 1913. This semi-direct transfusion method still required close proximity of donor and patient. To remove blood transfusion from the realm of surgeons, and to allow fractionation of blood products, anticoagulation of collected blood was necessary. In 1890, Arthus and Pagès in Switzerland had already shown that calcium was important for blood clotting. Pathologist Almroth Wright in London pointed out, in 1894,

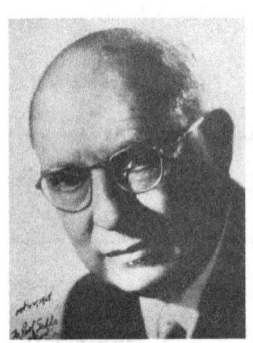

Lester Unger

Transfusion

that the soluble salts of several acids could prevent clotting indefinitely. He feared that the dose of citrate needed would cause convulsions. It took 20 years before further advances were made. In 1914, almost simultaneously in three countries, citrate-anticoagulated blood was introduced. Albert Hustin (1882-1967) in Brussels BE performed the first indirect transfusion on March 27, 1914, about four months before the start of World War I. His anticoagulation solution contained citrate and glucose. Over the next year, Louis Agote (1868-1954) in Buenos Aires AG, and Richard Weil (1876-1917) in New York also performed transfusions, with only citrate as anticoagulant. The latter also showed that blood could be stored for several days in an ice box and still be used. The Mayo Clinic (Rochester MN) reported on 1,000 transfusions (arm to arm, but perhaps indirect via citrated bottles) between 1915-1917, mainly under the leadership of thyroid surgeon John Pemberton (1887-1967).

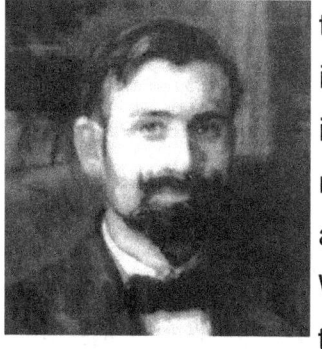

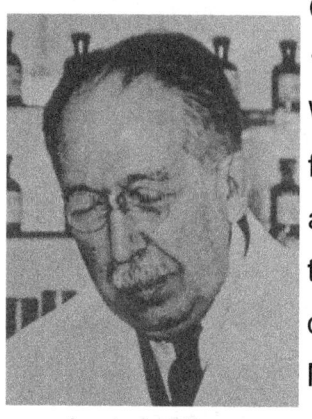

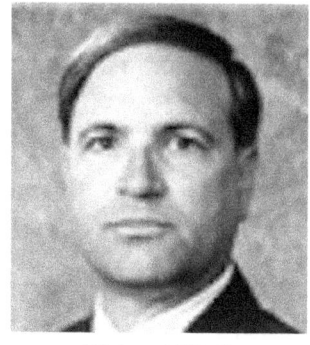

This came just in time for use in World War I. Military physician Oswald Robertson (1886-1963) was born in England, trained in the USA, and was

Blood is Life

now stationed in France with the volunteer Harvard Medical School Unit under the command of Roger Lee (1881-1964) at Base Hospital 5, near Béthune, in the British theater of war. They introduced a citrate-glucose solution to collect and store mainly blood-group-O blood in paraffin-coated glass bottles. The amount of solution was the same as the amount of blood collected. Robertson showed that the blood could be stored for 21 days. The large volume made it difficult to transport. Peyton Rous (1879-1970) and Turner in New York had already shown in 1916, with animal blood, that the supernatant could be removed, and they recommended this for blood transfusion; it received clinical acceptance more than a generation later. Oswald Robertson performed his first transfusion in the summer of 2017. Actually, Roger Lee and his colleague, surgeon Beth Vincent, probably already had performed a transfusion on April 23, 1915 in Paris. To make the war-time transfusion story even more confusing, Canadian army physician Lawrence Robertson (no relation) also used blood transfusions, with direct transfusion and no crossmatch. His first transfusion took place in October 1915. By 1918, on the Western front, each casualty-clearing station transfused about 50-100 units of citrated blood per day.

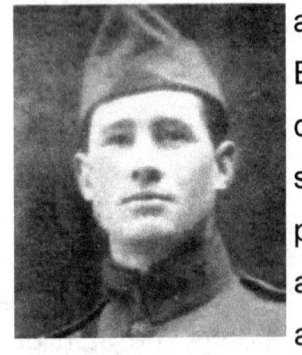

Oswald Robertson

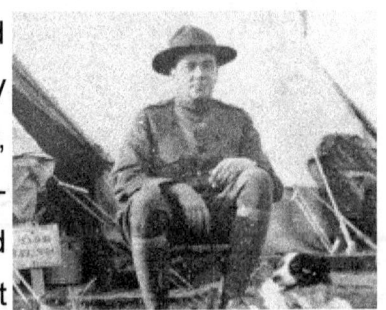

Roger Lee in France

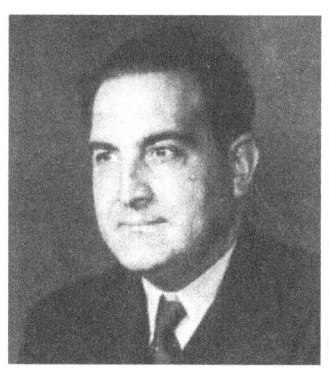

Transfusion

During the Spanish Civil War (1936-1939), Frederic Durán i Jordà (1905-1957) established a blood bank in Barcelona in 1936. The Republican army collected 9,000 liters of blood in citrate-glucose solution in 2.5 years and divided it into 300 ml units for transfusion. Canadian surgeon Norman Bethune (1890-1939) stressed the importance of prompt transfusion during his volunteer service for the loyalist government in Spain, and then in China (1938-1939), where he died from septicemia after an operation.

Frederic Durán i Jordà

The secretary of the British Red Cross had established the first blood-donor service already in 1921. This London Blood Transfusion Service was free of charge and typed volunteers. It became part of the British Red Cross in 1926. Similar systems were introduced in other countries (France, Germany, Austria, Belgium, Australia and Japan). The start of World War II led to an enormous activity on the blood transfusion front, especially in England. Frederic Durán i Jordà had fled to England in 1939, and with Janet M Vaughan (1899-1993) he created a system of national blood banks. With the threat of war, four large blood depots were set up around the country. The Galton Laboratory Serum Unit was moved from London to Cambridge (*p.101*) to produce blood-group typing sera. Volunteer donors of known blood type had been "on call" already for many years, and now "repeat donors" were volunteering to donate to the regional centers. When it was shown that blood could be stored for as long as 38 days, whole blood shipments to the European theater of war started in 1944. By then, John Loutit (*p.223*) and Patrick Mollison (*p.323*) had introduced their acid-citrate-dextrose (ACD) solution with 70 ml to 450 ml blood for 3-4 weeks of storage. In 1957, citrate phosphate-dextrose (CPD) was introduced by John Gibson and colleagues in Boston MA, which extended the storage time from 21 to 28 days; officially the storage time still remained 21 days. The National Blood Transfusion Service was established in England in 1946,

In 1937, Cook County Hospital organized the first hospital-based blood bank in the USA, but kept the blood in citrate for only 7-10 days, creating a lot of wastage. The Mayo Clinic claimed that they already had a functioning blood bank by 1935! In 1940, "*Blood for Britain*" was started in New York hospitals. The units were exported to Britain as dried plasma. African American surgeon Charles Drew (1904-1950) was in charge of the effort. He became the first Director of the American Red Cross. He resigned in 1942, when the army insisted that blood from black donors be separated from blood from white donors. That discriminatory policy lasted until 1950.

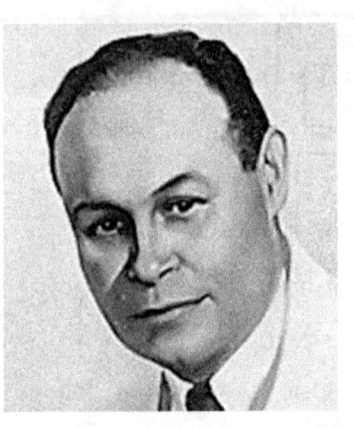

Charles Drew

Transfusion

In the Soviet Union, a completely different approach was chosen in the early 1930's. Cadaveric blood was collected from fatally stricken victims of acute cardiac arrest or severe trauma. Alexander Bogdanov (1873-1928), a polymath and active revolutionary, had spent several years in prison, after receiving his medical degree and before the 1917 Revolution. He persuaded Stalin to start a Blood Transfusion Institute in 1926, the first in the world. He also believed in improvement of the human race by exchanging blood between individuals. He himself died from a hemolytic transfusion reaction after his 12th exchange transfusion, despite a negative crossmatch. His philosophy of "stimulating" blood transfusions lived on in Russia into the 1990's, but nowhere else. Yet, the centralization of transfusion services was important for the country. Surgeon Sergei Yudin (1891-1954) reported in 1937 on 1,000 transfusions of cadaver blood, that had been stored for 3 weeks or more. Six years before his death, he was arrested by the KGB and exiled to Siberia. After Stalin's death, he was released, but he died a year later from myocardial infarction. The use of cadaver blood continued in the Soviet Union. Large volumes of blood could be obtained from a single donor. Norman Bethune had also used cadaver blood during the Civil War in Spain.

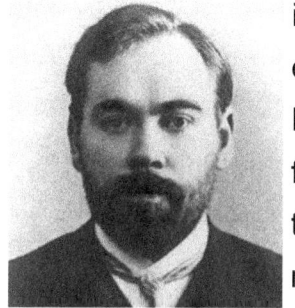

Alexander Bogdanov

Sergei Yudin

Blood groups

Leonard Landois (*p.38*) documented that blood incompatibility exists between species in 1875. Jules Bordet (*p.38*) found, 20 years later, that hemolysins were produced after xenogeneic transfusions. Paul Ehrlich (*p.49*) reported that part of these hemolysins already exist before the xenogeneic transfusion in 1900. The next year, Karl Landsteiner (1868-1943) (*p.321*) demonstrated that incompatibility also can exist between the red cells and serum of healthy, non transfused, humans. This was the start of the field of *immunogenetics*, the study of genetically determined polymorphisms with immunological techniques. Two years earlier in London, Samuel Shattock (1852-1924), - born Samuel Betty but changing his name at age 30 to prevent the family name Shattock from going extinct (!) -, had reported the clumping of normal red cells by serum from patients with pneumonia: "irregular rouleaux" formation. He ascribed it to the disease, not to blood-group differences. Landsteiner was aware of Shattock's observations, but wanted a more thorough analysis. He studied the reactions between the red cells and sera of 22 associates, all healthy. He saw that certain sera would agglutinate the red cells of certain other people. He divided the samples into three groups: A, B and C. Serum of A clumped B cells, serum of B clumped A cells, and serum C clumped both A and B red cells. C cells were not clumped by either A or B serum. In the same 3-page paper, he also reported that these iso-agglutinins tolerated drying and redissolving. Clearly not what some might call *"the smallest publishable unit"*! He felt that his observations might assist to explain "various consequences of therapeutical blood transfusion". The next year, two of his pupils confirmed his findings in 155 cases. They also found 4 people who had no agglutinins in their serum, but whose red cells were agglutinated by sera A, B, and C: the fourth blood group. Despite these observations, it took 10 years before their importance led to major changes in transfusion therapy! In the USA, medical literature in German was not very well read; in Europe, clinical and basic science were still far apart. Landsteiner's technique masked the reaction of warm "incomplete" antibodies against other blood groups (Rh, Kell and several others).

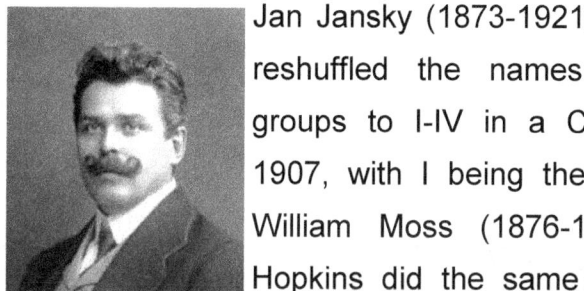

Jan Jansky (1873-1921) in Prague CZ reshuffled the names of the blood groups to I-IV in a Czech journal in 1907, with I being the most frequent. William Moss (1876-1957) at Johns Hopkins did the same in 1910, but his numbering was the opposite, with I the least frequent. In 1927, the Landsteiner naming was accepted as A, B, AB, and O, after he had relocated to New York. The Moss numbering persisted in the USA, Britain and France until World War II. Jansky's numbering was used in those years in the rest of Europe.

Jan Jansky

William Moss

Blood is Life

Ludwik Hirszfeld (1884-1954) and his boss Emil von Dungern (1867-1961) in Heidelberg GE, established the Mendelian inheritance of blood groups in 1909; they labeled them A, B and O (instead of C). To make the naming even more complex, Hirszfeld talked about "null" (zero), not O ("ohne"=without). Landsteiner then chose O. Mathematician Felix Bernstein (1878-1956) in Halle-Wittenberg GE detailed the exact manner of inheritance in 1924: multiple alleles at one locus The gene was found to be located on the long arm of chromosome 9 (1980-1990). This gene encodes glycosyltransferase, an enzyme that modifies the carbohydrate content of red blood-cell antigens (1978).

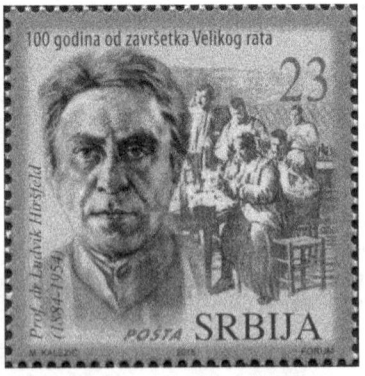

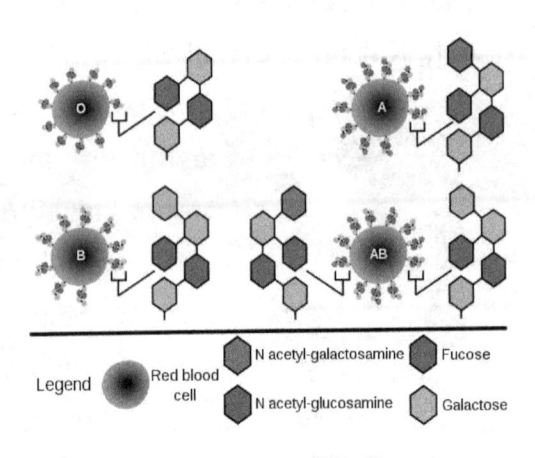

Serbian stamp from 2018 honoring Ludwik Hirszfeld

The ABO system

Not until 1927 were other blood group recognized. Then, Landsteiner and Philip Levine (1900-1987) in New York, sought additional blood groups by injecting rabbits with different human red cells. They discovered blood group M, its allele N, and a new agglutinin, which they called P. The next year they determined the three genotypes MM, MN, and NN, and the phenotypes M, MN and N.

Antibodies against these phenotypes were rarely associated with hemolytic reactions, and therefore were of no real importance for cross matching.

A far more important antigen was discovered by Levine and Stetson in New York in 1939. They studied an unusual hemolytic reaction in a 25-year old group-O woman transfused with her husband's group-O blood. The cross-match turned out to be positive. The woman had just delivered a stillborn child with *erythroblastosis fetalis*, the cause of which was unknown. The year before, Ruth Darrow in Chicago IL had described a case of this "icterus gravis (erythroblastosis) neonatorum". Levine reasoned that the infant had inherited an antigen from the father that was foreign to the mother. During the same years, Landsteiner and Alexander Wiener (1907-1976) had discovered a new antibody, by immunizing rabbits and guinea pigs with blood of rhesus monkeys. This antibody agglutinated not only rhesus monkey red cells, but also red cells from 86% of Caucasians in New York. Parallel experiments with Levine's serum showed identical distributions. Rh factor and anti-Rh were thus established.

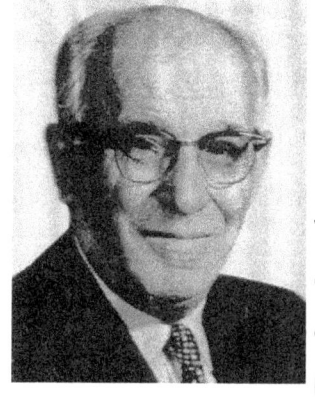

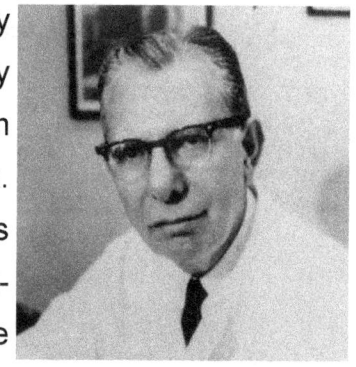

Philip Levine

Alexander Wiener

It turned out to be a dominant factor. Wiener and Peters found that the anti-Rh was indeed the cause of intragroup hemolytic reactions, and of clear clinical significance. Anti-Rh could not easily be detected in the blood of Rh-negative people. These antibodies were "incomplete" (Race, 1944) or "blocked" (Wiener, 1944). Louis Diamond (1902-1999) and Abelson in Boston MA found the next year, that this anti-Rh produced easily visible agglutination with a thick drop of blood on a warm slide. The Coombs test *(p.103)* made it even easier to detect these antibodies. Soon several alleles were discovered: Wiener defined six, Russell Race (1907-1984) in Cambridge UK had seven alleles. Geneticist/statistician Ronald Fisher (1890-1962) in Cambridge UK, worked out the logical scheme for the Rh three sets of alleles: C and c, D and d, E and e. The most common was D, and d was never found. Wiener had developed his own nomenclature (rh^{W1}, rh^{X}, *etc.*), but this one was too difficult to remember. Much later, DNA testing revealed two linked genes, the *RHD* gene which produces a single immune specificity (anti-D), and the *RHCE* gene with multiple specificities. Both genes are located on the short arm of chromosome 1. It turned out that both Fisher-Race (3 genes) and Wiener (1 gene) had been incorrect. In the 1940-50's, many additional blood groups were discovered, such as Lewis (1946, Arthur Mourant), Kell (1946, Robin Coombs), Duffy (1950, Marie Cutbush), Kidd (1951), and Ii (1956, Wiener). The "Bible" on blood groups became *Blood Groups in Man* by the husband-and-wife team of Robert

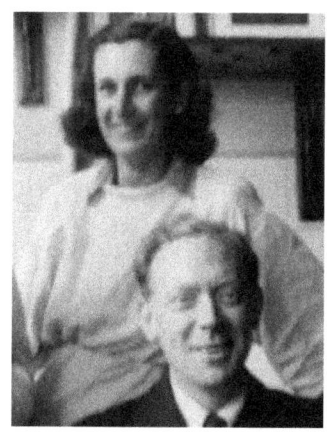

Race and Ruth Sanger (1916-2001) in London; the first edition appeared in 1950.

A fascinating issue was the distribution of the various blood groups over the world. In 1919, the Hirszfelds (Ludwik and his wife Hanka) reported their results of the blood-group typing of 8,000 soldiers on the Macedonian front. Western Europeans were mainly A and O, but Eastern Europeans and Asians frequently had blood group B. Similar differences were found for blood group Rh(D), with very few Rh(D) negatives among Blacks and Asians in New York City.

Nice theories can be formulated about the cause of the polymorphism. Diseases are among the more interesting theories. The organism of the plague (*P. pestis*) has an antigen similar with the human H antigen (on O red cells). Since group O individuals were not able to make anti-H, they were at higher risk of the plague in endemic areas, such as Mongolia, Turkey *etc.* (1960, Vogel and colleagues). Similar claims were made for smallpox: the virus has antigenic similarity to group A agglutinogen, suggesting increased virulence in group A individuals. Interestingly, now during the COIVD-19 pandemic, early studies also suggested more aggressive disease in group A individuals!

Blood products

Direct transfusions by necessity concerned full blood. When anticoagulants became available and allowed indirect transfusion, in the early decades of the 20th century, fractionation of collected blood became a possibility. Protein chemist Edwin Cohn (1892-1953) in Boston introduced the fractionation of plasma during World War II. He worked out the techniques for isolating the serum albumin fraction of plasma, which was essential for maintaining the osmotic pressure in blood vessels. The transfusion of purified albumin was responsible for saving many thousands of soldiers from shock. Cohn's group prepared units of 100 ml of concentrated (25%) serum albumin in a cylindrical can. This unit was calculated to increase plasma volume by approximately 500 ml. Even though the US Navy wanted only albumin, Cohn developed systems to use every component of donated blood through the American Red Cross, similar with the observations of Mollison about red cells during the London "blitz" (*p.323*).

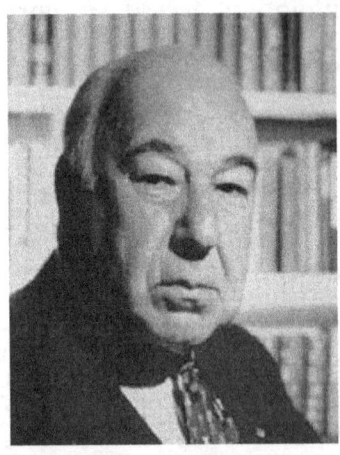

Edwin Cohn

Red cells

Most of the red-cell transfusions given during and after World War II, were "packed red cells" units. The blood unit is spun in a centrifuge and the plasma is taken off. With the additive CPD, adenine and pH control, the red-cell unit can be kept at refrigerated temperature for up to 45 days. Older units lose part of their 2,3-diphosphoglycerate (2,3-DPG) levels, and may carry oxygen less well. In hematology practice, virtually all red-cell transfusions can be achieved with packed cells since the 1960's. Many surgeons and some pediatricians still like to hold on to fresh whole blood. Whereas in industrialized countries most red-cell transfusions are given to patients over 65 years of age, in low income countries the majority go to children under 5 years of age. Historically, most red-cell transfusions were ordered as two units, but in the most recent decade ordering of one unit at a time is often recommended (*e.g.*, Nicole Guinn, Durham NC, 2017). When red-cell units need to be kept for more prolonged periods of time, cryopreservation with glycerol as cryoprotectant was introduced in 1963 by Charles Huggins (1930-1990), a surgeon in Boston. Storage at -80°C or less makes the red cells maintain their viability indefinitely. Obviously, glycerol has to be removed by washing before use, a cumbersome procedure. It is an good option for patients lacking high-incidence antigens who have developed allo-antibodies.

Platelets

William Duke (*p.43*), who introduced the first bleeding-time test, gave fresh blood to 3 bleeding patients with thrombocytopenia in 1910. Among them was a 20-year-old man with mucocutaneous bleeding and a platelet count of 6,000/mm^3. He was given a "large" amount of fresh blood, which stopped the bleeding and raised his platelet count to 123,000/mm^3! Blood was obtained in those days with steel needles and collected through uncoated rubber tubing into glass bottles; not quite the environment for platelets to survive. It had become clear during the war, that plastic surfaces and silicone-coated surfaces maintained the shape and function of platelets much better. Emil Freireich (*p.146*), then a young physician at NCI (Bethesda, MD), working with Gordon Zubrod (1914-1999) and Emil Frei (*p.142*) on childhood leukemia, described how he started using the recently introduced plastic collection bags shortly after 1955. He found out that platelets collected after blood had remained for 2 days at 4°C, were not very functional. He then showed, in a little randomized study, that use of fresh blood was much better. The group then helped develop 2 collection bags in a closed system. This allowed to collect 1 unit of blood, separate the platelet-rich plasma, return the red cells, and then collect the second unit of blood and repeat the separation and return. This way 2 units of platelet-rich plasma could be obtained.

Bleeding from thrombocytopenia induced by cancer chemotherapy was the most frequent indication. Initially, platelets were obtained from very fresh whole blood of ABO and Rh(D) compatible donors. Approximately 0.6×10^{11} platelets could be harvested from a single unit of blood. Most centers obtained first platelet-rich plasma by a centrifugation step, followed by further centrifugation to concentrate the platelets ("soft" spin technique). Other centers (mainly in Europe) made a buffy-coat first, followed by resuspension in plasma and a gentle centrifugation step ("hard" spin technique). The "hard" spin method left fewer white cells in the transfusion product. With both techniques, a transfusion would contain platelets from at least 4 units of blood (up to 8). The introduction of blood-cell separators by medical technologist Herb Cullis (1938-2020) of Fenwal, in 1972, completely changed platelet transfusion therapy. Instead of "random" platelets, "pheresis" platelets from a single donor became the norm (apheresis from Greek αφαίρεσίς=take away). About 6×10^{11} platelet can be collected from a single donor apheresis. The yield of a platelet transfusion can be calculated by the corrected count increment (*CCI*): post-transfusion platelet count – pre-transfusion count x BSA / number of platelets infused. After 1 hour, one hoped for an increment to about 20,000/mm^3, but mostly the CCI was less, due to platelet damage, age of the platelets, and bleeding. Platelets are stored at 20-22°C (Scott Murphy (1936-2006);1969) in gas-permeable plastic in synthetic media, under constant agitation on a shaker platform for a maximum of 5-7 days. Until the 1990's, a platelet count under 20,000/mm^3 in patients without sufficient platelet production, was used as the trigger to transfuse platelets

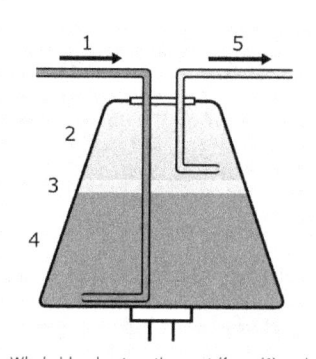

Whole blood enters the centrifuge (1) and separates into plasma (2), leukocytes (3), and erythrocytes (4). Selected components are then drawn off (5).

Apheresis method

prophylactically. In the 1990's, the threshold level was decreased to 5-10,000/mm^3 without evidence of harm. Higher thresholds were used for patients in sepsis or with massive bleeding. New guidelines have suggested when to use platelets prophylactically ("pre-emptively"), and when only therapeutically.

Granulocytes.

The risk of severe bacterial or fungal infections is dramatically increased for patients who have very low neutrophil counts (<500/mm^3, with extreme risk at <100/mm^3). Once it had been shown that platelet levels could be increased by platelet transfusion, it was logical to try the same method for granulocytes. The density of leukocytes was a problem, since it was more difficult to separate them from red cells. At first, Freireich and his colleagues at the NCI tried leukocytes from patients in the chronic phase of CML with white-cell counts >300,000/mm^3. They were able to collect $3 \times 10^9 - 2 \times 10^{11}$ granulocytes from these 11 "donors" for transfusion into children with ALL. As a complication, 3 of the 35 recipients developed temporary Ph'+ allografts.

In order to be able to collect sufficient (2×10^{10}-10^{11}) granulocytes from healthy donors, the NCI and IBM together built the continuous-flow blood-cell separator (NCI-IBM 2990) in 1963. IBM engineer George Judson was especially interested, since his 17-year-old son had been diagnos-

NCI-IBM 2990

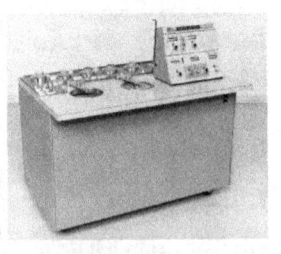

ed with leukemia; Judson took a leave of absence to work on the project. Hydroxyethyl starch (HES) was added to cause rouleaux formation of the red cells to enhance the leukocyte separation. Etiochonalone injections doubled the granulocyte count of the donor, although they sometimes caused fever. A median of 2×10^{10} granulocytes could now be obtained from healthy donors. The bowl and tubing had to be cleaned and sterilized between uses. In 1979, an improved continuous blood-cell separator was introduced as the "IBM 2997" with disposable plastic ware.

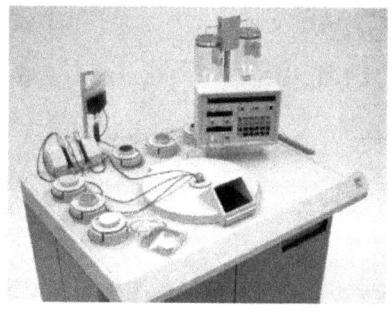

IBM 2997

Important contributions to the field of granulocyte transfusions were made by Ronald Strauss (b.1940) in Iowa City IA. He reported a beneficial effect of granulocyte transfusions for infected neutropenic patients in more than half the controlled studies, particularly when the transfused dose was $>10^{10}$ granulocytes. Treatment of the donors with filgrastim obviously increased the granulocyte dose collected. Yet, the introduction of better antibiotics, the occurrence of pulmonary complications *(p.320)*, and newer randomized studies in Europe and the USA, which did not prove benefit, either prophylactically or therapeutically (Juan Gea y Banacloche; Phoenix AZ, 2017), decreased their use. Perhaps for some patients (*e.g.*, persistent candida infection in severe neutropenia despite proper antifungal therapy), granulocyte transfusions may still have a place.

Overall though, granulocyte transfusions are something of the recent past.. The apheresis machines are now mainly used for collection of platelets and peripheral-blood stem cells (*p.232*).

Infectious complications

Many infectious organisms can be transferred by transfusion of blood products.

Bacterial hazards have been known since the early days of blood transfusion. Among the first was *Treponema Pallidum*, the spirochete that causes syphilis. The first report was in 1915 by dermatologist John Fordyce (1858-1925) in New York, two years after bacteriologist Paul Uhlenhuth (1870-1957) in Strasbourg GE (now FR) had shown the transfer of blood of infected patients into animals. By 1935, Hugh Morgan in Nashville TN had collected 16 cases. In 1939, James McCluskie in Glasgow UK proudly stated that cases had been found in the USA and continental Europe, but none so far in England; he then reported 3! By 1941, a total of 138 cases had been reported, probably an undercount considering the number of infected people and the difficult diagnosis of post-transfusion syphilis. In their 1941 publication, Eichenlaub and colleagues in Washington DC believed that donated blood stored for 4 days at 4°C would no longer transfer the spirochete. Later studies showed that highly

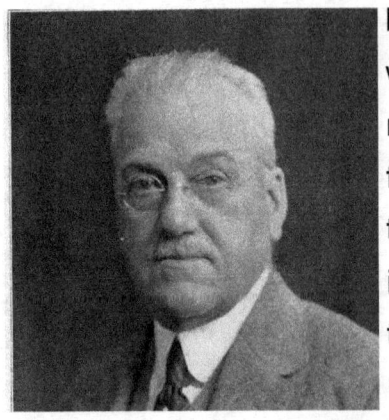

John Fordyce

contaminated blood was infectious for up to 5 days. To prevent transmission, McCluskie suggested the use of cadaveric blood (*p.295*). This did not really take off in England! Cases in the industrialized world rapidly decreased after the introduction of testing, but the transfer of *Treponema pallidum* with blood transfusion continues to be a concern in West Africa.

Other bacterial infections are rare and often associated with the storage temperature. With sterile single-use plastic bags the risk of bacterial contamination of red-cell units is low (<0.5 per million), but with re-usable glass bottles it clearly was higher. For platelet products, which are stored at 20-22°C, the risk was definitely higher at 1:2,000-5,000. Introduction of bacterial testing of platelet products in the 1990's, brought the risk down to 1:15,000. By the year 2000, the risk of a septic transfusion reaction from a culture negative single-donor platelet unit was 1:50,000. Lyme disease, caused by *Borrelia burgdorferi,* can potentially also be transmitted by blood transfusion, but no cases had been reported as of 2018. The rapid clearance of this spirochete from the circulation makes the transmission from an asymptomatic donor unlikely.

Parasitic infections caused by infected transfusion products are quite rare outside regions with active malaria. *Plasmodium* parasites are easily transferable, even from donors who do not have symptoms yet. With

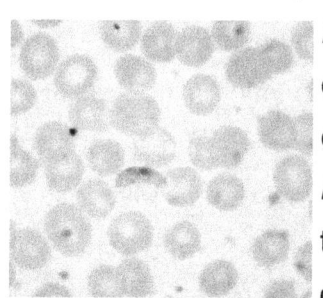

Plasmodium falciparum

increased travel, even in non-endemic regions cases may occur. The first case of transfusion-related malaria was reported by Woolsey in 1911, after transfusion into a patient with pernicious anemia. A more recent case was in 2003 in Houston TX. This patient, with acute renal failure, received 2 units of packed cells, but developed fever and mental confusion after 17 days. Blood cultures were negative, but a blood smear demonstrated *P. falciparum* parasites. One of the blood donors had arrived from Ghana two years earlier. He denied having any febrile illness during the last 12 months. His blood smear and PCR test were negative, but he had elevated titers of antibodies. *P. falciparum* can persist for at least one year before being completely cleared; for *P. vivax* that is 3 years and for *P. malariae* perhaps even decades. All *Plasmodium* species are able to survive in stored blood, even if frozen, and retain their viability for at least 7-10 days. In a review of transfusion-induced malaria in non-endemic areas in 2018, 100 cases were retrieved, with 54 occurring in the Americas and 38 in Europe. The incubation period varied from 19-64 days and the vast majority came from whole blood or red-cell transfusions.

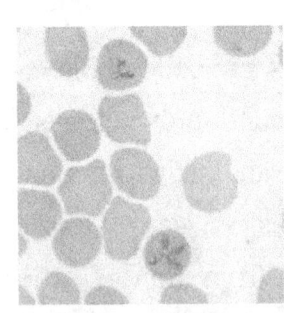

Babesiosis is a potentially life-threatening zoonotic infection most frequently caused by *Babesia microti* in the USA. The tick-borne disease is more common in the Northeastern and Midwestern USA, parts of Europe, and sporadic throughout the rest of the world in warm

Babesia microti

weather. Since the parasite lives inside the red blood cell, it can be transmitted by blood transfusion. The first transfusion induced babesiosis was reported in 1979. In recent years in New York, 1.4% of all cases of babesiosis were transfusion induced from asymptomatic blood donors. In fact, babesiosis is currently the most frequent transfusion-induced pathogen in the USA.

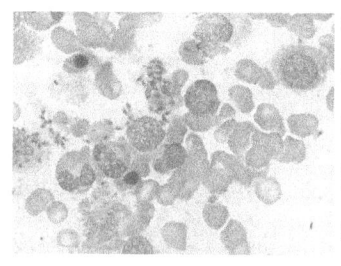

Leishmania donovani, the parasite causing kala azar, occurs mainly in South America, Africa, India, the Middle East, and southern and eastern Europe. It is one of the ten most neglected tropical diseases. Climate change and human migration are leading to expansion of the *leishmania* geographical range. The vast majority of visceral leishmania (kala azar) infections are asymptomatic, and transfusion from such donors may well transfer the infection. An obstacle to detecting the parasite in blood is their occurrence there in very low numbers. No reliable detection methods are available yet.

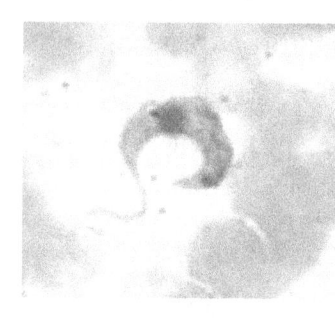

Leishmania donovani

Chagas disease occurs primarily in rural areas of Central and South America and is responsible for about 8,000 deaths per year. The disease, named after Brazilian physician Carlos Chagas (1879-1934), who discovered the causative parasite *Trypanosoma cruzi* in 1909, can

Trypanosoma cruzi

be easily transmitted by blood transfusion. Most patients with trypanosomiasis are asymptomatic and can spread the disease by blood donation. The first case was reported in 1952 by Pedreira de Freitas and colleagues in Brazil, but the possibility of transfusion-transmitted Chagas disease was raised already in 1936 by Mazza and colleagues in Argentina. The total number of cases is now between 400 and 800. Since 2005-2007, most blood in Europe and North America is being screened for *trypanosoma*.

Viral hazards have been even more dangerous for blood transfusion recipients than bacterial or parasitic infections. *Serum hepatitis* was the first blood-born disease recognized. The Sumerians reported the first cases of jaundice on clay tablets more than 4,000 years ago. The devil Ahhazu supposedly attacked the liver, the seat of the soul. Hippocrates, about 2,000 years later, described the features of epidemic jaundice, including some patients who died within 2 weeks. He used the name *icterus* (ικτέρος) for the first time. During the Middle Ages, patients with jaundice were considered "impure" and needed to be isolated, on instruction of Pope Zacharias, son of Polichronius (8th century). Infectious hepatitis was frequent during military campaigns, including the American Civil War. In World War II, hepatitis infections amounted to 16 million.

An outbreak of jaundice among shipyard workers in Bremen GE was reported by Lurman in 1885. Interestingly, the disease only occurred in people who had received a smallpox vaccine. He concluded that the source of infection was probably human lymph administered with the vaccine. The incubation period was 1-7 months. Many outbreaks were reported after intravenous injections of arsenic for syphilis or intramuscular injections of gold salts. Then in 1942, the US Navy had an outbreak of 56,000 cases following administration of a yellow-fever vaccine. Studies in several countries confirmed the transmissibility of two distinct forms of hepatitis between 1942 and 1950: hepatitis A and B. Between 1964 and 1967, pediatrician Saul Krugman (1911-1995) in New York State inoculated children in a school for mentally retarded children with hepatitis (!!) and discovered that one type had an incubation period of 4-6 weeks, and the other of 9-13 weeks.

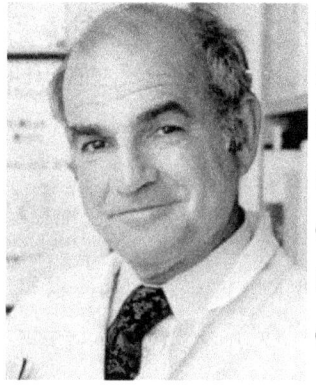

Barry Blumberg

In 1963, geneticist Baruch Blumberg (1925-2011) worked at the NIH (Bethesda MD) on the polymorphism of lipoproteins. He noticed in an immunodiffusion gel an unusual reaction between the serum of a poly-transfused hemophiliac and that of an Australian aborigine. He called it the *Australia antigen* (Au). When a lab technician, who had been Au-negative, developed jaundice and became Au-positive, follow-up studies prompted the connection between Au antigen and viral hepatitis. Blumberg received the 1976 Nobel prize in Physiology/ Medicine for his discovery. In 1968, virologist Alfred Prince (1928-2011) in New York showed, with immuno-electrophoresis, a serum antigen specifically associated with post transfusion hepatitis: the serum hepatitis (SH) antigen. Au and SH proved to be identical. Electron microscopy showed virus-like particles. David Dane (1923-1998) in London identified the 42nm particle, the HB virion, in 1970. Subtypes of the virus were reported later. The virus was shown to have an HBsAg coat, an inner core (HBc antigen), and a new soluble antigen HBe, found by Lars Magnius in Gothenburg SW. Kazuo Okochi in Tokyo JA established the association between the Au/SH antigen in blood donors and post transfusion hepatitis in 1972. The antigen was renamed HBs antigen and its detection in donor blood became mandatory. The protective role of anti-HBs immunoglobulin was confirmed (after needle-stick exposure, *etc.*). Blumberg filed a patent for a vaccine generated from high HBs-antigen plasma. Virologist Philippe Maupas (1939-1981) in Tours FR also developed an HBs vaccine in 1976. When Pierre Tiollais (b.1934) in Paris had cloned HBV in 1979, mass production of the recombinant hepatitis B vaccine became possible in 1985.

In 1974, both the NIH and Alfred Prince's New York groups noted that most cases of post-transfusion hepatitis were in fact HBs negative and hepatitis-A negative (*non-A, non-B hepatitis*). The disease could be transmitted to chimpanzees. Electron-microscopy studies revealed an enveloped virus (Daniel Bradley, b.1941;1985). Collaboration between Bradley's CDC (Atlanta GA) and the NIH groups allowed the team at Chiron Corp (Emeryville CA) to identify the first epitope of the hepatitis-C (HCV) envelope in 1989. HCV (a single-strand-positive RNA, 9,6 kb, flavivirus) and its

Transfusion

nuclear structures were then rapidly identified. An HCV vaccine is still under development. The incidence of transfusion-associated hepatitis decreased at the NIH markedly from 33% before the introduction of a HBs Ag test to 0.3% after the introduction of anti-HCV tests in 1994.

While the HCV story was developing in the 1970's to early 1980's, a new disease exploded among blood recipients. In 1981, opportunistic infections and Kaposi sarcoma were found among gay men in New York and California: *Acquired Immune Deficiency Syndrome* (AIDS). In late 1982, the first cases of AIDS in patients with hemophilia A were observed; the clotting factor concentrates were the only possible source. The next year, a multi-transfused infant developed AIDS and a single platelet donor had developed AIDS 10 months after the donation. Within 10 years, at least 10,000 cases of transfusion-associated AIDS had developed from before the introduction of an anti-HIV screening assay in 1985. Among all AIDS in children, transfusion accounted for 12%. Approximately 90% of severe hemophiliacs in the USA were HIV-infected before 1981. In Europe, the incidence was much lower, partly because the donor pools of factor-VIII concentrates were much smaller (or non-existent because of use of cryoprecipitate). In 1983, Luc Montagnier

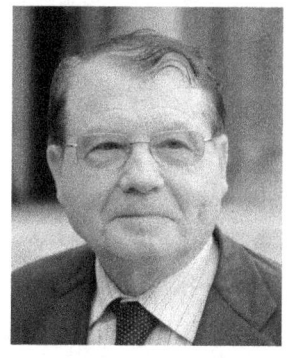

Luc Montagnier

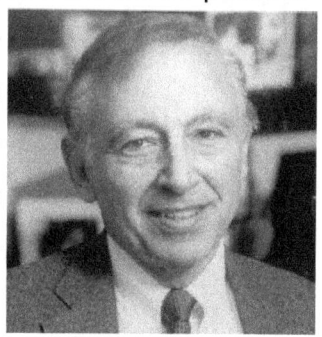

Robert Gallo

(1932-2022) in Paris, and in 1984 Robert Gallo at the NIH, isolated a T-lymphotropic retrovirus: *Human Immunodeficiency Virus* (HIV). Within a year, an assay for anti-HIV was licensed and used to test all transfusion products. In 2000, a nucleic acid screening test for HIV-RNA was introduced. The risk of transfusion-transmitted HIV decreased to 1 in 2 million. The blood-bank community has been blamed for slow reaction to the exploding epidemic in 1982-1984, but that is obviously easy in hindsight. Luc Montagnier shared in the 2008 Nobel prize in Physiology/Medicine.

West Nile Virus is another flavivirus. It is transmitted through mosquito bites and its primary hosts are birds (*e.g.*, American robin, crow, blue jay). The virus was recovered in Uganda in 1937, in Italy in 1998, and in North America in 1999. The first cases of transfusion-transmitted West Nile Virus in the USA date from 2002. Nucleic-Acid Testing (NAT) was introduced in 2003 and approved in 2005. In 2009, 145 prospective donors tested positive. In 2019, despite negative screening, a probably low viral load donor led to a platelet transfusion induced fatality in a heart-transplant recipient.

Non-infectious complications

The first clinical transfusions had a mortality of about 50%; partly because of the condition of the patient, partly because of the transfusion itself (*p.285-289*). The introduction of blood groups by Landsteiner (*p.296*) permitted pre-transfusion compatibility testing and decreased the risk of transfusion death due to ABO mismatch. Over the next 50 years, many new blood groups were discovered, and the Coombs test *(p.103)* continued to improve the safety of red cell transfusions.

Hemolytic transfusion reactions remained relatively frequent with a mortality of about 1 per 1,000 transfusions (Alexander Wiener, 1943). Even by the year 2000, hemolytic transfusion reactions occurred in 1 in 76,000 transfusions with a mortality of 1 in 1.8 million units transfused. Most of the deaths come from mis-identifying blood samples, components or patients; half of the errors occur outside the blood bank. National patient identification systems in Sweden and Finland almost completely eliminated mis-collected samples. Without such a system, the risk of mis-labelling is many times (1,000x?) greater than of clinically significant viral transmission.

The nearly universal use of packed red-cell units markedly decreased the risk of acute hemolysis by passively acquired antibody. Fresh frozen plasma is restricted to ABO compatible donors and hemolysis by non-ABO antibodies is unusual. Mismatched platelet transfusions may still cause hemolysis because of mismatched plasma.

Delayed hemolytic transfusion reactions are more common, but typically less severe. Fever, drop in hemoglobin, and mild jaundice often go unrecognized after hospital discharge. In sickle-cell anemia these reactions have been severe and sometimes fatal (Diamond, 1980). Newer molecular technologies are helping with that problem (Wendell Rosse, 1990).

Non-hemolytic (febrile) transfusion reactions continued to be frequent even when ABO-compatible blood was transfused. In 1957, Thomas Brittingham and Hugh Chaplin Jr in St. Louis MO, demonstrated that these febrile reactions in multi-transfused patients occurred when the buffy coat (*i.e.*, leukocytes) was left, but not when the buffy coat had been removed. Their results suggested that the reactions were caused by leukocytes. Herbert Perkins (1919-2013) in San Francisco CA, subsequently calculated in 1966, that the minimum number of leukocytes to cause a fever reaction varied between 0.25 and 25×10^9, and that the amount of temperature spike was dependent on the leukocyte number and the rate of infusion. A large amount of work in the field of prevention of non-hemolytic transfusion reactions was done by George Eernisse (1923-2000) and Anneke Brand (1946-2021) in Leiden NL, and by the group of Joghem van Loghem (1914-2005) in Amsterdam. The latter group introduced a commercial cotton-wool filter to remove leukocytes from red-cell units in 1972. Eernisse and Brand focused on platelet transfusions and demonstrated that leukocyte removal from transfused platelet and red-cell units, not only prevented febrile transfusion reactions, but also allo-

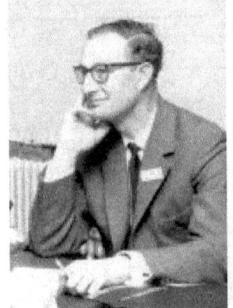

George Eernisse

Joghem van Loghem

immunization leading to platelet refractoriness (1981). In fact, in Leiden all patients with hematological diseases received only leukocyte-poor blood products by 1975. This practice spread rapidly over Europe, but far more slowly across the Atlantic. Charles Schiffer (Baltimore MD) and colleagues performed a randomized trial of leukocyte-depleted platelet transfusions in 1983, to decrease allo-immunization. Their conclusion was that leukocyte-depletion did not help, even though fewer patients who received leukocyte-depleted platelets became allo-immunized (p=0.07). My conclusion would be that this study was under-powered to show the actual benefit. The introduction of commercial filters, *e.g.*, the Pall Leukotrap® filter in 1988, slowly led to increased leukocyte depletion of cellular blood products in the USA.

Graft-versus-Host Disease (GvHD) after blood transfusion can occur whenever the postulates of Billingham (*p.225*) are fulfilled: 1) The infused product must contain immunologically active cells; 2) The recipient must have important transplantation antigens that are lacking in the donor; and 3) The recipient must be incapable of rejecting the donor cells, at least during the immediate period after infusion. Such situations may well exist: recipients may be incapable of rejecting the transfused T-lymphocytes, because of inborn immune deficiency (SCID, Wiskott-Aldrich syndrome; Seemayer, Montreal CN 1980), unusual HLA overlap with transfusions donated by homozygous family members (Michael Thaler, Tel Aviv IS, 1989), or medical immune suppression (fludarabine (*p.208,235*), stem-cell transplantation, acute leukemia treatment). Transfusion-induced GvHD was a serious complication with a mortality of close to 90%! Leukocyte depletion of blood products will likely decrease the incidence of GvHD, but the standard therapy was to irradiate the blood product with at least 1,500- 2,500 cGy. This irradiation does not damage the blood product (not even granulocytes !), but will prevent the donor T-lymphocytes from proliferating. Several pathogen-reduction technologies have been shown to be about as effective as γ-irradiation.

Transfusion-related acute lung injury (**TRALI**), originally called "noncardiogenic pulmonary edema", was described for the first time by Thomas Brittingham in St. Louis MO in 1957; he was able to provoke it by injecting blood containing leuko agglutinins into a research subject. Over the next 25 years, occasional cases were reported, and in 1970 it was postulated that leuko-agglutinins to HLA and non-HLA antigens were etiologic. In 1985, Mark Popovsky (b.1951) and Breanndan Moore (1944-2009) reported 5 cases and reviewed a total of 36. In three of their cases, the leuko-agglutinins corresponded with the HLA antigens of the recipient. It is currently the leading cause of transfusion-related death. Its incidence is 1 in 1,500-5,000 in the USA, 1 in 10,000-100,000 in Canada, and 1 in 8,000 – 1,000,000 in Europe. Anti-HLA class I or II or anti-granulocyte antibodies can cause TRALI, when transfused into patients with the cognate antigens. An alternative model of TRALI implicates the neutrophil as the effector cell. Recipient neutrophils are activated by a lipophilic priming activity (lyso-PCs) in the transfused product, while these recipient neutrophils are adherent to the pulmonary microvascular-endothelial cells. Prevention might consist of disqualifying donors with HLA antibodies from plasma or platelet donation. Multiparous females would fall into this category. This policy, however, would remove 25% of the entire donor pool! Using younger blood products (red cells less than 14 days and platelets less than 2 days) would markedly decrease the accumulation of neutrophil-activating agents.

Karl Landsteiner *was born in Vienna AT in 1868. He studied Medicine at the University there, followed by 2 years of chemistry study with Emil Fischer in Berlin, and in Munich and Zürich SU. He returned to Vienna to the Hygienic Institute and worked on the nature of antibodies. From 1897-1908 he was at the Pathology Institute of the university, working on serology, bacteriology, virology, and pathological anatomy. In 1900, he found out that the blood of two people on contact agglutinates and the next year that this agglutination was caused by serum. With blood from coworkers, he identified 3 blood groups: A, B, and C (later called O). He also showed that blood transfusion between persons of the same blood type did not lead to hemolysis, whereas this did occur between people of different blood types. This led to the first*

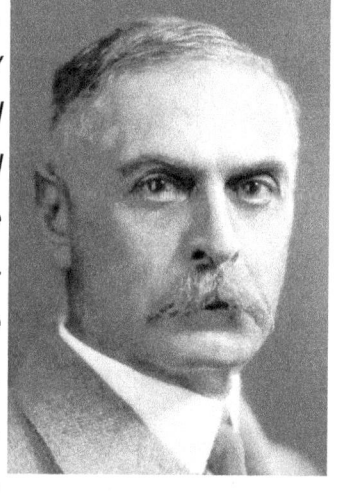

successful blood transfusion in 1908 in New York. (p.289). When much larger numbers of people were tested, Ludwik Hirszfeld and Emil von Dungern in Heidelberg GE established in 1908 the heredity of the ABO groups and found the fourth group: AB. Landsteiner also studied the poliomyelitis virus, and showed that the disease could be transferred to monkeys. Furthermore, he found the Donath-Landsteiner antibodies in syphilis.

Because the inhabitants of Vienna were starving after the end of World War I, Landsteiner and his family moved to The Hague NL in 1919, and he became a pathologist in a hospital there. Even though their nutritional situation was better, their financial situation remained precarious, and he "moon-lighted" by preparing tuberculin for a pharmacist. In 1923, he moved to the Rockefeller Institute in New York at the invitation of Simon Flexner. He continued his work on immunity and discovered blood groups M, N, and P, together with Philip Levine. A later discovery were irregular anti-A agglutinins. Rhesus monkey red cells had produced an agglutinin similar to the human M antigen in immunized guinea pigs. This antibody recognized 39 of 45 human blood specimens. Studies of mothers of erythroblastosis fetalis patients established the Rhesus blood group system. He received the Nobel prize in Physiology/Medicine for his discoveries in 1930. He retired in 1939, but kept a small laboratory at the Institute. He died in 1943 from a heart attack.

Transfusion

Patrick Loudon ("Pat") Mollison *was born in London in 1914. He did his medical training at St. Thomas' Hospital and graduated in 1938. During World War II, he was first a young doctor at the South London Blood Supply Depot, where he worked on blood preservation and storage. His group discovered that red cells preferred a slightly acidified solution: ACD (acid citrate dextrose). During the bombing of London, he learned that packed red cells were also helpful, not just the plasma. In 1943, he entered the Royal Army Medical Corps and he served in Germany (e.g., liberation of Bergen Belsen concentration camp) and Burma. After the war, he joined Hammersmith Hospital to resume his research, particularly on hemolytic anemia in newborns. He moved to St. Mary's hospital in 1960 as the Director of the Medical Research Council's Blood Transfusion Research Unit, which then became the Experimental Hematology Unit. He became Professor of Hematology in 1962. In 1951 he published the first edition of* Blood Transfusion in Clinical Medicine, *soon considered the "Bible" of blood transfusion. The book went through 6 subsequent editions with him as sole editor, and then three more editions with Marcela Contreras and Paul Engelfriet as co-editors. The 11th edition became "Mollison's Blood Transfusion in Clinical Medicine". He retired in 1979 and died in 2011 at the age of 97.*

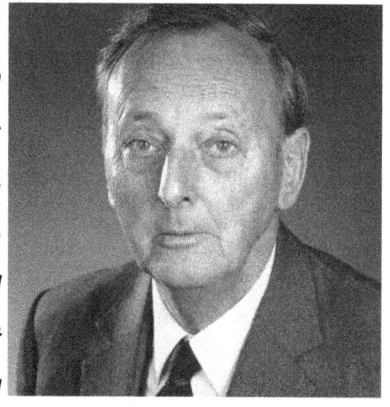

Nobel Prize laureates (Physiology/Medicine) in the field of Hematology

1901	Emil von Behring	serum therapy
1908	Ilya Mechnikov, Paul Ehrlich	cellular and humoral immunity
1912	Alexis Carrell	vascular sutures, transplantation
1919	Jules Bordet	discoveries in immunity
1930	Karl Landsteiner	blood groups
1934	George Whipple, George Minot, William Murphy	liver therapy for anemia
1944	Henrik Dam, Edward Doisy	vitamin K
1960	Frank Macfarlane Burnett, Peter Medawar	acquired immunological tolerance
1972	Gerald Edelman, Rodney Porter	chemical structure of antibodies
1974	Albert Claude, Christian de Duve	lysosomes
1975	David Baltimore, Howard Temin	reverse transcriptase
1976	Baruch Blumberg	Australia antigen
1980	Jean Dausset	HLA (human leukocyte antigens)
1984	Georges Köhler, César Milstein	monoclonal antibodies
1987	Susuma Tonegawa	antibody diversity
1990	Don Thomas	bone-marrow transplantation
1996	Peter Doherty, Rolf Zinkernagel	cell-mediated immune defense
2008	Francoise Barré-Sinoussi, Luc Montagnier	Human Immunodeficiency virus
2012	John Gordon, Shinya Yamanaka	mature cells becoming pluripotent
2020	Harvey Alter, Michael Houghton, Charles Rice	hepatitis-C virus

CONCLUSIONS

Blood diseases have a long history, but the medical discipline Hematology did not take off until studies of peripheral blood became possible in the mid-to-late 19th century. Bone marrow examination during life became possible less than a century ago. Studies of bone-marrow proliferation and stem cells date from after World War II.

The science of hematology has been quite international. Increasing international travel has markedly increased our understanding, but also the risks, of hematological diseases. Especially hematology in the USA has benefited from international migration, often forced by conditions in Tsarist Russia and Nazi Germany. It shows once again the valuable contribution of immigrants to most countries. This holds true for Cornelis Drebbel (*p.23*), Ilya Mechnikov (*p.135*), Karl Landsteiner (*p.321*), as well as for Bill Dameshek (*p.188*), Max Wintrobe (*p.83*) and Ernest Beutler (*p.85*).

Different fields of interest have existed in the history of hematology. The late 19th century was typified by increasing knowledge about the peripheral blood (Paul Ehrlich, Giulio Bizzozero, Georges Hayem), the early chemistry of red blood cells (Otto Warburg, Emil Fischer, Felix Hoppe-Seyler) and coagulation (Alexander Schmidt). Between 1900 and 1910, the chemistry of red-blood cells and the first hereditary anemia (hereditary spherocytosis) were studied, and phagocyte function was elucidated (Ilya Mechnikov). The second decade saw the introduction of indirect blood transfusion (Karl Landsteiner), the discovery of sickle-cell anemia, and the first studies of neutrophil physiology and of the reticuloendothelial system (Ludwig Aschoff). From 1920-1930, additional types of hereditary anemia (thalassemia) were reported and treatment of pernicious anemia was introduced and improved. The last decade before World-War II saw coagulation (Paul Morawitz) and serum-protein studies (Arne Teselius) take off. The World-War-II period had major effects on blood transfusion, and also introduced cancer chemotherapy (nitrogen mustard). After the war had ended, stem-cell biology became prominent, mainly based on the dangerous effects of radiation. Coagulation research rapidly improved (Armand Quick). Antibody research started (Örjan Ouchterlony, Astrid Fagraeus). In the 1950's, many fields expanded: G6PD deficiency (Ernest Beutler), multiple myeloma (Isadore Snapper), non-Hodgkin's lymphoma (Henry Rappaport), acute leukemia, myeloproliferative disorders (William Dameshek). Then in the 1960's, much attention was paid to Hodgkin's disease (Henry Kaplan), chronic myelogenous leukemia (Peter Nowell), HLA-typing (Jon van Rood) and platelet disorders. In the next decade, immunology, lymphoma, acute leukemia (classification and therapy), aplastic anemia (Bruno Speck) and stem-cell transplantation (Don Thomas) stood at the forefront. The 1980's saw the widespread use of monoclonal antibodies (George Köhler, Cesar Milstein) for diagnosis, the understanding of B-cell variety and the first attempts at gene transfer. In the 1990's, integration of morphology,

Conclusions

cytogenetics, FISH and PCR technology led to new classifications of leukemia (WHO) and malignant lymphoma (REAL). Stem-cell transplantation from matched unrelated donors, and with mobilized peripheral blood as stem-cell graft, became important. In the first decade of the 21st century, tyrosine-kinase inhibitor imatinib replaced allogeneic stem cell transplantation as primary therapy for CML (Brian Druker) and CAR-T cells for B-cell malignancy were introduced, The most recent decade is typified by immunological therapy for many diseases (non-myeloablative stem-cell transplants, related partially mismatched donors, CAR-T cells), and by disease interference via receptors, antigens and pathways (imatinib, JAK and BTK inhibitors).

What have we learned since Wintrobe published his *"Blood. Pure and Eloquent"* in 1980? In 1980, many hematologists still oversaw the entire field of blood diseases, even though subspecialties already existed (malignancies, anemias, hemostasis, transfusion *etc*). The rapid expansion of immunological techniques for diagnosis and therapy of hematological malignancies started with the introduction of monoclonal antibodies. The advances in molecular biology produced new methods to diagnose and treat hematological malignancies, as well as some anemias. The improvements in chemotherapy were gradual and not revolutionary anymore. Pathway interruption is now becoming more important than cytotoxicity.

Stem-cell transplantation has undergone major changes since 1980. From a discipline with only bone marrow (autologous, syngeneic and HLA-identical sibling allografts), the introduction of peripheral blood stem cells, umbilical cord-blood cells, matched unrelated donors and haplo-identical related donors caused major changes.

Hemostaseology and transfusion medicine have had major ups (factor V Leiden), and a dramatic down with HIV-infected coagulation and transfusion products. The production of recombinant clotting products should have resolved such problems. International travel will continue to be a challenge.

Overall, the improvements over the most recent 40 years have been enormous. What does that promise for the next 40 years? A former Vice-President from Indiana repeated a Danish (Niels Bohr?) or Yogi Berra (?) quote: "Predictions are difficult, especially about the future". Whatever will happen, "Blood will still be a special juice", to update Goethe for the new century. To conclude with a corny explanation:

person 1: Blood is the most important organ in humans.
person 2: why?
person 1: the function of the heart is to pump blood around; of the lungs to provide oxygen to the blood; of the bowels and liver to feed the blood; and of the kidneys and liver to cleanse the blood.
person 2: and of the brain?
person 1: to think about blood.

===============

BIBLIOGRAPHY

American Society of Hematology *50th Anniversary Reviews*, 2008

Bain B — *Leukaemia Diagnosis. A guide to the FAB Classification*. Gower Medical Publishing, London, 1990

Bernard J, Bessis M, Binet JL — *Histoire Illustrèe de l'"Hèmatologie de l'antiquitè à nos jours*. Roger Dacoste, Paris, 1992

Bessis M, Brecher G — *Hemopoietic Dysplasias (Preleukemic States)*. Springer Verlag, Berlin, 1977

Dacie JV — *The Hemolytic Anaemias. Congenital and Acquired.* Churchill, London, 1954

Downey H — *Handbook of Hematology.* Hamilton Medical, London 1938

Forkner C — *Leukemia and Allied Disorders*. MacMillan, New York, 1938

Forman SJ, Blume KG, Thomas ED — *Bone Marrow Transplantation.* Blackwell, Oxford UK, 1994

Gall EA, Mallory TB — *Malignant Lymphoma. A clinico-pathologic survey of 618 cases. Amer J Pathol 1942; 18: 381-429*

Gersen SL, Keagle MB — *The Principles of Clinical Cytogenetics*. Humana Press, Totowa NJ, 1999

Good R A, Fisher D W — *Immunobiology.* Sinauer Assoc Inc, Stamford CT, 1971

Gunz F, Baikie AG — *Leukemia.* Grune & Stratton, New York, 3rd edition, 1974

Hart GD — Descriptions of blood and blood disorders before the advent of laboratory studies. *British Journal of Haematology* 2001; 115: 719-728

Hayhoe FGJ — *Leukaemia. Research and Clinical Practice.* Churchill, London, 1960

Blood is Life

Hemker HC, Loeliger EA, Veltkamp JJ — *Human Blood Coagulation.* Leiden University Press, Leiden NL, 1969

Hirschfeld H, Hittmair A — *Handbuch der allgemeine Hämatologie.* Urban & Schwarzenberg, Berlin, 1933

Jackson H, Parker F — *Hodgkin's disease and allied disorders.* Oxford University Press, New York, 1947

Jansen J — *From Mice to Men. A history of early Bone Marrow Transplantation,* Amsterdam NL, 2020

Kaplan H S — *Hodgkin's Disease.* Harvard University Press, Cambridge MA, 1972

Keynes, G — *Blood Transfusion.* Oxford Medical Publications, London, 1922

Marshall A H E — *An outline of the cytology and pathology of the reticular tissue.* Olive and Boyd, Edinburgh UK, 1956

Mathé G, Amiel JL, Schwarzenberg L — *Bone Marrow Transplantation and Leucocyte Transfusions.* C C Thomas Publishers, Springfield IL 1971

McCarthy L J — *The Modern Pioneers in Transfusion Medicine.* Indianapolis IN, 2020

Mollison P L — *Blood Transfusion in Clinical Medicine;* 4th edition. Blackwell, Oxford UK, 1967

Naegeli O — *Blutkrankheiten und Blutdiagnostik.* Von Velt, Leipzig GE, 1908

Nilsson IIM — *Haemorrhagic and Thrombotic Diseases,* John Wiley Publishers, Hoboken NJ, 1974

Packman CH — The spherocytic haemolytic anaemias. *British Journal of Haematology* 2001; 112 :888-899

Pappenheim A — *Atlas der Menschlichen Blutzellen* Gustav Fischer Verlag, Jena GE, 1905

Bibliography

Pemberton S	*The Bleeding Disease: Hemophilia and the Unintended Consequences of Medical Progress.* Johns Hopkins University Press, Baltimore MD, 2011
Piller GJ	Leukaemia – a brief historical review from ancient times to 1950. *British Journal of Haematology* 2001;112: 282-292
Rolleston H	The history of hematology. *Journal of the Royal Society of Medicine 27:* 1161-1178, 1934
Snapper I, Turner LB, Moscovitz HL	*Multiple Myeloma.* Grune & Stratton, New York, 1953
Steensma DP, Tefferi A	The myelodysplastic syndrome(s): a perspective and review highlighting current controversies. *Leukemia Res* 2003; 27: 95-120
Tefferi A	The history of myeloproliferative disorders: before and after Dameshek. *Leukemia* 2008; 22; 3-13
Terasaki P	*History of HLA: ten recollections.* UCLA Tissue Typing Laboratory, Los Angeles CA, 1990
Van Bekkum DW, De Vries MJ	*Radiation Chimaeras.* Logos Press, London, 1967
Vroman L	*Blood.* Natural History Press, Garden City, NY, 1967
Waldenström J	*Diagnosis and treatment of Multiple Myeloma.* Grune & Stratton, New York, 1970
Wintrobe MM	*Blood, pure and eloquent.* McGraw-Hill, New York,1980
Wintrobe MM	*Hematology: the Blossoming of a Science. A story of Inspiration and Effort.* Lea & Febiger, Philadelphia PA, 1985
Young NS, Reis P	A Century of Hematology. *Seminars in Hematology* 1999; vol 36, suppl 7

About the Author

Jan Jansen was born in 1949 in Enschede NL. He attended medical school at the Free University in Amsterdam (1967-1973), where one then still had to pass a test in Medical History. He trained in Internal Medicine and Hematology at the Free University and the State University Leiden. At the latter, he also obtained his PhD in 1979, for work on clinical and immunological aspects of hairy cell leukemia. These studies were mentored by Ralph van Furth (1929-2018), who co-authored the mononuclear phagocyte system (MPS; *p.132*), and Willy Hijmans (1921-2018), an authority on surface and cytoplasmic immunoglobulins (*p.213*). From 1980-1981, he spent a sabbatical with John Kersey (1938-2013; *p.237)* in Minneapolis MN, to study antigens on stem cells. His focus in Leiden had by then changed to bone-marrow transplantation (BMT). In 1984, he became Professor of Medicine and founding director of the BMT program of Indiana University, and in 1989 of Indiana Blood and Marrow Transplantation (*IBMT*), both in Indianapolis IN. After his retirement in 2012, he relocated to Santa Fe, NM to devote his time to the study of (medical) history.

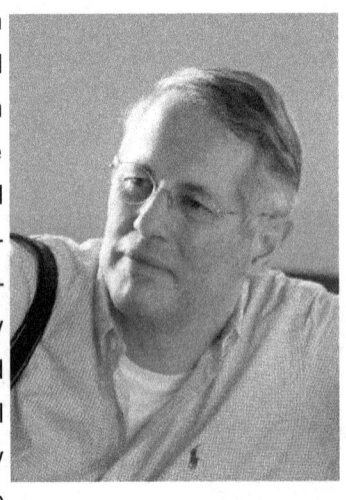

INDEX

List of countries and US states mentioned

AG	Argentina	HU	Hungary	NY	New York
AR	Arkansas	IL	Illinois	NZ	New Zealand
AT	Austria	IN	Indiana	OH	Ohio
AU	Australia	IO	Iowa	OR	Oregon
AZ	Arizona	IS	Israel	PA	Pennsylvania
BE	Belgium	IT	Italy	PO	Poland
CA	California	JA	Japan	PT	Portugal
CH	China	KY	Kentucky	RU	Russia
CN	Canada	LA	Louisiana	SP	Spain
CZ	Czech Republic	MD	Maryland	SU	Switzerland
		ME	Mexico	SW	Sweden
DC	District of Columbia	MI	Michigan	TA	Tanzania
		MN	Minnesota	TN	Tennessee
DE	Denmark	MO	Missouri	TU	Turkey
ES	Estonia	NC	North Carolina	TX	Texas
				UG	Uganda
FI	Finland	NI	Nigeria	UK	United Kingdom
FR	France	NJ	New Jersey		
GE	Germany	NL	Netherlands	VA	Virginia
GR	Greece	NM	New Mexico	WA	Washington State
		NO	Norway	WI	Wisconsin

333

Blood is Life

	page		
Abelson N M	300	Bence Jones H	214-215
ABVD chemotherapy	205	Bennett J H	26,137
Actuarius J	100	Bennett J M	145
Acquired hemolytic anemia	100-105	Bergsagel D E	219
Acute Lymphoblastic Leukemia (ALL)	141-147	Berk L	98
Acute Myelogenous leukemia (AML)	147-153	Bernard C	8,20,31,56
Acute promyelocytic leukemia (APL)	151-152	Bernard J	123,151,154, *169-171*,253
Adair G S	55	Bernard-Soulier syndrome	253
ADAMTS13	259	Bernstein F	298
Addis T	269	Bertina R M	283
Addison T	91,93,129,192	Bertino J R	150
Addison W	129,245	Bessis M	8,27,54,170
Adoptive immunotherapy	124	Bethune N	293,295
Adult T-cell leukemia/lymphoma (ATLL)	162-163	Beutler E	79,81,82,*85-87*, 160,166,181,326
Aggregometer	45	BFU-e, CFU-e	17
Agote L	291	Biermer M A	94
Agranulocytosis	131	Biggs R P	267,270
Aksoy M	108	Billingham R E	225,319
Albucasis	274	Binet J L	160
Allison A C	68	Björkman S E	174
Allwell N	218	Bizzozero	7,8,20,44,53,93, 246,255,266,280
Alving A S	79,82	Blaese M	73
Amos D B	39	Bland-Sutton J	76
Anagrelide	187	Blaud P	89
Anderson W F	73	Bleeding time	43
Andral G	100,272	Bloch C E	97
Ann Arbor staging system	202,206	Blood cell counting	30-33
Anti-lymphocyte globulin (ALG)	112	Blood cell separator	305-307
Anti-thrombin III	271-272	Block M	174
Anthony Nolan Register	229	Blokhin N	219
Aplastic anemia	106-120	Blumberg B S	313,314
Arinkin M J	10	Blundell J	287
Aristotle	261	Blume K	86,240
Arthus M	290	Boggs D R	232
Ashby W	41	Bogdanov A	295
Aschoff L	9,132,194,216,326	Bonadonna G	205-206
Askanazy M	182	Bone marrow biopsy	7,10-11
Assman H	182	Bone-marrow transplantation	14,63,72, 110, 115,119,179,*223-243*
L-asparaginase	141	Boorman K E	103
ATRA	152	Bordet J	38,263
Aubertin Ch	106	Born G V R	45
Autoimmune hemolytic anemia	100-105	Bortin M M	227
Australian antigen	313	Bounameaux Y	247
Babesiosis	310	Bouroncle B A	163
Babington B G	262	Boveri T H	35
Babylonian Talmud	4	Brackmann H H	276
Bach F H	40	Bradley D W	314
Bagby G	174	Bradley T R	16
Baltimore D	62	Brand A	318
Banti G	77	Braxton-Hicks J	289
Barlogie B	220,241	Brecher G	172
Barlow T	76	Brenner M K	233
Barnes D W H	225	Brentjens R J	209
Barrett AJ	179	Bright R	192
Bcr-abl	155	Brill N E	102,193
Becton Dickinson	34	Brinkhous K	47,248,267, 275,*283-284*
Beet E A	67,68		
Behring E A	50,94,133		

Index

British Comparative Thromboplastin 46
Brittingham T E 318,320
Brohm F 255
Broome J D 143
Brouet J C 163
Brown E A 82
Brown J H 290
Brown P K 131
Broxmeyer H E 115,234
Bruton tyrosine kinase (BTK) 161
Buchanan A 263
Buckner C D 239,243
BuCy 227
Burchenal J H 123,142
Burkhardt R 11
Burkitt D P 198,208
Burkitt's lymphoma 145,198,240
Cabot R C 91,92,185
Cadaveric blood 295,308
Caen J P 249,250
Cahn A 97
CALLA 144,145
Caminopetros J 59
Canellos G P 154,205,211
Carrel A 288
Carson E 266
Carson P E 81
Cartwright G E 84
Caspersson T 37
Castle W B 90,98
Catovsky D 121,146,165,167
Cazal P 148
CFU-c or CFU-GM 16
CFU-GEMM 17
CFU-s 15
CD (cluster of differentiation) 145
Chagas C R J 311
Chaplin H 318
Chargaff E 248
Chauffard A 75-76,101
Chen Z 152
Chervenick P A 232
Children.s Cancer Group (CCG) 143
CAR-T (Chimeric Antigen Receptor) 209-210,221,327
Chlorosis 88-89
Chloramphenicol 107
CHOP chemotherapy 208
Chronic Lymphocytic Leukemia (CLL) 156-161
Chronic Myelogenous Leukemia (CML) 153-156
Circumcision 4
Civin C I 233
Clarkson B D 150
Clowes G H A 95
CMOMC 15,16

Cohen J A 42
Cohn E J 302
Cohn Z A 132
Cohnheim J 129
Coller B S 250
Collins R 200
Conley C L 267
Colony-stimulating factor (CSF) 16
Constantinus Chlorus 57
Contreras M 323
Cooley T B 58,62
Coombs R R A 103,300
Coombs test 103
Copeland M M 216
Cordes W 78
Corner G W 58
Coulter W H 32-33
Crile G W 288
Croce C M 200
Cronkite E P 159, *172-173,*
Crosby W 82,117, *124-125*
Cullis H 305
Curie M S 13,108
Curtis A H 290
Cutbush M 300
Cytogenetics 35-37
CyTBI 227
Dacie J V 1 104,116,117, *120-122*
Dahlbäck B 282
Dameshek W 25,59,102,110,125,159, 177,180,181, *188-190,* 240,325,326
Dane D M S 314
Daniel M T 145
Darrow R 299
Dastre A 272
Dausset J B G J 39
David V C 290
Davie E W 271
De Duve C R M J 131
Dempsey E W 148
De Blainville H M D 263,278
Denis de Commercy P S 262
Denys H 255
Denys J B 285,286
De Senac J B 127
Desmopressin 277
De Vita V T 205, 211
De Vries H 35
De Vries M J 224
De Winiwarter H 35
Dexter T M 17
Diamond L K 110,300
Diamond W J 317
DIC (diffuse intravascular coagulation) 278-279
Dicke K A 238

Blood is Life

Di-dimer	47-48,279	Everett J L	159
Diggs L W	69	Ewald O	9,164
Di Guglielmo G A	176-177,186,187	Ewing J	197,216
Diocles	279	Extrinsic pathway	45-46,263-266
Direct transfusion	285-290,292	FAB classification	145,148,175
Dittrich W	33	Faber K	97
Dodd B E	103	Fabricius-Møller J	12,223
Döhle K G P	254	Factor V	265,283
Dolowy W C	143	Fagraeus A	134,216,326
Donath J	105	Falini B	166
Donath-Landsteiner antibody	104,322	Fanconi G	114
Donhauser J L	182	Farber S	142,196
Doniach D	99	Febrile transfusion reaction	318-319
Donné A F	31,137,245	Fefer A	239,243
Donnelly W J	164	Fenwick S	97
Donor lymphocyte infusions	228,235	Ferrata A	176,197
Doscherholmen A	99	Ferrebee J W	226,243
Douglas A S	267	Fessas P	62
Downey H	164	Fialkow P J	181-182
Drebbel C	23,325	Fibrometer	46
Dreissler L A	104	Finch C	93,243
Dreschfeld J	193	Firkin B G	251
Drets M E	37	Fisher A	35
Drew C R	294	Fisher E	66,80,322,325
Druker B J	155,327	Fisher R A	300
Dualistic	8	Flandrin G	145,171
Duhamel G	164	Flashman D H	158
Duke W W	42,303	Fleming A	130
Duran i Jordá F	293	Flemming W	35
Durie B G M	218	Flexner S	322
Easson E C	201	Fliedner T M	232
Eberth K J	246,280,281	Flint A	97,230
EBMT	237	Flow cytometry	34-36
Edelman G	213	Fludarabine	160,235,320
Eernisse G J	318	Fluorescent in-situ hybridization (FISH)	
Egeberg R O	281		37,149
Ehrich W E	134	Folic acid	95-96
Ehrlich P	8,21,26,29,38,*49-51*,	Folkers K A	96
	92,103,105,106,116,130,	Folli F	285
	133-134,139,157,285,296	Ford C E	14,36,224
Eichenlaub F J	308	Fordyce J A	308
Eijkman C	94	Forkner C E	140-141
Embryonic stem cells (ESC)	18	Fowler T	140
Embden G G	81	Fox H	195
Emmel V E	66	Frank E	255
Engelfriet C P	323	Frank M M	104
Engelhart J F P	55	Frei E	142,304
Enneking A M J	116	Freireich E J	146,236,304,306
Epstein E	186	Fulwyler M J	34
Erslev A J	111	Funk C	94
Erythroblastic islands	54	Funke O	9
Erythroblastosis neonatorum/fetalis		Furlan M	259
	299	Gaarder A	248
Essential thrombocythemia	186-187	Galen (of Pergamom)	5,7,88,100,128,279
Evans B D F	95	Galilei G	23
Evans R S	256	Gall E A	196
Evans M	18	Gall J G	37

Index

Gallo R C	163,316	Harousseau J L	241
Galton D A G	121,146,148,154,167	Harrington W J	255
Gässlen M	95	Harrington-Hollingsworth experiment	256
Gea y Banacloche J	307	Harris T N	134
Gee T S	150	Harrop G	80
Gene transfer	64,73	Hartert H	44
George J N	260	Harvey W	128
Geschickter C F	216	Hata S	50
Gianni A M	232	Hathaway W E	268
Gibson J G	294	Hay J	274
Gilbert R	201,204	Hayem G	8,21,31,*48-49*,53,89,101,
Gillespie E B	69,71		245, 248,266,269,280
Gilman A Z	12,204	Hayhoe F G J	148,165,167
Gladiators	3,285	Heath C W	90
Glanzmann E	249	Hedin S G	55,272
Glanzmann's thrombasthenia	249-251	Hegglin R	253
Glick B	134	Heinz R	79
Gloor W	140	Hellem A J	247
Gluckman E	115,234	Heller E L	183
Glucose 6 phosphate deficiency	78-83	Hematopoietic growth factors	
Glutathione (GSH)	81		111,113,131,178
Gmelin L	101	Hemocytometer	31-32
Göhde W	33	Hemolytic transfusion reaction	317-318
Goldman J	121,232,239	Hematocrit	30
Golomb H M	166	Hemoglobin	28-29,55-57
Good R A	134,217	Hemophilia A	5,274-277
Goodman J W	232	Hemophilia B (Christmas factor)	
Goodman L S	12,204		270,275,277
Gordon-Smith E C	121	Herrick J B	66
Gorer P A	39	Herzenberg L A	34
Gorin N C	238	Heuck G	182
Gowers W R	29,32,157	Hewson K	208
Gralnick H	146	Hewson W	25,53,127,133,156, 289
Granulocyte transfusion	235,306-307	Hijmans W	213
Gräsbeck A R G	98	Hijmans van den Bergh A	116
Gray S J	41	Hill J M	143
Greaves M	144	Hillestad L K	151
Greenberg P	178	Hippocrates	5,7,87,312
Greenberg P J	209	Hirschfeld H	139
Greenfield W S	194	Hirszfeld L	298,301,322
Grever M R	160	Hirschhorn R	132
Griffin J H	282	HIV/AIDS	276-277,315-316
Grijns C	94	HLA	39-41,51-52
Gross L	211	Hodgkin T	191-192
Grunke W	10	Hodgson G S	232
Guinn N R	303	Hoedemaker P J	98
Gunn R B	62	Hoffbrand A V	121
Gunz F W	180-181,186,190	Hoffmann E M	118
Gutterman J U	166	Hoogstraten B	219
Hagen P S	99	Hooke R	23
Hahn E V	69,71	Hooker R S	289
Hairy-cell leukemia (HCL)	163-167	Hookworms	91
Hairy cell variant	167	Hopff F	274
Ham T H	116	Hoppe-Seyler E F	9,55,80,325
Hamerton J L	36	Hörlein H	70
Hammersten O	262	Howard M A	251
H-antigens	39	Howell W H	271

Blood is Life

Hoyer L W	252	Kolb H J	228
Hsu T C	36	Körber H	60
Huggins C E	303	Korngold L	214
Hugues J	247	Krebs H A	81
Hünefeld F L	55	Krugman S	313
Hungerford D A	36,154	Kuessner B	104
Hunter J	261,272,278,280	Kundrat H	157,193,198
Hunter W	74,92	Kunkel H G	60
Hustin A	291	Kyle R A	213
Huygens C	24	Ladd W S	97
Hydroxyurea	63,72,154	Laemmli U K	78
IBMTR	237	Lajtha L	17
Idiopathic thrombocytopenic purpura		Lambotte-Legrand	68
(ITP)	254-257	Landois L	38,116,289,290,296
Induced pluripotent stem cells (IPSC)		Landsteiner K	38,105,296,298,*321-322*
	19	Lange J	88
Ingram V M	59,61,71	Langhans T	194
International Normalized Ratio (INR)		Large granular Lymphocyte leukemia	
	46		163
Intrinsic pathway	47,266-271	Larrabee R C	189
iron deficiency	87-91	Leder P	200
Itano H A	60,70	Lederer M	101
Iscove N N	16	Lee R I	292
Ivy A C	43	Lee S L	164
Jackson H	183,195,197	Lehman H	65
Jacobson L O	13,204,224	Lehmann H	28
Jamshidi, K	11	Leishmania (kala azar) 311	
Jansky J	297	Lejeune J	36
Janssen Z	23	Lennert K	199
Janus kinase (JAK) inhibitors	183,186	Leopold	158
Johannsen W L	35	Le Sourd L	247
Jones T W	266	Leukemia	25
Jorpes E	272	Levan A	36
Judson G T	306	Levine P	298,299,323
Juttner C A	232	Levine S A	97
Kahler O	217	Levitsky G A	35
Kaminski M	207	Levy R	207
Kaplan H S	196,202,204,*210-211*	Lewis S M	121-122
Karnofsky D	123	Lieutaud J	25,127,156
Kaufman M	18	Link K P	266
Kaznelson P	255	Linman J W	174
Keating M J	160	Lipari R	214
Kersey J H	237-238	Lippershey H	23
Kidd J G	143	Lissauer A	140
Kiel classification	199	List A F	179
Killmann S A	96	Lister J	266,288
Kimpton A R	290	Loeliger E A	46
Kinmonth J B	203	Lord Dawson of Penn 76	
Kinoshita T	119	Lorenz E	13,224
Kirkwood T	46	Loughran T P	163
Klein G	200	Louis P C A	127
Klemperer P	197	Loutit J F	103,225,294
Klima needle	10	Lower R	285,286
Knudtzon S	233	Lucarelli G	63
Koch R	49,94,130	Lugano classification 203	
Köhler A	24	Lukes R J	195,200
Köhler G	144,326	Lurman A	312

Index

Lüscher E F	247	Moldavan A	32
Lusher J M	277	Mollison P L	121,294,302, *323*
Lusitano A	254	Mononuclear phagocyte system (MPS) 132	
Luzzato L	117,119,121	Monophyletic	8
Lydon N B	155	Montagnier L	315-316
Lyme disease	309	Monteiro H	203
Lymphangiogram	203	Montgomery J	208
Lymphatic system	25	Moore M A S	17-18,114
Lyon M F	86	Moore S B	320
Lysosome	131	MOPP chemotherapy 205	
Lyso-PCs	320	Morawitz P	263-264,266,272, 281,326
Magendie F	53		
Magnius L O	314	Moreno Robins M	109,236
Maimonides	4	Moreschi C	103
Malassez L C	31	Morgan J H	308
Mallory T B	196	Morris L M	10
Malpighi M	23,24,261	Morrison M	223
Manhattan project	13	Moschkowitz E	257
Mannucci P	277	Moscovitz H L	217
Marchiafava E	115	Moss W L	297
Margolis J	268	Mourant A	300
Marmont A M	112,240	MUD (matched unrelated donor) 229-230	
Marschalkó T	216	Müller J	262
Martin G R	18	Mullis K	38
Martini M	230	Multipotent adult progenitor cells (MADC) 19	
Mathé G	112,*123-124*,226, 228,234,236	Murphy J B	134
		Murphy W P	91,94,98,99
Maupas P	314	Murphy S	305
Maximow A	8,10,21, 231	Mustard gas	12
May R	253	Myelodysplastic syndrome (MDS) 174-179	
May-Hegglin anomaly	253-254	Myeloma	214-221
May-Grünwald-Giemsa stain	27	Myeloproliferative disorder (Mypro) 180-188	
Mazza S M A	312	NADP	81
McCluskie J A W	308,309	Naegeli O	8,54,75,139,140,147
McCulloch E A	14	Nasse C F	274
McElwain T J	219,241	Nathan D	62
Mcfarlane R G	251,267	National Marrow Donor Program (NMDP) 229	
McIntyre W	215	Neel J V	67
McLean J	272	Neutrophil alkaline phosphatase (NAP) 153	
Mechnikov I I	50,129, *135-136*,325	Neumann F E C	7,9,18, *20-21*, 53, 93,133,138,147,182
Medawar P B	39,225	Nicholson-Weller A 118	
Megaloblasts	92,93	Nilsson I M	252
Mendel G	35	Nitrogen mustard	12,141
Metcalf D	16,17,21	Nomarski G	25
Meulengracht E	77	Nowell P C	36-37,154,326
Meyerhof O F	81	Noyes W D	109,236
Michelli F	115	Nurden A T	249,250
Microscopy	23-28,137	Nussenzweig V	118,144,199
Mielke C H	43	O'Brien J R	45
Miletich J	282	Ohno S	82,86,181
Mills C A	278	Okochi K	314
Milstein C	144,326	Ollgaard E	248
Milstone J H	267,273	Osgood E E	14,109,154,223
Minkowski O	74	Osler W	141,185,245
Minot G R	90,91,94,97,251	Osmotic fragility	75
Moake J L	258		

339

Blood is Life

Ottesen J	131	Primary myelofiborisis (PMF or MMM)	182-184
Otto J C	5,274	Prince A	313,314
Ouchterlony O	212,326	Prolymphocytic leukemia	167
Owren P A	247,264-265	Protein C	265,281-283
Pagès C	290	Prothrombin time (PT)	45
Pagniez P	247	Pusey W A	201
Painter T S	35	Pythagoras	78,83
Pall Leukotrap filter	319	Quick A J	45,251,264,326
Pappenehim A	8,21,139,157-158,197,216	Race R R	103,300,301
Paracelsus	128	Radiation	12,13,15,137,143,154, 201-203,223-227,230
Pardue M L	37	Radiation chimaera	224-225
Parker F	183,195,197	Rai K R	159
Parkes-Weber F	185	Ramon y Cajal S	215
PARMA study	240	Ranvier L A	133
Partial thromboplastin time (aPTT)	47,267	Rappaport H	194,198,326
Patek A J	269	Ratnoff O D	267-268
Pauling L	60,69	REAL classification	200,327
Pavlovsky A	270	Reed D M	194-195
Payne R O	40	Reed-Sternberg cell	194-196
Pedreira de Freitas J L	312	Reichert K	28
Pekelharing C A	262	Reiman F	90
Pemberton J deJ	291	Reschad H	139
Pepper W	93	Reticulo-endothelial system (RES)	9,132,139,194
peripheral blood stem cells (PBSC)	10,231-233	Reverse transcriptase	62
Perkins H A	318	Rheingold J J	174
pernicious anemia	91-100	Rich A	134
Perlzweig W A	216	Rich M L	107
Perutz M	56,60,71	Richardson J	129
Peters H S	300	Richter's syndrome	159
Peters M V	201-204	Rietti F	58
Philadelphia chromosome (Ph')	37,154-155	Rituximab	207,257
Phlebotomy	5	Roads C P	174
Pike B L	16	Robertson L B	292
Pillemer L	116	Robertson O H	291
Pinkel D	142-143	Robinson W A	16
Pinkus F	157,190	Romanovsky D	27
Piomelli S	63	Röntgen W	201
plasma cell	134,215-216	Roosevelt E	111
Plasmodium (malaria)	65,68,309	Rosenberg S A (Stanford)	205,211
Platelet transfusions	303-306	Rosenberg S A (NCI)	209
Plato	261	Rosenthal N	164
Pluznik D H	16	Roskam J	43,247
PNH	111, 114,115-120	Rosse W F	117-118,318
Polycthyemia vera	184-186	Rotimi C N	65
Polycythemia vera study group	185	Roulet F C	194
Polymerase chain reaction (PCR)	38,149	Rous F P	292
Ponfick E	290	Rowley J	155,200
Pool J G	275	Royston I	161
Popovsky M A	320	Rush B	88
Porotic hyperostosis	57,88	Russell M H	202
Potter F	285	Rye conference	196,202
Powles R L	219,241	Saarni M I	174
		Sachs D H	235
		Sachs L	16

Index

Sadelain M	209	Sternberg C	158,194
Sahli H	29	Stetson S R E	299
Salmon S	218	Stockman R	89
Samwick A A	223	Storb R	237,241
Sanger R A	301	Strauss R G	307
Sanchez-Medal I	110	Stretton A O	58,61
Santesson C G	108	Strober S	235-236
Santos G	227	Strübing P	115-116
Sartorius J A	257	Sultan C	145
Satterlee H S	289	Sun H D	150
Schiffer C A	318	Sutton W	35
Schilling R F	99	Svedberg T	212
Schilling-Torgau V	9,139,147	Swammerdam J	23,278
Schimmelbusch C	246	Sweet D	34
Schmidt A	262,267,271,325	Sydenham T	89,128
Schmitz J A	115	Sydenstricker V P	67,71
Schmorl C G	182	Sykes M	235
Schofield F W	265	Sylvius F	278,280
Schönlein J L	274	Symmers D	194
Schrek R	164	Takatsuki K	162
Schretzenmayr A	223	Talpaz M	154
Schwartz M	99	Tallquist T W	29
Schwartz S O	102	Taylor K	99
Seegers W H	263,271,282	T-cell depletion	226,237
Seemayer T A	319	Tefferi A	176
Senn N	201	Temin H M	62
Serum hepatitis	310-313	Terasaki P I	40
Seshadri R S	165	Teselius A	210,326
Seyfarth C	10	Thalassemia	57-64
Sézary A	162	Thaler M	319
Sézary syndrome	162	Thackrah C T	30,261
Shakespeare W	7,88	Thomas D	143
Shattock S G	296	Thomas E D	226,227,237, 243-244,326
Shaw H B	76		
Shaw M A	37	Thomson J A	18,19
Sherman I J	69	Thromboelastography (TEG) 43	
Shriner D	65	Thrombophilia	279-281
Shulman L E	258	Thrombopoietic (TPO) 247	
Sickle cell anemia	65-73	Thrombosis	277-281
Slavin S	236	Ti Huang	279
Smadel J E	107	Till J E	15
Smith H P	263,264,281,284	Tiollais P J R N	314
Smith T	92	Tiselius A	212
Smithers D W	202	Tjio J H	36
Snapper I	217-218,323	Total body irradiation (TBI) 13	
Snell G	39	Total therapy ALL	141-142
Solly S	214	Tissue plasminogen activator (t-PA) 271	
Sörensen S	92		
Soulier J P	253	TRALI	320-321
Southern E	37	transfusion GvHD	317-318
Speck B	112,179,229,326	Trentin J J	225
Spherocytosis	72-77	Treponema pallidum (syphilis) 306	
Spiers A S	121	Tricot G J	175
Steensma D	176	Trypanosoma cruzi (Chagas disease) 309	
Stem cells	10,12,18,		
Stenflo J	282	Tsai H M	259
Sterling K	41	TTP	255-256

Blood is Life

Tubiana M	203	Wachstein M	153
Tuddenham E	269	Waldenstrom J	105,212-213
Türk W	28,158,185	Waller A V	129
Turnbull H M	197	Wallenius G	60
Turner J R	290	Wang Y	231
Turner L B	215	Wang Z Y	152
Turpin R A	36	Warburg O H	55,80,81,325
Uhlenhuth P	308	Warfarin	266
Ultmann J E	258	Washington G	88
Umbilical cord blood cells (UCB)		Wasserman L	185
	233-234	Watson J	71
Unger L J	290	Weatherall D J	62
Uphoff D E	13	Weber E H	10
Upshaw J D	258	Weber G	70
Van Bekkum D W	15,224	Weigert K	29,49
Van den Berghe H	176	Weil R	291
Van Creveld S	248,270	Weisenburger D D	200
Van Furth R	132	Weismann G	132
Vanlair C F	74	Weiss H J	252
Van Leeuwen A A	51	Welch W H	280
Van Leeuwen E F	276	Werlhof P G	254-255
Van Leeuwenhoek A	24,,53,245	Westerman-Jensen needle	11
Van Loghem J	318	West Nile virus	316
Van Rood J J	39,*51-52*,326	Whipple G H	58,91,92
Vaquez L	106,184	WHO classification	149,176-178,327
Vaughan J M	293	WHO hemoglobin color scale	29
Vecchio F	60	Widal G F	48,101
Velpeau A J M	137	Wiener A S	299,300,317
Verfaillie, C	19	Wilkinson J F	116
Vermylen C	72	Wllks S	93,192
Vierordt K	31	Wills L	95
Vilter R	97	Wilson C	74
Vinca Nuclear reactor	226	Wintrobe M M	30,59,*83-85*,107
Vincent B	292		134,177,255,325,327
Virchow R	7,8,20,26,53,128,	Wiseman R	280
	129,130,138,157,	Wislocki G B	148
	168-169, 193,262,280	WMDA	243
Vitetta E	144,199	Woodward R B	96
Vogel F H	301	Woolsey G	310
Vogel J	101	Working formulation	200
Voltaire Masius J B N	74	Worlledge S	121
Von Behring E A	50	Wren C	285
Von Bunge G	89	Wright A E	269,290
Von Dungern E	298	Wright D H	198
Von Goethe J W	3	Wright J H	216,246
Von Jaksch R	57	Wright's stain	27
Von Manteuffel Z	269	Wynter W E	76
Von Mering J	97	X-chromosome silencing	86
Von Nägeli K W	35	Yam L T	164
Von Noorden C V	89	Yamanaka S	19
Von Recklinghausen F D	129	Yudin S S	295
Von Rusitzky J	215	Young N S	114
Von Waldeyer-Hartz H W G	35,215	Yunis A A	107
Von Willebrand E A	251	Zahn F W	44,281
Von Willebrand factor (VWF)		Zernicke F	25
	253,258-259,275	Zubrod G	304
Von Witzleben H D	216	2,3 DPG	303
Vroman L	268		

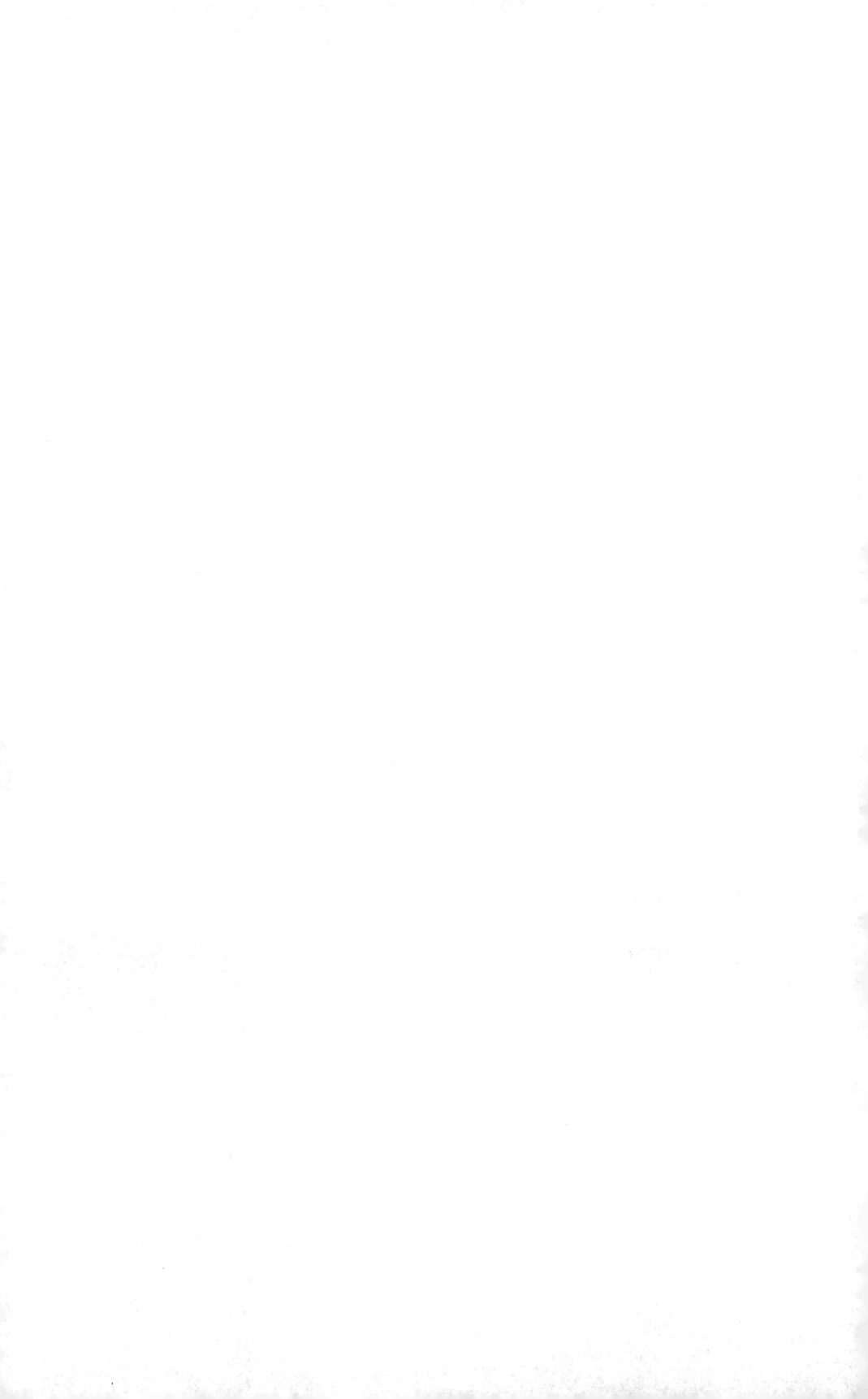

CPSIA information can be obtained
at www.ICGtesting.com
Printed in the USA
LVHW080322260522
719743LV00011B/361

9 781638 480532